T0332641

Immunology of
Gastrointestinal Disease

IMMUNOLOGY AND MEDICINE SERIES

IMMUNOLOGY
SERIES · SERIES · SERIES · SERIES AND SERIES · SERIES · SERIES · SERIES
MEDICINE

Volume 19

Immunology of Gastrointestinal Disease

Edited by
T. T. MacDonald

Department of Paediatric Gastroenterology
St. Bartholomew's Hospital
London, UK

Series Editor: K. Whaley

KLUWER ACADEMIC PUBLISHERS
DORDRECHT / BOSTON / LONDON

Distributors

for the United States and Canada: Kluwer Academic Publishers, PO Box 358, Accord Station, Hingham, MA 02018-0358, USA
for all other countries: Kluwer Academic Publishers, Distribution Center, PO Box 322, 3300 AH Dordrecht, The Netherlands

British Library Cataloguing-in-Publication Data

Immunology of gastrointestinal disease. – (Immunology and medicine; v.19)
  I. MacDonald, Tomas T.   II. Series
  616.33079

  ISBN 0792389611

Library of Congress Cataloging-in-Publication Data

Immunology of gastrointestinal disease/edited by T. T. MacDonald.
     p.   cm. — (Immunology and medicine series; v. 19)
  Includes bibliographical references and index.
  ISBN 0-7923-8961-1 (casebound)
  1. Gastrointestinal system—Diseases—Immunological aspects. I. Series
  [DNLM: 1. Gastrointestinal Diseases—Immunology.   2. Gastrointestinal
  System—Immunology.   W1 IM53BI v. 19/W1 100 I343]
  RC802.I457   1992
  616.3'3079—dc20
  DNLM/DLC
  for Library of Congress   91-35387
                                                                        CIP

Contents

CONTENTS

Series Editor's Note

The interface between clinical immunology and other branches of medical practice is frequently blurred and the general physician is often faced with clinical problems with an immunological basis and is expected to diagnose and manage such patients. The rapid expansion of basic and clinical immunology over the past two decades has resulted in the appearance of increasing numbers of immunology journals and it is impossible for a non-specialist to keep apace with this information overload. The *Immunology and Medicine* series is designed to present individual topics of immunology in a condensed package of information which can be readily assimilated by the busy clinician or pathologist. The present volume gives comprehensive coverage of the immunology of the gastrointestinal tract and the immunological basis of gastrointestinal disease.

K. Whaley, Glasgow
December 1991

Preface

Gastrointestinal diseases present a considerable problem in human medicine in terms of both morbidity and mortality. The aim of this book is to cover the breadth of the different immunological disorders of the gut with special reference to the immunopathological and protective mechanisms. By providing the key features of the particular disease, this book will be of general interest to clinicians, scientists and students with an interest in the gastrointestinal tract.

The current status of research into toxin-secreting pathogens, *Campylobacter*, *Giardia* and HIV is covered. The immunological features of idiopathic inflammatory gut diseases such as Crohn disease and intractable diarrhoea are featured, as are diseases where the cause is known, such as gluten in coeliac disease. The mechanism of the genesis of the flat mucosa is discussed. Finally, there are the iatrogenic diseases of the gut such as graft-versus-host disease and small bowel allografts.

Consideration is also given to the immune mechanisms and lesions in the gut of patients with parasitic nematode infections, which due to their prevalence in the tropics are important diseases in human terms. Basic background on the immune apparatus in the intestine is also discussed, as is the mechanism by which immune cells migrate and lodge in the intestinal mucosa in normal and diseased intestine. The effects of inflammation on intestinal permeability are also discussed in detail.

List of Contributors

C. P. BRAEGGER
Universitätskinderklinik
University of Zürich
Steinwiesstrasse
CH-8032 Zürich
Switzerland

P. BRANDTZAEG
Laboratory for Immunohistochemistry
and Immunopathology (LIIPAT)
Institute of Pathology
University of Oslo
The National Hospital
Rikshospitalet
N-0027 Oslo 1
Norway

N. BROUSSE
Service d'Anatomie et de Cytologie
Pathologiques
Hopital Necker–Enfants Malades
149 rue de Sèvres
75743 Paris Cedex 15
France

D. CANIONI
Service d'Anatomie et de Cytologie
Pathologiques
Hopital Necker–Enfants Malades
149 rue de Sèvres
75743 Paris Cedex 15
France

N. CERF-BENSUSSAN
INSERM U 132
Hopital Necker–Enfants Malades
149 rue de Sèvres
75743 Paris Cedex 15
France

E. S. COOPER
Tropical Metabolism Research Unit
University of the West Indies
Mona, Kingston 7
Jamaica, West Indies

B. CUENOD
Service de Gastroentérologie et Nutrition
Hopital Necker–Enfants Malades
149 rue de Sèvres
75743 Paris Cedex 15
France

T. S. HALSTENSEN
Laboratory for Immunohistochemistry and
Immunopathology (LIIPAT)
Institute of Pathology
University of Oslo
The National Hospital
Rikshospitalet
N-0027 Oslo 1
Norway

R. V. HEATLEY
Department of Medicine
St James's University Hospital
Leeds LS9 7TF
UK

L. HELGELAND
Laboratory for Immunohistochemistry and
Immunopathology (LIIPAT)
Institute of Pathology
University of Oslo
The National Hospital
Rikshospitalet
N-0027 Oslo 1
Norway

LIST OF CONTRIBUTORS

M. F. HEYWORTH
Cell Biology Section (151E)
VA Medical Center
4150 Clement Street
San Francisco, CA 94121
USA

J. HOLMGREN
Department of Medical Microbiology and
Immunology
University of Göteborg
Guldhedsgatan 10
S-413 46 Göteborg
Sweden

P. G. ISSACSON
Department of Histopathology
University College and Middlesex School
of Medicine
University Street
London WC1E 6JJ
UK

S. JALKANEN
Department of Medical Microbiology
Turku University
Kiinamyllynkatu 13
SF-20520 Turku
Finland

K. KETT
Laboratory for Immunohistochemistry and
Immunopathology (LIIPAT)
Institute of Pathology
University of Oslo
The National Hospital
Rikshospitalet
N-0027 Oslo 1
Norway

T. T. MACDONALD
Department of Paediatric Gastroenterology
St Bartholomew's Hospital
West Smithfield
London EC1A 7BE
UK

I. S. MENZIES
Department of Chemical Pathology
St Thomas's Hospital
London SE1 7EH
UK

A. M. MOWAT
Department of Immunology
University of Glasgow
Western Infirmary
Glasgow G11 6NT
UK

E.-O. RIECKEN
Medical Clinic, Department of
Gastroenterology
Klinikum Steglitz
Hindenburgdamm 30
1000 Berlin 45
Germany

M. SALMI
Department of Medical Microbiology
Turku University
Kiinamyllynkatu 13
SF-20520 Turku
Finland

S. SARNACKI
Départmente de Chirurgie Experimentale
Hopital Necker–Enfants Malades
149 rue de Sèvres
75743 Paris Cedex 15
France

E. SAVILAHTI
Children's Hospital
University of Helsinki
SF-00290 Helsinki
Finland

J. SPENCER
Department of Histopathology
University College and Middlesex School
of Medicine
University Street
London WC1E 6JJ
UK

A.-M. SVENNERHOLM
Department of Medical Microbiology and
Immunology
University of Göteborg
Guldhedsgatan 10
S-413 46 Göteborg
Sweden

M. W. TURNER
Molecular Immunology Unit
Institute of Child Health
30 Guilford St
London WC1N 1EH
UK

R. ULLRICH
Medical Clinic, Department of Gastroent.
Klinikum Steglitz
Hindenburgdamm 30
1000 Berlin 45
Germany

LIST OF CONTRIBUTORS

J. L. VINEY
Lymphocyte Molecular Biology Laboratory
Imperial Cancer Research Fund
Lincolns Inn Fields
London WC2A 3PY
UK

N. ZEITZ
Medical Clinic, Department of
Gastroenterology
Klinikum Steglitz
Hindenburgdamm 30
1000 Berlin 45
Germany

J. A. WALKER-SMITH
Academic Department of Paediatric
Gastroenterology
Queen Elizabeth Hospital for Children
Hackney Road
London E2 8PS
UK

1

The cells and tissues of the gastrointestinal tract

J. L. VINEY and T. T. MACDONALD

INTRODUCTION

The cells and tissues of the gastrointestinal immune system provide protection from the external environment at a site which is potentially extremely vulnerable to infection, since only a single epithelial layer separates the gut lumen and the tissues. Large numbers of leukocytes are present throughout the gut as single cells in the lamina propria and epithelium, and as aggregates in lymphoid follicles. For the most part the antigenic stimulus for the induction of the gut lymphocyte populations appears to be food and microorganisms that are present in the lumen of the intestine. In infection and allergy there are changes, not only in the gut structure, but in the cellular infiltrate in the intestinal mucosa, suggesting that local immune reactions may be involved in the pathogenesis of intestinal disease. The aim of this chapter is to describe the basic cellular and structural components of the mucosal immune system, abnormalities of which are the subject of the ensuing chapters.

STRUCTURE AND CELLULAR COMPOSITION OF THE GUT-ASSOCIATED LYMPHOID TISSUE

Peyer's patches

Throughout the small intestine there are areas of organized lymphoid tissue overlying the muscularis mucosa, forming Peyer's patches (PP), as first described by de Peyer in 1667. Peyer's patches are structurally similar in human and rodents, and similar aggregates of lymphoid tissues have also been described in the gut of other species (e.g. sheep, cattle, swine and dogs).

Human PP can be easily identified as small round blebs from the mucosal surface and distinguished from the surrounding villi, particularly in tissue from the terminal ileum. At birth there are approximately 100 PP throughout the length of the small intestine, most of which are in the ileum. By adolescence this number has more than doubled to around 225–300 PP, before decreasing with increasing age, so that the small intestine from an aged individual is likely to have roughly the same number of Peyer's patches as at birth[1]. PP have anatomical features which distinguish them from other secondary lymphoid tissues, the most obvious of which is the lack of a defined capsule or afferent lymphatics. PP have a well-defined cellular zonation and are usually composed of a follicle centre surrounded by a mantle of small lymphocytes which merges into the mixed-cell zone of the dome. The dome area also contains plasma cells, dendritic cells, macrophages and centrocyte-like B cells which infiltrate the overlying epithelium[2]. In addition, PP are characterized by the presence of a specialized epithelium without crypts or villi (follicle-associated epithelium – FAE), which facilitates the transmission of antigen from the gut lumen. The FAE is composed of cuboidal epithelial cells interspersed with few goblet cells, and there is no secretory component[3]. This is unlike the epithelium covering the crypts and villi, which is composed of columnar cells which contain secretory component, and which are interspersed with numerous goblet cells. The FAE is also characterized by the presence of specialized M cells, so called because of the presence of short irregular microfolds on their luminal aspect[4]. Since M cells are deficient in cytoplasmic acid phosphatase and microvillus-associated alkaline phosphatase[5], and are HLA-DR − [3], it is unlikely that they play a role in classical antigen presentation. However, since M cells are noted for the presence of numerous tubules, vesicles and vacuoles in the apical cytoplasm, this is a likely translocation system which allows for the direct sampling of antigen from the gut lumen by pinocytosis[6]. Antigen is transported through the epithelium and presented to immunocompetent cells in the underlying area. Small T and B lymphocytes, plasma cells, macrophages and dendritic cells populate the subepithelial layer, emphasizing that this site is important in antigen recognition[7,8]. In rodents the M cells of the FAE have been shown to transport inert particles such as horseradish peroxidase[9,10], and microorganisms such as reovirus[11], rotavirus[12] and poliovirus[13] through the FAE to the underlying subepithelial layer. Although most attention has centred on M cells in the FAE of PP, it is likely that HLA-DR + epithelial cells in the dome epithelium may also have a role in antigen processing or presentation.

B cells and plasma cells

Human PP contain large numbers of B cells. The narrow mantle zone surrounding the follicle centre is composed of cells expressing surface IgM or IgD. The B cells which surround the mantle zone, B cells in the mixed cell zone of the dome and B cells in the epithelium, do not express IgD but express surface IgM or IgA[2]. One of the major differences between human and rodent PP is that, in humans, sIgD + cells appear to be restricted to a

2

narrow zone around the follicle centre, whereas in rodents sIgD+ cells are abundant in the dome region and the dome epithelium as well as surrounding the follicle centres[14]. The majority of cells with abundant cytoplasmic immunoglobulin of all isotypes, excluding IgD, are present in the dome region of PP[15]. Interestingly, less than half of the cIgG+ cells found in the dome region are J-chain positive, in contrast to the lamina propria where the majority of cIgG+ cells are J-chain positive[15]. There are also cells with cIgA, cIgM and IgG in the T cell zone surrounding the high endothelial venules (HEV)[2]. There are few IgA plasma cells in PP[16], although PP themselves are the source of IgA plasma cell precursors that migrate to, and subsequently populate, the lamina propria[17,18].

T cells

The greatest density of CD3+ T cells can be found surrounding the HEV in the interfollicular zones[2]. There are also numerous T cells surrounding the follicle centre (Fig. 1.1) in the mixed-cell zone of the dome, and clusters of CD3+ cells have been identified particularly adjacent to M cells in the subepithelial dome region[19]. The majority of human PP CD3+ T cells also bear CD4. The number of CD4+ cells present in the FAE of PP is increased compared to the number of CD4+ cells in the villous epithelium[3].

Accessory cells

In humans, B cells, activated T cells, dendritic cells and macrophages in the PP are Class II positive, emphasizing that PP are a site active in antigen presentation and immune recognition. Numerous non-lymphoid HLA-DR+ cells with cytoplasmic processes are present in the dome area of human PP, as well as in the T cell zones. These macrophage-like cells under the dome epithelium and in the epithelium itself are heterogeneous[20]. Most HLA-DR+ cells in the dome region of the PP are likely to be dendritic cells, whereas HLA-DR+ cells in the interfollicular zones are likely to be interdigitating cells[21]. The dome epithelium itself is HLA-DR+ and thus may also be capable of presenting antigen to the numerous lymphoid cells within and adjacent to the epithelium. The presence of dendritic cells in the mixed-cell zone of the dome underlying the Class II negative M cells indicates that most antigen presentation in PP takes place in the dome region.

The role of PP in IgA responses

The relationship between PP and the secretory IgA response was first demonstrated by Craig and Cebra in 1971[17], who showed that PP contained a rich source of cells that were able to adoptively transfer an IgA response when injected into irradiated recipients. Furthermore, compared to B cells from the spleen, PP contain a high frequency of B cells which, having

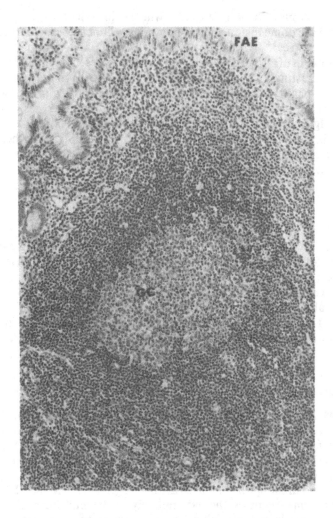

Figure 1.1 The Peyer's patch. Organized aggregates of lymphoid follicles forming PP are frequently observed in the intestine. The specialized FAE covering the dome region of the PP contains fewer goblet cells than the villous epithelium. ×30

undergone istotype switching, are committed to secreting IgA[22]. It has also been shown that antigenic stimulus from the gut triggers the B cell commitment to making IgA[22]. The role of the T cell in the IgA response has also been studied in some detail. Compared to T cells from the spleen, PP T cells are able to induce greater IgA responses in B cells co-stimulated with LPS[23]. Other studies have also suggested the existence of autoreactive 'switch' cells in Peyer's patches, which are capable of driving surface IgA− B cells to become surface IgA+[24]. The significance of these cells *in vivo* is still not fully understood. There has been a great deal of interest recently in the role of cytokines in driving the IgA response; however, it is beyond the scope of this chapter to cover these data.

Organized lymphoid tissue of the colon

Organized lymphoid follicles, similar to the PP in the small intestine, can be identified in the colon of humans and rodents. Human colonic lymphoid follicles were first described by Dukes and Bussey in 1926[25], who reported that there were approximately eight follicles per cm^2 of colonic mucosa in children, and this decreased to three per cm^2 in old age. The number of follicles is greater in the rectum than in the colon. These lymphoid follicles produce points of discontinuity along the length of the large intestine by residing just below the muscularis mucosa. The cellular composition of colonic lymphoid follicles is indicative of this being an active antigen-processing site. Although these structures often do not have a germinal centre, they are characterized by a central B cell zone, surrounded by a T cell zone containing interdigitating cells[26]. In addition, colonic lymphoid follicles have a specialized dome epithelium containing M cells, similar to the specialized FAE overlying PP in the small intestine[26].

The appendix

The human appendix is characterized by numerous lymphoid nodules separated by regions of lamina propria, into which the glandular crypts penetrate. The distribution of cell types and the zonal arrangement is very similar to that seen in PP. The lymphoid nodules have a reactive follicle centre, surrounded by a narrow mantle of sIgM +, IgD − B cells which merge with the mixed-cell zone beneath the epithelium. The T cell zone lies mostly between the follicle centre and muscularis mucosa, with CD4+ cells predominating over CD8+ cells. The FAE, which contains T and B cells, is often HLA-DR$^+$. Lysozyme-containing macrophages are uncommon in the dome region, so most of the HLA-DR+ cells with cytoplasmic processes are likely to be dendritic cells[14]. In the dome region, and in the region immediately adjacent to the follicles, IgG plasma cells predominate, whereas the majority of plasma cells in the lamina propria between follicles are IgA-secreting[15].

The tonsils

The first organized lymphoid structures exposed to dietary and bacterial antigens are the nasopharyngeal and palatine tonsils at the pharynx/mouth junction. The palatine tonsil is covered in squamous epithelium, whereas the nasopharyngeal tonsil has patches of ciliated columnar and squamous epithelium[27]. The epithelium is densely infiltrated with lymphocytes and forms deeply penetrating crypts into the lymphoid tissue. There are numerous follicles in tonsillar tissue, each of which have germinal centres surrounded by a mantle zone of T and B cells. One of the major differences between tonsil lymphoid tissue and other gut-associated follicles is that most of the plasma cells express IgG[27]. Of the IgA plasma cells in tonsils, the majority express IgA1, rather than IgA2 which is more characteristic of mucosal surfaces[28].

The lamina propria

The lamina propria is the region of tissue between the epithelium and the muscularis mucosa, comprising a villous core over which epithelial cells migrate from the crypt to the villous tip. Large numbers of plasma cells, T and B lymphocytes, macrophages and granulocytes populate the lamina propria, together with smooth muscle cells and fibroblasts, thus forming the basic gut structure of villi and crypts. Lymphocyte migration into the lamina propria of the gut from the blood is mediated by specialized vessels at the base of the villi[29,30]. Lamina propria lymphocytes bear homing receptors which selectively bind to the mucosal lymphoid high endothelium[30,31]. The lamina propria lymphoid infiltrate is not totally dependent on antigen since lymphoid cells are present in fetal gut, although numbers do increase after birth[32]. Plasma cells are antigen-dependent, however, since at birth these cells are absent[33].

B cells and plasma cells

The lamina propria is densely infiltrated with lymphocytes, approximately half of which are B cells. Small B cells comprise 15–45% of total mononuclear cells[34], most of which are sIgA +, although sIgM +, sIgG + and sIgD + cells are also found [35-37]. There are no IgA + cells in human fetal small intestine (Fig. 1.2). In the normal intestine there are numerous plasma cells, most of

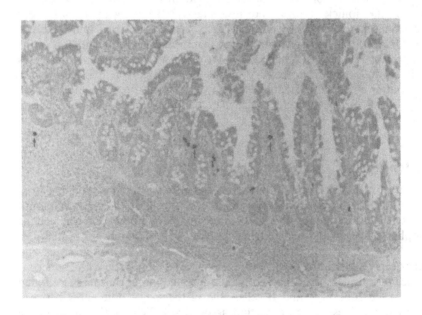

Figure 1.2 IgA + cells in human neonatal small intestine. Human neonatal small intestine was stained by immunohistochemistry for IgA + cells. Very few positively stained cells can be seen. × 26

6

which are located near the crypts. In humans, IgA plasma cells constitute approximately 30% of the total mononuclear cells in the intestinal lamina propria (Fig. 1.3), and 80% of the total plasma cells[28,38-41]; hence the major immunoglobulin isotype in intestinal secretions is IgA[28,42]. Over half of the IgA plasma cells in the gut secrete IgA2[37,38]. This is in contrast to lymph nodes where most of the secreted IgA is IgA1. Of the remaining plasma cells, approximately 20% secrete IgM and only a very small number (3-5%) secrete IgG[37,38]. Plasma cells of the IgD or IgE isotype are rarely seen. Most of the IgA in intestinal secretions is dimeric[43], binding specifically via J chain/secretory component interactions at the basolateral surface of crypt epithelial cells, then being actively transported into the lumen[44].

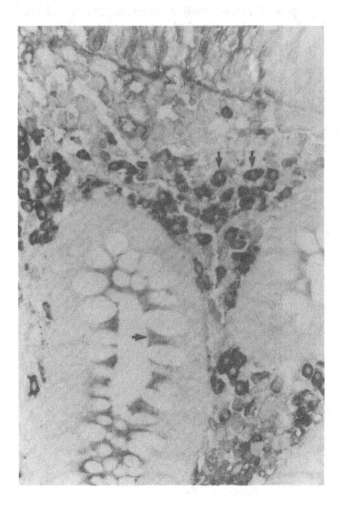

Figure 1.3 IgA plasma cells in human colon. Densely stained IgA plasma cells can be observed in the lamina propria of the large intestine. Note also the IgA staining at the apex of the epithelial cells which represents IgA being actively transported across the epithelium. ×75

T cells

CD3+ cells comprise approximately half of the lymphocytes in the lamina propria (Fig. 1.4). The majority of these T cells in both the small and large intestine[45-48] are CD4+. In humans most of the T cells in the lamina propria[49-51] are HLA-DR− and IL-2R−. However, equal numbers of these T cells stain with CD45RA and CD45RO, indicating that at least some may be memory cells[41,52,53]. T cells bearing the $\alpha\beta$ TcR are most prominent in the lamina propria, with virtually no $\gamma\delta$ cells.

Accessory cells

In the lamina propria of human small intestine the majority of HLA-DR+ cells are small and stellate-shaped with the characteristics of dendritic cells[49],

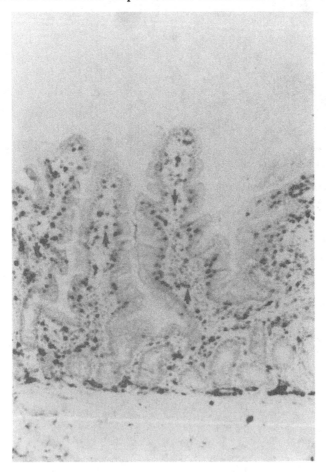

Figure 1.4 CD3+ T cells in normal human lamina propria. Numerous T cells can be observed throughout the lamina propria (arrowed), as well as in the epithelium. ×30

suggesting that the majority of DR+ cells in the small intestine are antigen-presenting cells. The appearance of these cells in the mucosa is antigen-independent[53,54]. In the large intestine, however, the majority of DR+ cells are strongly acid phosphatase- and esterase-positive, but weakly ATPase-positive, characteristic of phagocytic cells[49]. It should be emphasized, however, that the distinction between the macrophage and dendritic cell types in the gut is vague and controversial.

Intraepithelial lymphocytes

Intraepithelial lymphocytes (IEL) are usually situated just above the basal lamina, amongst the epithelial cells covering the crypts and villi (Fig. 1.5). The position of these lymphocytes is unique, since they are separated from

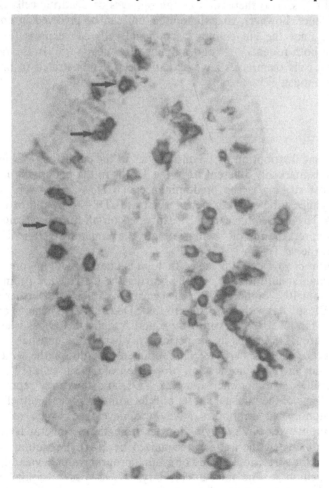

Figure 1.5 CD3+ T cells in normal human intestinal epithelium. Numerous basally situated CD3+ intraepithelial lymphocytes can be identified within the columnar epithelium. ×75

the antigenic load of the gastrointestinal lumen only by tight junctions between the epithelial cells. The number of IEL reflects the degree of antigenic stimulation from the gut lumen. IEL are most numerous in the small intestine, with fewer in the colon and virtually none in the stomach or oesophagus. Ultrastructural studies have revealed lymphocytes entering and leaving the epithelium from and into the underlying lamina propria[55]. Most of the experimental work on the basic biology of IEL has been done in rodents.

B cells and accessory cells

Unlike the lamina propria, where there are numerous small B lymphocytes and plasma cells, the epithelium of humans and rodents is completely devoid of these cell types. Also there are no macrophages or dendritic cells. There is some evidence, however, that the epithelium can be involved in antigen presentation since the gut columnar epithelial cells can express Class II molecules in both rodents[56-58] and humans (Fig. 1.6)[21,59,60]. In the rat the gut epithelial cells themselves have actually been demonstrated to process and present antigen[61-64].

T cells

The phenotypic distribution of T lymphocytes in the epithelium of humans and rodents is markedly different from the T cells in the underlying lamina propria. Most striking is the predominance of CD8+ cells over CD4+ cells[45-47]. In mice, although the majority of IEL are CD8+, only approximately half express Thy1, an antigen usually expressed on all murine T cells[65,66]. These cells express the $\alpha\beta$ TcR[67]. Interestingly, the remaining CD8+, Thy1− IEL express the $\gamma\delta$ TcR[68].

The tropism of $\gamma\delta$ T cells for the epithelium is unexplained. In contrast to mice, in human small intestine, T cells bearing the $\alpha\beta$ TcR are prominent, with only about 10% of the CD3+ cells bearing $\gamma\delta$ TcR[69-71]. Further study of murine IEL subsets with antibodies to the CD8α and CD8β chains reveals that CD8+, Thy1+ IEL co-express the α and β chains of CD8 as is usually seen on mature CD8+ cells in the periphery, whereas the unusual CD8+, Thy1− cell type expresses a CD8$\alpha\alpha$ homodimer. In addition, the same may be true for human IEL, since a small proportion of CD3+ cells (12%) also express the CD8$\alpha\alpha$ homodimer and lack CD5, and thus may represent a human analogue of the unusual subset of cells found in rodent epithelium[72]. Recently, monoclonal antibodies have been developed which recognize mucosal lymphocytes but not lymphocytes from the peripheral lymphoid tissues. In human gut the antigen recognized by HML-1 is found almost exclusively on the surface of IEL and on lamina propria lymphocytes adjacent to the epithelium[47]. The mouse corollary, M290, has a similar tissue distribution[73]. Interestingly, both monoclonal antibodies immunoprecipitate molecules of similar apparent molecular weight from human and mouse IEL, although the antibodies themselves are species-specific.

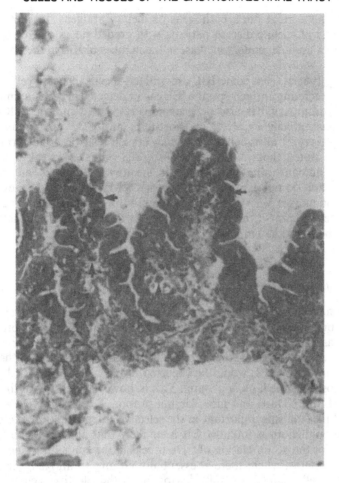

Figure 1.6 HLA-DR expression on normal human epithelial cells. All of the villous epithelial cells and numerous accessory cells in the lamina propria are HLA-DR+. ×75

Role of IEL in the epithelium

Despite an abundance of descriptive reports on IEL there is a notable paucity of functional studies. Recently, however, it has been proposed that $\gamma\delta$ TcR+ IEL may have a role in surveillance of epithelial surfaces and be involved in the first lines of defence protecting the mucosa from the external environment[74,75]. IEL do not have NK activity or NK surface markers. Neither do they respond well to mitogens, although sheep red cell fragments augment their proliferative response presumably via CD2[76-78]. Approximately equal proportions of IEL express the different isoforms of the leukocyte common antigen, CD45RA and CD45RO, indicating that at least some cells may be memory cells[41,53,72]. It is generally assumed that, because the frequencies of IEL vary in different conditions, the number of IEL in some way reflects immune responsiveness to enteric antigens, whether it be the antigens of the normal flora, pathogens or dietary antigens. In support of this, challenge of coeliac disease patients with graded doses of gluten does indeed cause a dose-dependent increase in the number of IEL in the proximal jejunum[79].

It is likely that at least some IEL are antigen-specific effector cells, since lymphokine-secreting antigen-specific IEL can be detected in parasite-infected mice[80]. In addition, it has also been demonstrated that murine TcR-$\alpha\beta$+ IEL are constitutively cytolytic in short-term anti-CD3 mAb redirected cytotoxicity assays[68], although the frequency of such cells was not determined. It should be noted that $\gamma\delta$ TcR + IEL showed only very weak cytolytic activity. In humans mucosal T cells in healthy individuals are rarely HLA-DR + and do not express IL2 receptors[49]. Many normal IEL express the activation marker VLA-1, which is a receptor for laminin and collagen[81]. This surface receptor presumably enables IEL to cross the basement membrane between the lamina propria and epithelium.

Origin and fate of IEL

The origin and fate of IEL have been the subject of much controversy. The immediate precursors of IEL are likely to be derived from the lamina propria, since increased numbers of IEL are always accompanied by increased lymphocyte density in the lamina propria[82]. If migration into the epithelium was a random event, IEL would be expected to have the same distribution of T cell subsets as the lamina propria. This is, however, clearly not the case as most IEL are CD8 + and most lamina propria T cells are CD4 +. The factors and mechanisms important in the selective entry/retention of CD8 + cells in the epithelium is unknown. It is unlikely that antigen is the factor responsible for the accumulation of CD8 + cells in the epithelium since even in the human fetus, where there is essentially no foreign antigen, there are more CD8 + cells than CD4 + cells[32]. More likely the selective accumulation of CD8 + IEL reflects the ability of different T cell subsets to traverse the basement membrane, reflected by the distribution of extracellular matrix protein receptors on the surface of lymphocytes.

In mice it has been clearly demonstrated that IEL can arise from the bone marrow without the need for thymus processing. This phenomenon is demonstrated by the presence of IEL in congenitally athymic mice[83], and in mice which have been thymectomized, irradiated and reconstituted with bone marrow[84,85]. These cells are Thy1 −, CD8 + IEL expressing the $\gamma\delta$ TcR[67,86]. In addition there is another population of cells which is dependent on the presence of a thymus and antigenic stimulation from the gut lumen. These cells arise from precursor cells within the PP and migrate via the MLN and thoracic lymph back to the mucosal epithelium[87,88]. These cells are the conventional Thy1 +, CD8 + IEL expressing the $\alpha\beta$ TcR[67,86].

Although it is not an idea which has sustained much interest in recent years, it has been proposed that some IEL may represent effete lymphocytes dying within the epithelium. There is some histological evidence from early studies in mice[89,90] and humans[91,92] that lymphocytes in the epithelium show features associated with cells undergoing apoptosis. Recent evidence in mice demonstrates that $\gamma\delta$ TcR+ IEL rapidly and selectively die by apoptosis *in vitro*[93]. Recently, apoptosis has been identified as the mechanism by which self-reactive thymocytes are eliminated[94,95]. Since it is well documented that $\gamma\delta$ TcR+ IEL can arise in the absence of thymic and antigenic influence and express functional $\gamma\delta$ TcR, these observations may have important implications for the possible development of $\gamma\delta$ TcR+ cells at extrathymic sites. Furthermore, there is some preliminary evidence that $\gamma\delta$ IEL may be able to productively rearrange their TcR genes and express $\gamma\delta$ TcR on their cell surface without thymic influence[96,97].

References

1. Cornes, J. S. (1965). Number, size and distribution of Peyer's patches in the human small intestine. Part 1: The development of Peyer's patches. *Gut*, **6**, 225–229; Part 2: The effect of age on Peyer's patches. *Gut*, **6**, 230–3

2. Spencer, J., Finn, T. and Isaacson, P. (1986). Human Peyer's patches: an immunohistochemical study. *Gut*, **27**, 405–10

3. Bjerke, K. and Brandtzaeg, P. (1988). Lack of relation between expression of HLA-DR and secretory component (SC) in follicle-associated epithelium of human Peyer's patches. *Clin. Exp. Immunol.*, **74**, 270–5

4. Owen, R. L. and Jones, A. L. (1974). Epithelial cell specialisation within human Peyer's patches: an ultrastructural study. *Gastroenterology*, **66**, 189–203

5. Owen, R. L., Apple, R. T. and Bhalla, D. K. (1986). Morphometric and cytochemical analysis of lysosomes in rat Peyer's patch follicle epithelium: their reduction in volume fraction and acid phosphatase content in M cells compared to adjacent enterocytes. *Anat. Rec.*, **216**, 521–7

6. Bye, W. A., Allan, C. H. and Trier, J. S. (1984). Structure, distribution and origin of M cells in Peyer's patches of mouse ileum. *Gastroenterology*, **86**, 789–801

7. Parrott, D. and Ferguson, A. (1974). Selective migration of lymphocytes within mouse small intestine. *Immunology*, **26**, 571–88

8. Bhalla, D. K. and Owen, R. L. (1983). Migration of T and B lymphocytes to M cells in Peyer's patch follicle epithelium. An autoradiographic and immunocytochemical study in mice. *Cell. Immunol.*, **81**, 105–17

9. Bockman, D. and Stevens, W. (1977). Gut associated lymphoepithelial tissue: Bidirectional transport of tracer by specialised epithelial cells associated with lymphoid follicles. *Reticuloendothelial Soc.*, **21**, 245–54

10. Owen, R. L. (1977). Sequential uptake of horseradish peroxidase by lymphoid follicle epithelium of Peyer's patches in normal unobstructed mouse intestine: an ultrastructural study. *Gastoenterology*, **72**, 440–51.

11. Wolf, J. L., Rubin, D. H., Finberg, R., Kaufman, R. S., Sharpe, A. H., Trier, J. S. and Fields, B. N. (1981). Intestinal M cells: a pathway for entry of reovirus into host. *Science*, **212**, 471–2.

12. Dharakul, T., Riepenhoff-Talty, M., Albini, B. and Ogra, P. (1988). Distribution of rotavirus antigen in intestinal lymphoid tissues: potential role in development of the mucosal immune response to rotavirus. *Clin. Exp. Immunol.*, **74**, 134–9

13. Sicinski, P., Rowinski, J., Warchol, J. B., Jarzabek, Z., Gut, W., Szczygiel, B., Bielecki, K. and Koch, K. (1990). Poliovirus type I enters the human host through intestinal M cells. *Gastroenterology*, **98**, 56–8

14. Spencer, J., Finn, T. and Isaacson, P. (1986). A comparative study of the gut-associated lymphoid tissue of primates and rodents. *Virchows Arch.*, **51**, 509–519

15. Bjerke, K. and Brandtzaeg, P. (1986). Immunoglobulin- and J chain-producing cells associated with lymphoid follicles in the human appendix, colon and ileum, including Peyer's patches. *Clin. Exp. Immunol.*, **64**, 432–41

16. Faulk, W., McCormick, J., Goodman, J., Yoffey, J. and Fudenberg, H. (1971). Peyer's patches: morphological studies. *Cell. Immunol.*, **1**, 500–20

17. Craig, S. W. and Cebra, J. J. (1971). Peyer's patches: an enriched source of precursors for IgA producing immunocytes in the rabbit. *J. Exp. Med.*, **134**, 184–200
18. Husband, A. J. and Gowans, J. L. (1978). The origin and antigen-dependent distribution of IgA containing cells in the intestine. *J. Exp. Med.*, **148**, 1146–60
19. Bjerke, K., Brandtzaeg, P. and Fausa, O. (1988). T cell distribution is different in follicle associated epithelium of human Peyer's patches and villous epithelium. *Clin. Exp. Immunol.*, **74**, 270–5
20. Sminia, T., Wilders, M., Janse, E. and Hoefsmit, E. (1983). Characterisation of non-lymphoid cells in Peyer's patches of the rat. *Immunobiology*, **164**, 136–43
21. Spencer, J., Finn, T. and Isaacson, P. (1986). Expression of HLA-DR antigens on epithelium associated with lymphoid tissue in the human gastrointestinal tract. *Gut*, **27**, 153–7
22. Gearhart, P. J. and Cebra, J. J. (1979). Differentiated B lymphocytes: potential to express particular antibody variable and constant regions dependent on site of lymphoid tissue and antigen load. *J. Exp. Med.*, **149**, 216–25
23. Elson, C. O., Heck, J. A. and Strober, W. (1979). T cell regulation of murine IgA synthesis. *J. Exp. Med.*, **149**, 632–43
24. Kawanishi, H., Ozato, K. and Strober, W. (1985). The proliferative response of cloned Peyer's patch switch T cells to syngeneic and allogeneic stimuli. *J. Immunol.*, **134**, 3586–91
25. Dukes, C. and Bussey, H. J. R. (1926). The number of lymphoid follicles of the human large intestine. *J. Pathol. Bacteriol.*, **29**, 111–16
26. O'Leary, A. D. and Sweeney, E. C. (1986). Lymphoglandular complexes of the colon: structure and distribution. *Histopathology*, **10**, 267–83
27. Korsrud, F. R. and Brandtzaeg, P. (1980). Immune systems of human nasopharyngeal and palatine tonsils: histomorphometry of lymphoid components and quantification of immunoglobulin producing cells in health and disease. *Clin. Exp. Immunol.*, **39**, 361–70
28. Crago, S., Kutteh, W., Moro, I., Allansmith, M., Radl, J., Haaijman, J. and Mestecky, J. (1984). Distribution of IgA1-, IgA2-, and J chain-containing cells in human tissues. *J. Immunol.*, **132**, 16–18
29. Miller, D., Rahman, M., Tanner, R., Mathan, V. and Baker, S. (1969). The vascular architecture of the different forms of small intestinal villi in the rat. *Scand. J. Gastroenterol.*, **4**, 477–82
30. Jeurissen, S., Duijvestein, A., Sontag, Y. and Kraal, G. (1987). Lymphocyte migration into the lamina propria of the gut is mediated by specialised HEV-like blood vessels. *Immunology*, **62**, 273–7
31. Jalkanen, S., Nash, G., Toyos, L., MacDermott, R. and Butcher, E. (1989). Human lamina propria lymphocytes bear homing receptors and bind selectively to mucosal lymphoid high endothelium. *Eur. J. Immunol.*, **19**, 63–8
32. Spencer, J., Dillon, S., Isaacson, P. G. and MacDonald, T. T. (1986). T cell subclasses in human fetal ileum. *Clin. Exp. Immunol.*, **65**, 553–56
33. Perkkio, M. and Savilahti, E. (1980). Time of appearance of immunoglobulin-containing cells in the mucosa of the neonatal intestine. *Paediatr. Res.*, **14**, 953–55
34. MacDonald, T. T., Spencer, J., Viney, J., Williams, C. and Walker-Smith, J. A. (1987). Selective biopsy of Peyer's patches during ileal endoscopy. *Gastroenterology*, **93**, 1356–62
35. Tseng, J. (1982). Expression of immunoglobulin isotypes by lymphoid cells of mouse intestinal lamina propria. *Cell. Immunol.*, **73**, 324–36
36. Tseng, J. (1983). Expression of immunoglobulin isotypes by lymphoid cells isolated from the lamina propria of mouse small intestine. *Ann. N Y Acad. Sci.*, **409**, 885–6
37. Brandtzaeg, P., Kett, K., Rognum, T., Soderstrom, R., Bjorkander, J., Soderstrom, T., Petrussen, B. and Hanson, L. (1986). Distribution of mucosal IgA and IgG subclass-producing immunocytes and alterations in various disorders. *Monogr. Allergy*, **20**, 179–94
38. Crabbe, P., Carbonara, A. and Heremans, J. (1965). The normal intestinal mucosa as a major source of plasma cells containing γA-globulin. *Lab. Invest.*, **14**, 235–48
39. Crabbe, P. and Heremans, J. (1966). The distribution of immunoglobulin containing cells along the human gastrointestinal tract. *Gastroenterology*, **51**, 305–16
40. Weisz-Carrington, P., Schrater, A., Lamm, M. and Thorbecke, G. (1979). Immunoglobulin isotypes in plasma cells of normal and athymic mice. *Cell. Immunol.*, **44**, 343–51
41. Brandtzaeg, P., Halstensen, T., Kett, K., Krajki, P., Kvale, D., Rognum, T., Scott, H. and Sollid, L. (1989). Immunobiology and immunopathology of human gut mucosa: humoral

14

immunity and intraepithelial lymphocytes. *Gastroenterology*, **97**, 1562–82
42. Ginsberg, A. (1971). Alterations in immunologic mechanisms in diseases of the gastrointestinal tract. *Dig. Dis.*, **16**, 61–81
43. Kett, K., Brandtzaeg, P. and Fausa, O. (1988). J chain expression is more prominent in immunoglobulin A2 than in immunoglobulin A1 colonic immunocytes and is decreased in both subclasses associated with inflammatory bowel disease. *Gastroenterology*, **94**, 1419–25
44. Brandtzaeg, P., Sollid, L., Thrane, P., Kvale, D., Bjerke, K., Scott, H., Kett, K. and Rognum, T. (1988). Lymphoepithelial interactions in the mucosal immune system. *Gut*, **29**, 1116–30
45. Janossy, G., Tidman, N., Selby, W., Thomas, J. and Granger, S. (1980). Human T lymphocytes of inducer and suppressor phenotypes occupy different microenvironments. *Nature*, **288**, 81–4
46. Selby, W., Janossy, G., Goldstein, G. and Jewell, D. (1981). T lymphocyte subsets in human intestinal mucosa: the distribution and relationship to MHC-derived antigens. *Clin. Exp. Immunol.*, **44**, 453–8
47. Cerf-Bensussan, N., Jarry, A., Brousse, N., Losowska Grospierre, B., Guy-Grand, D. and Griscelli, C. (1987). A monoclonal antibody (HML-1) defining a novel membrane molecule present on human intestinal intraepithelial lymphocytes. *Eur. J. Immunol.*, **17**, 1279–85
48. Selby, W., Janossy, G., Bofill, M. and Jewell, D. (1983). Lymphocyte subpopulations in human small intestine: the findings in normal mucosa and in the mucosa of patients with coeliac disease. *Clin. Exp. Immunol.*, **52**, 219–28
49. Selby, W., Poulter, L., Hobbs, S., Jewell, D. and Janossy, G. (1983). Heterogeneity of HLA-DR positive histiocytes in human intestinal lamina propria: a combined histochemical and immunological analysis. *J. Clin. Pathol.*, **36**, 379–84
50. Selby, W., Janossy, G., Bofill, M. and Jewell, D. (1984). Intestinal lymphocyte subpopulations in inflammatory bowel disease: an analysis by immunohistological and cell isolation techniques. *Gut*, **25**, 32–40
51. Hirata, I., Berrebi, G., Austin, L., Keren, D. and Dobbins, W. (1986). Immunohistological characterisation of intraepithelial and lamina propria lymphocytes in control ileum and colon and in inflammatory bowel disease. *Dig. Dis. Sci.*, **31**, 593–603
52. Moore, K. and Nesbitt, A. (1987). Functional heterogeneity of CD4 + T lymphocytes: two subpopulations with counteracting immunoregulatory functions identified with the monoclonal antibodies WR16 and WR19. *Immunology*, **61**, 159–65
53. Harvey, J., Jones, D. and Wright, D. (1989). Leucocyte common antigen expression on T cells in normal and inflamed human gut. *Immunology*, **69**, 13–17
54. Spencer, J., MacDonald, T. T. and Isaacson, P. (1987). Heterogeneity of non-lymphoid cells expressing HLA-D region antigens in human fetal gut. *Clin. Exp. Immunol.*, **67**, 415–24
55. Toner, P. and Ferguson, A. (1971). Intraepithelial cells in the human intestinal mucosa. *J. Ultrastruct. Res.*, **34**, 329–44
56. Scott, H., Solheim, B., Brandtzaeg, P. and Thorsby, E. (1980). HLA-DR-like antigens in the epithelium of the human small intestine. *Scand. J. Immunol.*, **12**, 77–82
57. Barclay, A. and Mason, D. (1982). Induction of Ia antigen on rat epidermal cells and the gut epithelium by immunological stimuli. *J. Exp. Med.*, **156**, 1665–9
58. Mayrhofer, G., Pugh, C. and Barclay, A. (1983). The distribution, ontogeny and origin in the rat of Ia-positive cells with dendritic morphology and of Ia antigen in epithelia, with special reference to the intestine. *Eur. J. Immunol.*, **13**, 112–22
59. Trejdosiewicz, L., Malizia, G., Badr-el-Din, S., Smart, C., Oakes, D., Southgate, J., Howdle, P., Janossy, G., Poulter, L. and Losowsky, M. (1987). T cell and mononuclear phagocyte populations of the human small and large intestine. *Adv. Exp. Med. Biol.*, **216**, 465–73
60. MacDonald, T. T., Weinel, A. and Spencer, J. (1988). HLA-DR expression in human fetal intestinal epithelium. *Gut*, **29**, 1342–48
61. Bland, P. and Warren, L. (1986). Antigen presentation by epithelial cells of the rat small intestine I. Kinetics, antigen specificity and blocking by anti-Ia antisera. *Immunology*, **58**, 1–7
62. Bland, P. and Warren, L. (1986). Antigen presentation by epithelial cells of the rat small intestine. II. Selective induction of suppressor T cells. *Immunology*, **58**, 9–14
63. Bland, P. and Whiting, C. (1989). Antigen processing by isolated rat intestinal villous enterocytes. *Immunology*, **68**, 497–502
64. Steiniger, B., Falk, P., Lohmuller, M. and van der Meide, P. (1989). Class II MHC antigens in the rat digestive system. Normal distribution and induced expression after interferon-gamma treatment *in vivo*. *Immunology*, **68**, 507–13

65. Parrot, D., Tait, C., MacKenzie, S., Mowat, A., Davies, M. and Micklem, H. (1983). Analysis of the effector functions of different populations of mucosal lymphocytes. *Ann. N Y Acad. Sci.*, **409**, 307–20
66. Dillon, S. and MacDonald, T. T. (1984). Functional properties of lymphocytes isolated from murine small intestinal epithelium. *Immunology*, **52**, 501–9
67. Viney, J. L., MacDonald, T. T. and Kilshaw, P. J. (1989). T cell receptor expression in intestinal intraepithelial lymphocyte subpopulations of normal and athymic mice. *Immunology*, **66**, 583–87
68. Viney, J. L., Kilshaw, P. J. and MacDonald, T. T. (1990). Cytotoxic $\alpha\beta+$ and $\gamma\delta+$ T cells in murine intestinal epithelium. *Eur. J. Immunol.*, **20**, 1623–26
69. Spencer, J., Isaacson, P., Diss, T. and MacDonald, T. T. (1989). Expression of disulphide-linked and non-disulphide-linked forms of the T cell receptor $\gamma\delta$ heterodimer in human intestinal intraepithelial lymphocytes. *Eur. J. Immunol.*, **19**, 1335–38
70. Groh, V., Porcelli, S., Fabbi, M., Lanier, L., Picker, L., Anderson, T., Warnke, R., Bhan, A., Strominger, J. and Brenner, M. (1989). Human lymphocytes bearing T cell receptor $\gamma\delta$ are phenotypically diverse and evenly distributed throughout the lymphoid system. *J. Exp. Med.*, **169**, 1277–94
71. Halstensen, T. S., Scott, H. and Brandtzaeg, P. (1989). Intraepithelial T cells of the TcR$\gamma\delta+$, CD8$-$ and Vδ1/Jδ1$+$ phenotypes are increased in coeliac disease. *Scand. J. Gastroenterol.*, **30**, 665–72
72. Jarry, A., Cerf-Bensussan, N., Brousse, N., Selz, F. and Guy-Grand, D. (1990). Subsets of CD3$+$ T cell receptor ($\alpha\beta$ or $\gamma\delta$) and CD3$-$ lymphocytes isolated from normal gut epithelium display phenotypical features different from their counterparts in peripheral blood. *Eur. J. Immunol.*, **20**, 1097–104
73. Kilshaw, P. and Baker, K. (1988). A unique surface antigen on intraepithelial lymphocytes in the mouse. *Immunol. Letters*, **18**, 149–54
74. Janeway, C. (1988). Frontiers of the immune system. *Nature*, **333**, 804–6
75. Janeway, C., Jones, B. and Hayday, A. (1988). Specificity and function of T cells bearing $\gamma\delta$ receptors. *Immunol. Today*, **9**, 73–6
76. Cerf-Bensussan, N., Guy-Grand, D. and Griscelli, C. (1985). Intraepithelial lymphocytes of human gut: isolation, characterisation and study of natural killer activity. *Gut*, **26**, 81–8
77. Ebert, E., Roberts, A., Brolin, R. and Raska, K. (1986). Examination of the low proliferative capacity of human jejunal intraepithelial lymphocytes. *Clin. Exp. Immunol.*, **65**, 148–57
78. Ebert, E. (1989). Proliferative responses of human intraepithelial lymphocytes to various T cell stimuli. *Gastroenterology*, **97**, 1372–81
79. Leigh, R., Marsh, M., Crowe, P., Kelly, C., Garner, V. and Gordon, D. (1985). Studies of intestinal lymphoid tissue IX. Dose-dependent, gluten-induced lymphoid infiltration of coeliac jejunal epithelium. *Scand. J. Gastroenterol.*, **20**, 715–19
80. Dillon, S., Dalton, B. and MacDonald, T. T. (1986). Lymphokine production by mitogen and antigen activated mouse intraepithelial lymphocytes. *Cell. Immunol.*, **103**, 326–8
81. Choy, M., Richman, P., Horton, M. and MacDonald, T. T. (1990). Expression of the VLA family of integrins in human intestine. *J. Pathol.*, **160**, 35–40
82. Monk, T., Spencer, J., Cerf-Bensussan, N. and MacDonald, T. (1988). Stimulation of mucosal T cells *in situ* with anti-CD3 antibody: location of the activated T cells and their distribution within the mucosal microenvironment. *Clin. Exp. Immunol.*, **74**, 216–22
83. Ferguson, A. and Parrott, D. (1972). The effect of antigen-deprivation on thymus dependent and thymus independent lymphocytes in the small intestine of mouse. *Clin. Exp. Immunol.*, **72**, 477–88
84. Fichtelius, K., Yunis, E. and Good, R. (1968). Occurrence of lymphocytes within the gut epithelium of normal and neonatally thymectomised mice. *Proc. Soc. Exp. Biol.*, **128**, 185–8
85. Mayrhofer, G. and Whately, R. (1983). Granular intraepithelial lymphocytes of the rat small intestine. I. Isolation, presence in T lymphocyte deficient rats and bone marrow origin. *Int. Arch. Allergy Appl. Immunol.*, **71**, 317–27
86. De Geus, B., van den Enden, M., Coolen, C. and Rozing, J. (1990). Localisation and phenotype of CD3 associated $\gamma\delta$ receptor expressing intestinal intraepithelial lymphocytes. *Thymus*, **14**, 31–41
87. Guy-Grand, D., Griscelli, C. and Vassali, P. (1978). The mouse gut T lymphocyte, a novel type of T cell: nature, origin and traffic in mice in normal and graft-versus-host conditions.

J. Exp. Med., **148**, 1661–77

88. McDermott, M., Horsewood, P., Clark, D. and Bienenstock, J. (1986). T lymphocytes in the intestinal epithelium and lamina propria of mice. *Immunology*, **57**, 213–18
89. Andrew, W. and Andrew, N. (1945). Mitotic division and degeneration of lymphocytes within the cells of intestinal epithelium in the mouse. *Anat. Rec.*, **93**, 251–77
90. Andrew, W. and Sosa, J. (1947). Mitotic division and degeneration of lymphocytes within cells of intestinal epithelium in young and adult white mice. *Anat. Rec.*, **97**, 63–97
91. Andrew, W. and Collings, C. (1946). Lymphocytes within the cells of intestinal epithelium in man. *Anat. Rec.*, **96**, 445–57
92. Shields, J., Touchon, R. and Dickson, D. (1969). Quantitative studies on small lymphocyte disposition in epithelial cells. *Am. J. Pathol.*, **54**, 129–45
93. Viney, J. L. and MacDonald, T. T. (1990). Selective death of T cell receptor $\gamma\delta$ + intraepithelial lymphocytes by apoptosis. *Eur. J. Immunol.*, **20**, 2809–12
94. Smith, C., Williams, G., Kingston, R., Jenkinson, E. and Owen, J. J. T. (1989). Antibodies to CD3/T cell receptor complex induce death by apoptosis in immature T cells in thymic cultures. *Nature*, **337**, 181–3
95. MacDonald, H. R. and Lees, R. (1990). Programmed death of autoreactive thymocytes. *Nature*, **343**, 642–4
96. Guy-Grand, D., Cerf-Bensussan, N., Malissen, B., Malassis-Seris, M., Briottet, C. and Vassalli, P. (1991). Two gut intraepithelial CD8 + lymphocyte populations with different T cell receptors: a role for the gut epithelium in T cell differentiation. *J. Exp. Med.*, **173**, 471–81
97. Rocha, B., Vassalli, P. and Guy-Grand, D. (1991). The Vβ repertoire of mouse gut homodimeric α CD8 + intraepithelial T cell receptor $\alpha\beta$ + lymphocytes reveals a major extrathymic pathway of T cell differentiation. *J. Exp. Med.*, **173**, 483–6

2
The mucosal immune system in inflammatory bowel disease

P. BRANDTZAEG, T. S. HALSTENSEN, L. HELGELAND and K. KETT

INTRODUCTION

Inflammatory bowel disease (IBD) is collectively used to include ulcerative colitis (UC) and Crohn's disease, which are generally considered as two different entities, although they have many common features. The aetiology is unknown and the initial lesion has not been clearly defined; but patchy necrosis of the surface epithelium, focal accumulations of leukocytes adjacent to glandular crypts, and an increased number of intraepithelial lymphocytes (IEL) and certain macrophage subsets have been described as putative early changes, especially in Crohn's disease[1,2].

Several attempts have been made to identify contributing initiating factors; there have thus been reports on a genetically determined mucin defect in UC[3] and increased intestinal permeability[4] and/or a defective mucosal immunoglobulin A (IgA) system[5] in Crohn's disease. The additional involvement of infective agent(s) in the latter, and autoimmunity in the former, disorder seems plausible on the basis of available information[1,2]. Localized tendency to thrombus formation, leading to multifocal intestinal infarction, has recently been proposed as a cause of early lesions in Crohn's disease[6]; but whether this is secondarily related to vascular complement activation[7] or procoagulant activity of activated endothelial cells and/or macrophages remains unknown. Altogether, however, there is considerable circumstantial evidence that hyperactivation of the mucosal immune system through various immuno-pathological mechanisms may cause the established IBD lesion.

THE NORMAL MUCOSAL IMMUNE SYSTEM

Secretory immunity

The generation of secretory antibodies protecting mucous membranes depends primarily on the local occurrence of IgA-producing immunocytes (plasma cells and blasts) in the absence of overt inflammation; 70–80% of all Ig-producing cells in humans are in fact located in the intestinal mucosa[8]. Exocrine tissues, and especially the gut, thus constitute quantitatively the most important mediator organ of specific humoral immunity.

Immunocytes adjacent to exocrine glands, such as the crypts of Lieberkühn, produce mainly polymeric IgA (poly-IgA = dimers and larger polymers). Such poly-IgA contains a disulphide-linked polypeptide called the 'joining' or J chain[9,10]; it can therefore be transported through the glandular epithelium along with J-chain-containing polymeric IgM (poly-IgM) via the poly-Ig receptor, which is constituted by the transmembrane secretory component or SC[8,9]. This receptor protein is produced by serous types of secretory epithelial cells such as the crypt cells in the gut[8,9]. Secretory immunity thus depends on an intimate interaction between the B-cell system and exocrine epithelia, resulting in the external transport of secretory IgA (SIgA) and secretory IgM (SIgM) (Fig. 2.1), the former normally being predominant because of the abundant local production of poly-IgA[8,9].

Immune regulation

The regulation of local humoral immunity is only partly understood. However, it normally results in the generation of a large number of early memory B-cell clones with prominent J-chain expression and preference for IgA production[9,10]. This is the basis for secretory immunity which gives rise to a 'first line' defence or immune exclusion mediated mainly by SIgA antibodies (Fig. 2.2). The abundance of locally produced IgA is probably also crucial for immunological homeostasis within the lamina propria. IgA antibodies lack potent effector functions such as complement activation and may therefore block non-specific biological amplification mechanisms triggered by locally produced or serum-derived IgG antibodies[11].

It would, in addition, be conducive to preservation of health to avoid hypersensitivity against harmless luminal antigens caused by excessive IgG and IgE responses or overactivated T lymphocytes eliciting cell-mediated immunity (Fig. 2.2). There is admittedly little direct evidence that such 'oral tolerance'[12] is induced to avoid undue mucosal tissue damage in humans[11]. However, it is most likely part of human local immune regulation because the vulnerable gut mucosa normally shows no inflammation, very few IgG-producing cells (Fig. 2.3), and little activation of T cells[13]. This is remarkable in view of the fact that there is always an influx of small amounts of intact dietary antigens after meals[11].

It is not clear how inductive and suppressive immunoregulatory mechanisms are achieved in the gut[8,10–12,14,15]. The local mucosal site with its lamina

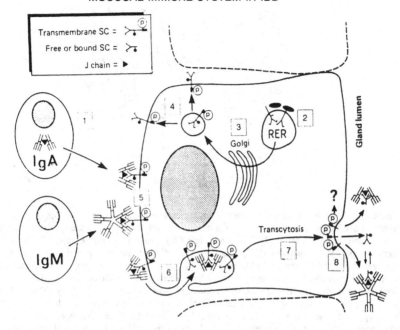

Figure 2.1 Model for local generation of secretory IgA (SIgA) and secretory IgM (SIgM). [1] Production of J-chain-containing poly-IgA and poly-IgM by mucosal plasma cells. [2] Synthesis and core glycosylation (——) of transmembrane SC (poly-Ig receptor) in rough endoplasmic reticulum (RER) of secretory epithelial cell. [3] Terminal glycosylation (—●) in Golgi complex. [4] Phosphorylation (P) at some later step. [5] Complexing of SC with J-chain-containing poly-Ig on the basolateral cell membrane. [6] Endocytosis of complexed and unoccupied SC. [7] Transcytosis of vesicles. [8] Cleavage and release of SIgA, SIgM, and excess free SC. The cleavage mechanism and the fate of the cytoplasmic tail of transmembrane SC are unknown (?). During the external translocation, covalent stabilization of the IgA-SC complexes regularly occurs (two disulphide bridges indicated in SIgA between SC and one of the IgA subunits), whereas an excess of free SC in the secretion serves to stabilize the non-covalent IgM-SC complexes (dynamic equilibrium indicated for SIgM). (Adapted from ref. 14)

propria and epithelium, the organized lymphoepithelial nodules, and the larger lymphoid aggregates such as the Peyer's patches (PP) are probably all involved in a complex interplay. The gut-associated lymphoid tissue (GALT) is increasingly being subjected to structural and functional studies to reveal its role in mucosal immunity[16,17]. Stimulated B cells representing precursors for the mucosal IgA immunocytes are unquestionably derived mainly from organized GALT such as the PP[11,18]. Also the numerous IEL, found especially in the small intestine, seem to originate mainly in PP and become primed by antigen there[8,14]. Most intestinal IEL are of the CD8 ('suppressor/cytotoxic') phenotype, in contrast to those found in the lamina propria, which are predominantly of the CD4 ('helper/inducer') phenotype (Fig. 2.2). Circumstantial evidence suggests that the CD8+ IEL normally may be involved in oral tolerance to non-replicating luminal antigens which do not bind to the gut epithelium[8,14].

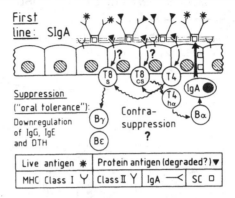

Figure 2.2 First line mucosal defence (immune exclusion) mediated by secretory antibodies, mainly of SIgA type. In addition, oral tolerance is induced to down-regulate systemic (phlogistic) types of immunity – that is, IgG (Bγ) and IgE (Bε) antibody responses and T-cell-mediated delayed type hypersensitivity (DTH) against non-adherent luminal protein antigens. CD8+ suppressor cells (T8s) are probably involved in oral tolerance, perhaps being stimulated by luminal antigens endocytosed and presented by epithelial cells in the context of MHC (or HLA) Class II molecules, or through an immunosuppressive circuit induced by CD4+ (T4) cells. Stimulated CD8+ contrasuppressor cells (T8cs) may release IgA-promoting helper cells (T4hα) from suppression so that a prominent mucosal IgA response can develop. Wavy arrows indicate immunoregulatory signals, straight or curved arrows molecular migration or biological effects. For further details, see ref. 8

IMMUNOPATHOLOGY OF THE MUCOSAL IBD LESION

T-cell alterations

Only small IBD-related mucosal alterations of the CD4+ to CD8+ T-cell ratios were noted in early studies[19], but a significant increase of CD4+ lymphocytes in the lamina propria of severely inflamed UC lesions was recently reported by others[20]. Interestingly, the same authors described a striking increase of CD4+ and a decrease of CD8+ cells in the epithelium compared with normal colon[20], perhaps reflecting an aberrant relationship between helper and suppressor cells.

There is discrepant information in the literature with regard to the functional properties of T cells isolated from IBD lesions[1,2,21,22]. However, the established Crohn lesion has been found to contain a significantly reduced proportion of naive T cells (CD45RA+), thus suggesting a preferential accumulation of antigen-primed memory cells[8,21]. This has been supported by a raised proportion of mononuclear cells with the early activation marker 4F2[23].

The presence of a large fraction of activated CD4+ T cells was recently also suggested by immunohistochemical staining for interleukin-2 (IL-2) receptor or CD25; this feature seemed to distinguish Crohn's disease from UC[24], as also borne out by different reactivity to IL-2 when mucosal mononuclear cells were tested *in vitro*[25] but not by the levels of soluble IL-2 receptor in serum[26,27].

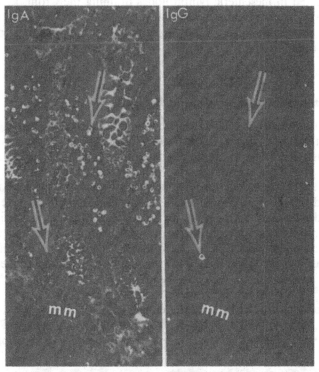

Figure 2.3 Two-colour immunofluorescence staining for IgA (*left panel*, green) and IgG (*right panel*, red) in same field from section of normal colonic mucosa. Examples of identical positions are indicated by arrows. Note striking predominance of IgA-producing plasma cells in lamina propria and selective uptake of IgA in surface and crypt epithelial cells (except goblet cells, which are negative). Muscularis mucosae (mm) and submucosa are virtually devoid of Ig-producing cells. Lumen at the top. (Magnification: ×140)

A remarkably intensified epithelial expression of HLA-DR in both UC and Crohn's disease indicates that various cytokines are released locally from activated T cells[28-31]. Both interferon-γ (IFN-γ) and tumour necrosis factor-α (TNF-α) are capable of enhancing epithelial HLA-DR on intestinal epithelium[32,33] but difficulties have been encountered in demonstrating production of the former cytokine in the IBD lesion[34]. Conversely, a raised number of cells producing TNF-α has been reported for both types of lesion, most strikingly in Crohn's disease[34]. The positive cells seemed to include both T lymphocytes and macrophages.

Much evidence thus suggests that mucosal T cells are particularly stimulated in Crohn's disease, which may be relevant to the granulomatous nature of this disorder. Further *in situ* characterization of the activated cells is nevertheless needed because recent two-colour flow-cytometric analyses have provided conflicting information; dispersed CD4 + and CD8 + mucosal T cells were reported to show fairly equal levels of stimulation, and there tended to be more activated T lymphocytes in UC than in Crohn's disease[35].

Preferential usage of the variable region T-cell receptor gene product Vβ8 has been noted in mesenteric lymph nodes draining the Crohn lesion; this could reflect a selective immune response but might also be ascribed to a polyclonal stimulatory effect of superantigen(s) or crossreacting epithelial autoantibodies[36].

Mucosal macrophages and dendritic cells

The monocyte-derived cell lineage contains remarkably heterogeneous subpopulations of accessory cells, including classical phagocytic macrophages and various types of dendritic antigen-presenting cells (APC). The latter are poorly phagocytic but express large amounts of HLA Class I and II molecules, which generally act as antigen restriction elements during stimulation of CD8 + and CD4 + T cells respectively. Monoclonal antibodies have greatly helped to dissect these subpopulations but the heterogeneity is bewildering, and probably reflects both developmental and functional overlap.

Dense accumulations of large macrophages, positive for CD4 and HLA Class II (Fig. 2.4), are found among the immunocytes just beneath the surface epithelium in normal gut mucosa, as well as in IBD lesions with intact epithelium[29,37-39]. Many of these cells show phenotypic features of both mature macrophages (RFD7 +) and dendritic cells (RFD1 +), and they can apparently function both as phagocytes and APC[40]. There are also RFD1 − scavenger macrophages with strong acid phosphatase and calprotectin

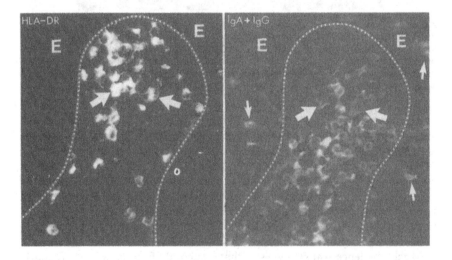

Figure 2.4 Two-colour immunofluorescence staining for HLA-DR (*left panel*, green) and IgA + IgG (*right panel*, red) in field including surface epithelium (E) at some distance from an ulcer (not shown) in the colonic mucosa of a patient with Crohn's disease. Note cluster of large DR-positive histiocytic cells between the epithelium and the dense immunocyte infiltrate. With rare exceptions (large arrows) the DR-positive cells are negative for IgA + IgG. Epithelium in this area is DR-negative and shows apical staining for IgA as sign of secretory activity (small arrows). The basement membrane zone is indicated by broken line. (Magnification ×260)

activity in the IBD lesions[41,42]. Some phenotypic alterations seem to be different in Crohn's disease and UC. Thus, the RFD9$^+$ (epithelioid-like) phenotype appears more frequently and is oftener aggregated in the former than latter disease[40]. This subset seems to be highly activated, as shown by enhanced respiratory burst. However, other mucosal macrophage subpopulations present in IBD can also be characterized as activated, both by their respiratory burst level, expression of IL-2 receptor, intercellular adhesion molecule 1 (ICAM-1), and production of TNF-α and IL-1[24,34,40,43,44]. It has been speculated, on the basis of in vitro experiments, that the combined release of IFN-γ and TNF-α from activated mucosal mononuclear cells may be directly involved in epithelial damage[45].

Are alterations of local immunity caused by break of oral tolerance?

Reduced immune exclusion because of a primary defect of the SIgA system does not seem to be generally involved in the pathogenesis of IBD[46], although a recent study suggested that mucosal production of IgA may be defective in apparently normal intestinal mucosa in Crohn's disease[5]. We have been unable to confirm this observation by measuring SIgA in jejunal secretion of such patients (Hvatum et al., unpublished data).

The normal mucosal down-regulation of systemic types of immune responsiveness to luminal antigens (Fig. 2.2) is apparently abrogated at some step in the IBD evolution, as suggested by activation of cell-mediated immunity (T cells and macrophages/APC) and a disproportionate although highly varying local over-production of IgG (Figs 2.5 and 2.6) seen in both Crohn's disease and UC[8,11,20,29,47-49]. Antigen feeding, combined with some sort of damage to the gut epithelium in experimental animals, seems to be incompatible with induction of oral tolerance[11]. The same is true when APC are excessively activated by stimuli such as muramyl dipeptide, oestrogen or a graft-versus-host reaction[12]. All these experimental situations apparently favour general overstimulation of CD4 + helper T cells[8,14], and may parallel events taking place in the pathogenesis of IBD (Fig. 2.7).

As discussed above, cytokines released from activated T cells and macrophages probably explain the increased epithelial HLA-DR expression seen in IBD; this aberrant biological phenomenon may also be involved in abrogation of oral tolerance. The density of Class II molecules involved in antigen presentation is important for the magnitude of immune responsiveness, and such molecules induced on human colonic epithelial cells by IFN-γ are functional in terms of being recognized by T cells[50]. Moreover, murine small intestinal villous epithelial cells are able to present soluble antigen in a Class II-restricted and stimulatory manner to CD4 + specific T helper cells[51]. A raised number of CD4 + cells in and beneath the epithelium in IBD lesions[20] may be further conducive to intensified B-cell activation and increased Ig production (Fig. 2.7). It has also been claimed that human intestinal epithelial cells normally activate preferentially CD8 + antigen non-specific suppressor cells, but that this function is inherently lacking for epithelium derived from IBD patients; their epithelial cells rather stimulate CD4 + antigen non-specific

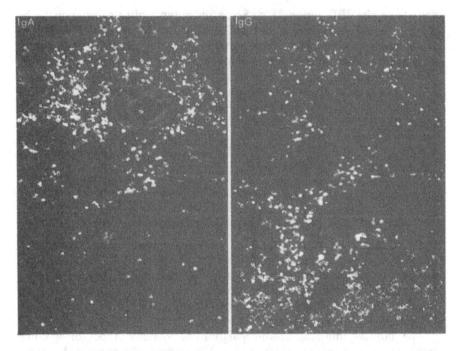

Figure 2.5 Two-colour immunofluorescence staining for IgA (*left panel*, green) and IgG (*right panel*, red) in same field from section of colonic mucosa from patient with active ulcerative colitis. Note striking predominance of IgG-producing plasma cell in the submucosa (at the bottom) and deeper layers of the mucosa, whereas IgA immunocytes are numerous in the luminal part of mucosa (at the top). The distorted crypt epithelium shows variable degrees of selective staining for IgA. (Magnification ×140)

helper cells and may thereby contribute additionally to abrogation of oral tolerance[52].

Altered local immunoglobulin production as a major immunopathological feature

The established mucosal IBD lesion is dominated by Ig-producing cells, both in UC (Fig. 2.5) and Crohn's disease. We and others have found that the mucosal IgA- and IgM-cell populations are increased several times, and that there is a disproportionate rise of IgG immunocytes (Fig. 2.6), depending on the severity of the lesion, both in Crohn's disease and in UC[8,11,20,29,47–49].

In addition to the dramatically raised proportion of IgG immunocytes, the IgA1-producing cells are increased to the extent that they become much more frequent than the IgA2 counterparts[53,54]. It is also noteworthy that J-chain expression is reduced[55,56], both in IgG and IgA1 cells, and to a lesser extent in IgA2 cells (Fig. 2.8). This change apparently reflects local accumulation of relatively mature B-cell clones because cytoplasmic J chain seems to be a marker of early memory clones which are able to 'home' to normal exocrine sites[9].

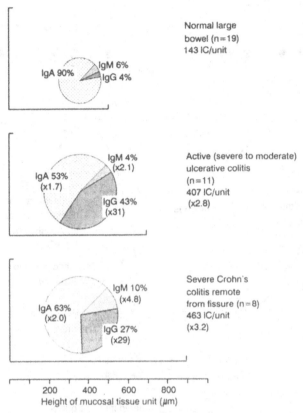

Figure 2.6 Pie charts of median numbers of Ig-producing immunocytes (IC) per intestinal mucosal tissue unit in severe Crohn's disease and active ulcerative colitis. The median percentage class distributions and increase factors (in parentheses) of the immunocyte populations compared with normal mucosa are also given. All tissue units are 500 μm wide (vertical axis) and the median height from the muscularis mucosae to the lumen (horizontal axis) for each specimen category is indicated (n = number of subjects). Data adapted from the authors' laboratory (ref. 48)

It seems, therefore, that the local humoral immune responses initially engage the poly-IgA (SIgA) system to enhance the 'first line' defence in IBD (Fig. 2.7). Later on, however, more and more features of systemic immunity evolve locally, associated with an increasing degree of inflammation. This development may be considered establishment of a 'second line' defence aiming at elimination of antigens massively penetrating into the mucosa; but the consequence is a substantial alteration of the local immunological homeostasis (Fig. 2.7).

Subclass pattern of the prominent local IgG response

IgG1 is clearly the dominating fraction of locally produced IgG in IBD; but it was originally suggested that, in relative terms, there is a preferential

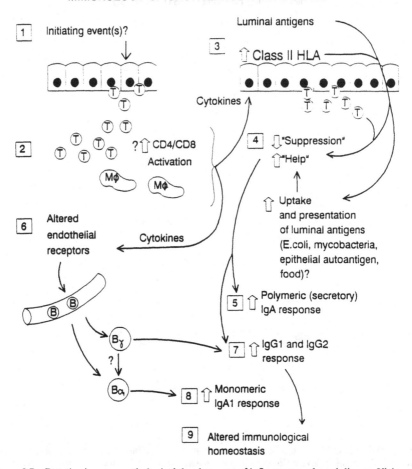

Figure 2.7 Putative immunopathological development of inflammatory bowel disease. Vicious immunostimulatory circle leading to altered homeostasis: [1] Initiating event(s) attracts T cells to the epithelium; [2] there is activation of T cells and macrophages and perhaps an increased proportion of CD4 + helper cells; [3] cytokines released from activated mononuclear cells induce epithelial HLA Class II expression; [4] Class II positive epithelium mediates enhanced uptake and presentation of luminal antigens and induces help rather than suppression; such abrogation of 'oral tolerance' will be accelerated if luminal antigens gain excessive access by some sort of epithelial breaching; [5] overstimulation initially gives rise to a secretory immune response; [6] cytokines from activated mononuclear cells induce altered endothelial receptor mechanisms which attract B cells belonging to the systemic immune system; [7] such extravasation, along with reduced suppression, gives rise to overproduction of IgG1 and IgG2 (the former being favoured in ulcerative colitis); [8] the IgG response is accompanied by preferential production of monomeric IgA1; [9] the changed relationship between secretory and systemic types of local immunity leads to altered immunological homeostasis favouring further inflammation, tissue damage, and immunostimulation. Key: ↑ = increased; ↓ = decreased; T = T cell; B = B cell; MΦ = macrophage. (Modified from ref. 8)

mucosal IgG2 response in Crohn's disease[57,58]; this notion has also been supported by subclass determinations in serum[59]. However, by comparing the colonic IBD response as determined immunohistochemically in our laboratory[58] with the subsequently established normal mucosal IgG-subclass

28

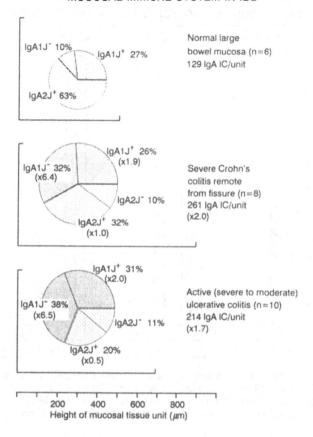

Figure 2.8 Pie charts of median numbers of IgA subclass-producing immunocytes (IC), with (J⁺) or without (J⁻) coexpression of J chain, per large bowel mucosal tissue unit in severe Crohn's disease and active ulcerative colitis. The median percentage distributions and increase factors (in parentheses) of the four IgA-cell subsets compared with normal mucosa are also given. Tissue units are defined as in Fig. 2.6. Data adapted from the author's laboratory (refs 48, 54 and 56)

pattern[60], it turns out that the mucosal IgG1- and IgG2-immunocyte subsets are fairly equally expanded on a relative basis in Crohn's disease (Fig. 2.9).

Re-evaluation of the data from MacDermott's laboratory on spontaneous IgG secretion by isolated mucosal mononuclear cells[57] likewise shows no convincing preferential overproduction of IgG2 in Crohn's disease (~39%) compared with the normal mucosal IgG2 response (~37%); the minor discrepancies between the two laboratories may well be explained by sampling variations. Conversely, the local IgG1 production is, on average, clearly favoured by UC as documented in a strikingly similar way by the two studies (Fig. 2.9); they were notably based on completely different methodology and performed on patients from Norway and the USA, respectively. In addition, this observation has recently been confirmed by an immunohistochemical investigation of Japanese patients, including both normal and non-IBD colitis controls[61].

29

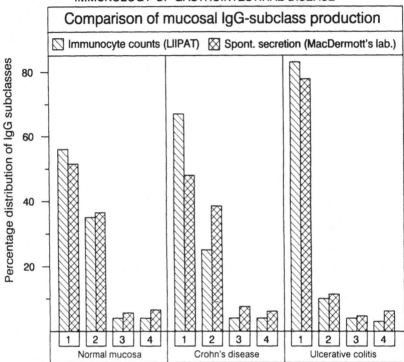

Figure 2.9 Median percentage subclass distribution of IgG production in normal colonic mucosa, Crohn's disease and ulcerative colitis. Comparison of data from two laboratories based on counts of IgG immunocytes (LIIPAT) and spontaneous IgG secretion by isolated mucosal mononuclear cells (MacDermott's laboratory). Adapted from refs 58 and 57, respectively

Our recent findings in monozygotic twins discordant with regard to IBD have, moreover, supported the idea that a genetic component contributes to the preferential IgG1-subclass response in UC[60]. The affected subjects were in an inactive phase of their disease, but the proportion of rectal IgG1 cells in UC was nevertheless significantly increased, and that of IgG2 cells decreased, compared with normal controls. In discordant twin pairs in whom the diseased twin had UC, the healthy ones also tended to have a raised IgG1-cell fraction and that of IgG2 cells was significantly reduced. Furthermore, the proportion of IgG1 cells in healthy and diseased UC twins showed a high degree of correlation, but this was not the case for the twin pairs discordant with regard to Crohn's disease.

PUTATIVE CONSEQUENCES OF ALTERED IMMUNOLOGICAL HOMEOSTASIS

The relatively mature B-cell clones accumulating and undergoing terminal differentiation to plasma cells in the IBD lesions may originate directly from the circulation because of altered endothelial recognition mechanisms[8]. At a certain level of activation, lymphoid cells show reduced expression of receptors for mucosal endothelium[62], and endothelial recognition determinants ('vascular addressins') are likewise subjected to modulation by cytokines such as IFN-γ[63]. Vascular addressins identified at inflammatory sites have in fact been shown to be different from those found in normal mucosal tissue[64].

An additional mechanism may be that mature B-cell clones expand locally; many of the IgA1-producing immunocytes are perhaps derived from J-chain-negative IgG precursors by sequential switching of heavy-chain genes[8]. A third possibility is generation of mature memory clones in overstimulated lymphoid follicles present in the gut wall. We have found, even in the normal state, that there is an IgG-predominant population of plasma cells with down-regulated J-chain expression adjacent to solitary lymphoid follicles and in the domes of PP[65]. It is possible that this population is expanded in IBD, perhaps as a result of ulceration of the follicle-associated epithelium, which in fact may represent an early lesion[1].

Significance of systemic types of immunity in the mucosa

The consequences of systemic types of humoral immunity generated in the IBD lesion are probably conflicting in terms of preservation of health. A 'second line' defence established within the gut wall (Fig. 2.7) may promote immune elimination and thereby limit dissemination of antigenic and possibly replicating agents[11]; but it will at the same time disturb the normal immunological homeostasis in the mucosa by inducing phlogistic and tissue-damaging immune reactions. Local down-regulation of J chain in IgA immunocytes[56] shifts the production from polymers to monomers[53,55], and this change may jeopardize secretory immunity. However, the overall production of poly-IgA seems to be quantitatively maintained in IBD because of the great total increase of mucosal IgA immunocytes (Fig. 2.8). Nevertheless, epithelial IBD lesions often show decreased SC expression[30,46], which results in patchy defects of SIgA (and SIgM) secretion[47] and thereby topically reduced immune exclusion. Moreover, the relative shift from local IgA2 to IgA1 production (Fig. 2.8) is probably unfavourable because the latter isotype is less resistant to proteolytic degradation and shows poorer antibacterial properties[66,67].

The local overproduction of IgG may be of paramount pathogenic significance because it consists mainly of the highly phlogistic IgG1 subclass, especially in UC (Fig. 2.9). Such IgG antibodies have potent capacity for immune elimination of foreign material by promoting phagocytosis and cytotoxicity, but they may also maintain inflammatory and tissue-damaging processes through complement activation and by arming of Fcγ receptor-bearing killer cells. IgG-antibody production against various faecal bacteria, and especially *Escherichia coli* strains, has been reported in several studies of IBD lesions[1,2,29]. Hybridoma generation of antibody-producing cells from mesenteric lymph nodes draining IBD lesions has suggested frequent specificites for *E. coli* and mycobacteria but not for food and autoantigens[68]. IgG autoantibodies to the colonic epithelium may nevertheless be produced locally, particularly in UC[69,70]. It seems, therefore, that persistent immunopathological reactions are maintained in IBD lesions by ubiquitous microbial components present in the gut lumen, but some antigens may be more important in Crohn's disease (? mycobacteria or other microorganisms) and others in UC (? epithelial autoantigens).

Mucosal complement activation

Some of the locally produced IgG may be directed against intestinal micro-organisms and epithelial antigen(s), as discussed above. Complement activation is likely to follow specific binding of such antibodies, particularly those of the IgG1 and IgG3 subclasses. Activation of the complement cascade can be identified by monoclonal antibodies to neo-epitopes in C3b (early component) and in the cytotoxic terminal complement complex (TCC). Our recent immunohistochemical studies revealed both activation products apically on colonic epithelial cells in patients with UC (Fig. 2.10). In addition, selective binding of the IgG1 subclass was often seen within these apical deposits, which were tissue-bound (not removed by extensive washing) and correlated well with the topical degree of mucosal inflammation[71].

These findings suggested that IgG1-mediated complement activation may be involved in autoimmune damage of the surface epithelium (Fig. 2.11). Perhaps this phenomenon has bearing on the previously identified 40-kD epithelial antigen recognized by tissue-bound IgG obtained from the UC

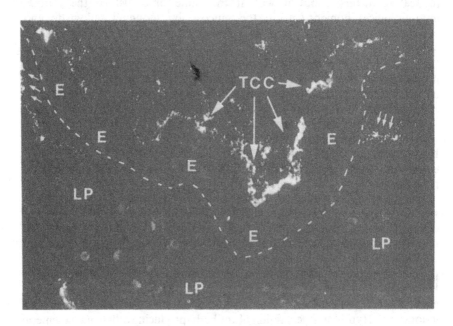

Figure 2.10 Immunofluorescence staining for TCC in colonic section from patient with active ulcerative colitis. Note intense deposition of activated complement (TCC, arrows) apically on the epithelium (E). TCC deposition in basement membrane zone (broken line) of lamina propria (LP) was observed only near disrupted epithelium (small arrows). (Magnification ×140)

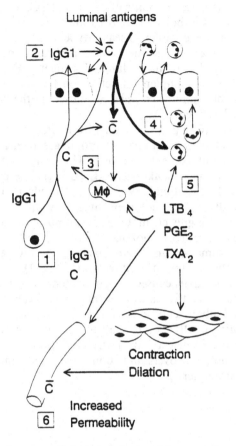

Figure 2.11 Putative immunopathological circle caused by mucosal complement activation: [1] IgG1 autoantibodies (in ulcerative colitis) and complement factors reach the luminal surface by leakage after local production or trasudation from vessels; [2] immune reactions lead to complement activation and subsequent epithelial damage; [3] luminal antigens form immune complexes and activated complement stimulates macrophages to produce complement factors and release biologically active metabolites of arachidonic acid; [4] immune complexes with activated complement mobilize numerous granulocytes (crypt abscesses) whose lysosomal enzymes and toxic products may further damage the epithelium; [5] mediators released from activated macrophages influence smooth muscles (spastic contractions) and give rise to vasodilation; [6] increased vascular permeability may also be directly induced by complement activation in vessel walls; further transudation of IgG antibodies and complement contributes to an immunopathological circle. Key: C = complement; $\bar{C}$ = activated complement; $M\Phi$ = macrophage; LTB_4 = leukotriene B_4; PGE_2 = prostaglandin E_2; TXA_2 = thromboxane A_2. Modified from ref. 8

lesion[72] and to which many UC patients have circulating IgG antibodies[73]. Moreover, a surprisingly large fraction of the IgG immunocytes in the lesion have recently been reported to produce autoantibodies, partly showing reactivity for the apical face of the colonic epithelium[70].

Luminal complement deposition was also observed in Crohn's disease but apparently not associated with epithelium-bound IgG[74]. We have, moreover, noted significantly increased amounts of C3b and TCC in submucosal blood vessels of active lesions in both UC and Crohn's disease[7]. This suggests an involvement of immune complex disease (type 3 hypersensitivity) in the pathogenesis, perhaps as a consequence of complement-mediated epithelial damage leading to undue influx of luminal antigens (Fig. 2.11). Findings suggestive of fluid phase complement activation have, moreover, indicated the presence of soluble immune complexes diffusely in the lamina propria of intensely inflamed UC specimens[71].

The anaphylatoxins (C3a and C5a) and TCC liberated during complement activation have been shown to stimulate macrophages to release prostaglandin E_2 (PGE$_2$) and thromboxane B_2 (TXB$_2$). The anaphylatoxins may also stimulate the production of leukotriene B_4 (LTB$_4$). The elevated levels of PGE$_2$, TXB$_2$, and LTB$_4$, found by various methods in UC lesions may therefore be a result of local complement activation[2,8]. Both LTB$_4$ and anaphylatoxin C5a are highly chemotactic for granulocytes and are probably involved in the massive mucosal mobilization of such cells seen in IBD (crypt abscesses); and lysosomal enzymes and toxic oxygen radicals released from these cells may further attack the epithelium (Fig. 2.11).

Break in the surface barrier caused by complement activation will obviously lead to bombardment of the underlying mucosal tissue with a battery of luminal antigens and subsequently intensify the immunopathological alterations. If epithelial breaching in IBD is the result of an initiating event – explained, for example, by a mucin defect[75] or a virus infection – abrogation of oral tolerance and immunological overstimulation with altered humoral homeostasis may be an early consequence.

CONCLUSIONS

Secretory immunity is the best-defined part of the mucosal immune system. This adaptive humoral defence mechanism depends on a fascinating cooperation between the secretory epithelium and the local plasma cells. These mucosal immunocytes produce preferentially dimers and larger polymers of IgA. Such poly-IgA, and also poly-IgM, contains J chain and can therefore become bound to epithelial SC which functions as a poly-Ig transport receptor. These microenvironmental molecular interactions are necessary for the generation of SIgA and SIgM.

There is abundant evidence that SIgA and SIgM antibodies perform immune exclusion in a first line defence, thereby counteracting microbial colonization and mucosal penetration of soluble antigens; but the relative contribution of poly-IgA is significantly down-regulated in IBD, as revealed by a strikingly decreased J-chain content of mucosal IgA immunocytes. Although the overall increase of the total mucosal immunocyte population probably compensates for the relatively reduced poly-IgA production, decreased SC expression in regenerating and dysplastic epithelium shows that the SIgA system is by no means intact in IBD. There is, moreover, a significant shift from the IgA2 to the IgA1 subclass, which is less resistant to proteolytic degradation. These changes, along with overactivation of T cells and macrophages, and a dramatic increase of IgG-producing cells, may reflect establishment of a second line local defence; this will, nevertheless, alter the local immunological homeostasis and jeopardize mucosal integrity.

Complement activation observed in relation to epithelium-bound IgG1 deposits in UC indicates that the surface epithelium is subjected to immunological attack. These luminal deposits regularly contain terminal cytotoxic TCC and often also C3b as a sign of persistent activation. Comparison of identical twins, discordant with regard to UC, suggests that the marked local IgG1 response seen in diseased mucosa may be at least partly genetically determined; an interesting possibility is that it represents an autoimmune (anti-epithelial) response. However, the initial event(s) eliciting immunopathology in IBD remains unknown. Abrogation of oral tolerance to luminal antigens has been suggested as a putative perpetuating mechanism, perhaps involving interactions between activated CD4+ T cells and epithelial cells with unduly intensified HLA Class II expression.

Acknowledgements

Studies in the authors' laboratory are supported by the Norwegian Cancer Society, the Norwegian Research Council for Science and the Humanities, and Anders Jahre's Foundation. We thank Professor O. Fausa, Medical Department A, the National Hospital, for providing much of the patient material.

References

1. Elson, C. O. (1988). The immunology of inflammatory bowel disease. In Kirsner, J. B. and Shorter, R. G. (eds), *Inflammatory Bowel Disease*. Philadelphia, PA: Lea & Febiger, pp. 97–164
2. MacDermott, R. P. and Stenson, W. A. (1988). Alterations of the immune system in ulcerative colitis and Crohn's disease. *Adv. Immunol.*, 42, 285–322
3. Tysk, C., Riedesel, H., Lindberg, E., Panzini, B., Podolsky, D. and Järnerot, G. (1991). Colonic glycoproteins in monozygotic twins with inflammatory bowel disease. *Gastroenterology*, 100, 419–23·
4. Olaison, G., Sjödahl, R. and Tagesson, C. (1990). Abnormal intestinal permeability in Crohn's disease. A possible pathogenic factor. *Scand. J. Gastroenterol.*, 25, 321–8
5. Marteau, P., Colombel, J. F., Nemeth, J., Vaerman, J. P., Dive, J. C. and Rambaud, J. C. (1990). Immunological study of histologically non-involved jejunum during Crohn's disease: evidence for reduced *in vivo* secretion of secretory IgA. *Clin. Exp. Immunol.*, 80, 196–201
6. Wakefield, A. J., Sawyerr, A. M., Dhillon, A. P., Pittilo, R. M., Rowles, P. M., Lewis, A. A. M. and Pounder, R. E. (1989). Pathogenesis of Crohn's disease: multifocal gastrointestinal infarction. *Lancet*, 2, 1057–62
7. Halstensen, T. S., Mollnes, T. E. and Brandtzaeg, P. (1989). Persistent complement activation in submucosal blood vessels of active inflammatory bowel disease: immunohistochemical evidence. *Gastroenterology*, 97, 10–19
8. Brandtzaeg, P., Halstensen, T. S., Kett, K., Krajči, P., Kvale, D., Rognum, T. O., Scott, H. and Sollid, L. M. (1989). Immunobiology and immunopathology of human gut mucosa: humoral immunity and intraepithelial lymphocytes. *Gastroenterology*, 97, 1562–84
9. Brandtzaeg, P. (1985). Role of J chain and secretory component in receptor-mediated glandular and hepatic transport of immunoglobulins in man. *Scand. J. Immunol.*, 22, 111–46
10. Mestecky, J. and McGhee, J. R. (1987). Immunoglobulin A (IgA): Molecular and cellular interactions involved in IgA biosynthesis and immune response. *Adv. Immunol.*, 40, 153–245

11. Brandtzaeg, P., Baklien, K., Bjerke, K., Rognum, T. O., Scott, H. and Valnes, K. (1987). Nature and properties of the human gastrointestinal immune system. In Miller, K. and Nicklin, S. (eds), *Immunology of the Gastrointestinal Tract*, pp. 1–85. (Boca Raton, FL: CRC Press)

12. Mowat, A. M. (1987). The regulation of immune responses to dietary protein antigens. *Immunol. Today*, **8**, 93–8

13. MacDonald, T. T. (1990). The role of activated T lymphocytes in gastrointestinal disease. *Clin. Exp. Allergy*, **20**, 247–52

14. Brandtzaeg, P., Sollid, L., Thrane, P., Kvale, D., Bjerke, K., Scott, H., Kett, K. and Rognum, T. O. (1988). Lymphoepithelial interactions in the mucosal immune system. *Gut*, **29**, 1116–30

15. Strober, W. and Sneller, M. C. (1988). Cellular and molecular events accompanying IgA B cell differentiation. *Monogr. Allergy*, **24**, 181–90

16. Brandtzaeg, P. and Bjerke, K. (1990). Immunomorphological characteristics of human Peyer's patches. *Digestion*, **46** (Suppl. 2), 262–73

17. McGhee, J. R., Mestecky, J., Elson, C. O. and Kiyono, H. (1989). Regulation of IgA synthesis and immune response by T cells and interleukins. *J. Clin. Immunol.*, **9**, 175–99

18. Mestecky, J. (1987). The common mucosal immune system and current strategies for induction of immune responses in external secretions. *J. Clin. Immunol.*, **7**, 265–76

19. Selby, W. S., Janossy, G., Bofill, M. and Jewell, D. P. (1984). Intestinal lymphocyte subpopulations in inflammatory bowel disease: an analysis by immunohistological and cell isolation techniques. *Gut*, **25**, 32–40

20. Kobayashi, K., Asakura, H., Hamada, Y., Hibi, T., Watanabe, M., Yoshida, T., Watanabe, N., Miura, S., Aiso, S. and Tsuchiya, M. (1988). T lymphocyte subpopulations and immunoglobulin-containing cells in the colonic mucosa of ulcerative colitis: a morphometric and immunohistochemical study. *J. Clin. Lab. Immunol.*, **25**, 63–8

21. James, S. P. (1988). Cellular immune mechanisms in the pathogenesis of Crohn's disease. *In vivo*, **2**, 1–8

22. Fiocchi, C. (1989). Mucosal immunity and inflammation. *Ital. J. Gastroenterol.*, **21**, 81–90

23. Pallone, F., Fais, S., Squarcia, O., Biancone, L., Pozzilli, P. and Boirivant, M. (1987). Activation of peripheral blood and intestinal lamina propria lymphocytes in Crohn's disease. *In vivo* state of activation and *in vitro* response to stimulation as defined by the expression of early activation antigens. *Gut*, **28**, 745–53

24. Choy, M. Y., Walker-Smith, J. A., Williams, C. B. and MacDonald, T. T. (1990). Differential expression of CD25 (interleukin-2 receptor) on lamina propria T cells and macrophages in the intestinal lesions in Crohn's disease and ulcerative colitis. *Gut*, **31**, 1365–70

25. Kusugami, K., Youngman, K. R., West, G. A. and Fiocchi, C. (1989). Intestinal immune reactivity to interleukin 2 differs among Crohn's disease, ulcerative colitis, and controls. *Gastroenterology*, **97**, 1–9

26. Mahida, Y. R., Gallagher, A., Kurlak, L. and Hawkey, C. J. (1990). Plasma and tissue interleukin-2 receptor levels in inflammatory bowel disease. *Clin. Exp. Immunol.*, **82**, 75–80

27. Mueller, C. H., Knoflach, P. and Zielinski, C. C. (1990). T-cell activation in Crohn's disease. Increased levels of soluble interleukin-2 receptor in serum and in supernatants of stimulated peripheral blood mononuclear cells. *Gastroenterology*, **98**, 639–46

28. Selby, W. S., Janossy, G., Mason, D. Y. and Jewell, D. P. (1983). Expression of HLA-DR antigens by colonic epithelium in inflammatory bowel disease. *Clin. Exp. Immunol.*, **53**, 614–18

29. Brandtzaeg, P. (1985). Immunopathology of Crohn's disease. *Ann. Gastroenterol. Hepatol.*, **21**, 201–20

30. Rognum, T. O., Elgjo, K., Fausa, O. and Brandtzaeg, P. (1982). Immunohistochemical evaluation of carcinoembryonic antigen, secretory component, and epithelial IgA in ulcerative colitis with dysplasia. *Gut*, **23**, 123–33

31. Fais, S., Pallone, F., Squarcia, O., Biancone, L., Ricci, F., Paoluzi, P. and Boirivant, M. (1987). HLA-DR antigens on colonic epithelial cells in inflammatory bowel disease: I. Relation to the state of activation of lamina propria lymphocytes and to the epithelial expression of other surface markers. *Clin. Exp. Immunol.*, **68**, 605–12

32. Sollid, L. M., Gaudernack, G., Markussen, G., Kvale, D., Brandtzaeg, P. and Thorsby, E. (1987). Induction of various HLA class II molecules in a human colonic adenocarcinoma cell line. *Scand. J. Immunol.*, **25**, 175–80

33. Kvale, D., Brandtzaeg, P. and Lövhaug, D. (1988). Up-regulation of the expression of secretory component and HLA molecules in a human colonic cell line by tumour necrosis

factor-α and gamma interferon. *Scand. J. Immunol.*, **28**, 351–57

34. MacDonald, T. T., Hutchings, P., Choy, M-Y., Murch, S. and Cooke, A. (1990). Tumour necrosis factor-alpha and interferon-gamma production measured at the single cell level in normal and inflamed human intestine. *Clin. Exp. Immunol.*, **81**, 301–5

35. Schreiber, S., Nash, G. S., Schloemann, S., Bertovich, M., Gamero, J. and MacDermott, R. P. (1990). Activation of human lamina propria mononuclear cells in inflammatory bowel disease. In MacDonald, T. T., Challacombe, S. J., Bland, P. W., Stokes, C. R., Heatley, R. V. and Mowat, A. M. (eds), *Advances in Mucosal Immunology*, pp. 675–80 (Lancaster: Kluwer)

36. Posnett, D. N., Schmelkin, I., Burton, D. A., August, A., McGrath, H. and Mayer, L. F. (1990). T cell antigen receptor V gene usage. Increases in Vβ8$^+$ T cells in Crohn's disease. *J. Clin. Invest.*, **85**, 1770–6

37. Selby, W. S., Poulter, L. W., Hobbs, S., Jewell, D. P. and Janossy, G. (1983). Heterogeneity of HLA-DR-positive histiocytes in human intestinal lamina propria: a combined histochemical and immunohistological analysis. *J. Clin. Pathol.*, **36**, 379–84

38. Hume, D. A., Allan, W., Hogan, P. G. and Doe, W. F. (1987). Immunohistochemical characterisation of macrophages in human liver and gastrointestinal tract: expression of CD4, HLA-DR, OKM1, and the mature macrophage marker 25F9 in normal and diseased tissue. *J. Leukoc. Biol.*, **42**, 474–84

39. Allison, M. C., Cornwall, S., Poulter, L. W., Dhillon, A. P. and Pounder, R. E. (1988). Macrophage heterogeneity in normal colonic mucosa and in inflammatory bowel disease. *Gut*, **29**, 1531–38

40. Mahida, Y. R. and Jewell, D. P. (1990). Respiratory burst capacity of human intestinal macrophage subpopulations. In MacDonald, T. T., Challacombe, S. J., Bland, P. W., Stokes, C. R., Heatley, R. V. and Mowat, A. M. (eds), *Advances in Mucosal Immunology*, pp. 701–6 (Lancaster: Kluwer)

41. Seldenrijk, C. A., Drexhage, H. A., Meuwissen, S. G. M., Pals, S. T. and Meijer, C. J. L. M. (1989). Dendritic cells and scavenger macrophages in chronic inflammatory bowel disease. *Gut*, **30**, 484–91

42. Rugtveit, J., Scott, H., Halstensen, T. S., Fausa, O. and Brandtzaeg, P. (1991). Macrophage subsets in inflammatory bowel disease (IBD): increased fraction of KP1$^+$L1$^+$ cells. (Abstract No. 37-14) 11th Meeting, European Federation of Immunological Societies, Helsinki, Finland

43. Malizia, G., Calabrese, A., Cottone, M., Raimondo, M., Trejdosiewicz, L. K., Smart, C. J., Oliva, L. and Pagliaro, L. (1991). Expression of leukocyte adhesion molecules by mucosal mononuclear phagocytes in inflammatory bowel disease. *Gastroenterology*, **100**, 150–9

44. Mahida, Y. R., Wu, K. and Jewell, D. P. (1989). Enhanced production of interleukin 1-β by mononuclear cells isolated from mucosa with active ulcerative colitis or Crohn's disease. *Gut*, **30**, 835–8

45. Deem, R. L., Shanahan, F. and Targan, S. R. (1991). Triggered human mucosal T cells release tumour necrosis factor-alpha and interferon-gamma which kill human colonic epithelial cells. *Clin. Exp. Immunol.*, **83**, 79–84

46. Brandtzaeg, P. and Baklien, K. (1977). Intestinal secretion of IgA and IgM: a hypothetical model. In *Immunology of the Gut*. Ciba Foundation Symposium 46, pp. 77–108 (Amsterdam: Elsevier/Excerpta Medica/North-Holland)

47. Brandtzaeg, P., Baklien, K., Fausa, O. and Hoel, P. S. (1974). Immunohistochemical characterization of local immunoglobulin formation in ulcerative colitis. *Gastroenterology*, **66**, 1123–36

48. Baklien, K. and Brandtzaeg, P. (1975). Comparative mapping of the local distribution of immunoglobulin-forming cells in ulcerative colitis and Crohn's disease of the colon. *Clin. Exp. Immunol.*, **22**, 197–209

49. Baklien, K. and Brandtzaeg, P. (1976). Immunohistochemical characterization of local immunoglobulin formation in Crohn's disease of the ileum. *Scand. J. Gastroenterol.*, **11**, 447–57

50. Lundin, K. E. A., Sollid, L. M., Bosnes, V., Gaudernack, G. and Thorsby, E. (1990). T-cell recognition of HLA class II molecules induced by gamma-interferon on a colonic adenocarcinoma cell line (HT29). *Scand. J. Immunol.*, **31**, 469–75

51. Kaiserlian, D., Vidal, K. and Revillard, J-P. (1989). Murine enterocytes can present soluble antigen to specific class II-restricted CD4$^+$ T cells. *Eur. J. Immunol.*, **19**, 1513–16

52. Mayer, L. and Eisenhardt, D. (1990). Lack of induction of suppressor T cells by intestinal epithelial cells from patients with inflammatory bowel disease. *J. Clin. Invest.*, **86**, 1255–60

53. MacDermott, R. P., Nash, G. S., Bertovich, M. J., Mohrman, R. F., Kodner, I. J., Delacroix, D. L. and Vaerman, J. P. (1986). Altered patterns of secretion of monomeric IgA and IgA subclass 1 by intestinal mononuclear cells in inflammatory bowel disease. *Gastroenterology*, **91**, 379–85

54. Kett, K. and Brandtzaeg, P. (1987). Local IgA subclass alterations in ulcerative colitis and Crohn's disease of the colon. *Gut*, **28**, 1013–21

55. Brandtzaeg, P. and Korsrud, F. R. (1984). Significance of different J chain profiles in human tissues: generation of IgA and IgM with binding site for secretory component is related to the J chain expressing capacity of the total local immunocyte population, including IgG and IgD producing cells, and depends on the clinical state of the tissue. *Clin. Exp. Immunol.*, **58**, 709–18

56. Kett, K., Brandtzaeg, P. and Fausa, O. (1988). J-chain expression is more prominent in immunoglobulin A2 than in immunoglobulin A1 colonic immunocytes and is decreased in both subclasses associated with inflammatory bowel disease. *Gastroenterology*, **94**, 1419–25

57. Scott, M. G., Nahm, M. H., Macke, K., Nash, G. S., Bertovich, M. J. and MacDermott, R. P. (1986). Spontaneous secretion of IgG subclasses by intestinal mononuclear cells: differences between ulcerative colitis, Crohn's disease, and conrols. *Clin. Exp. Immunol.*, **66**, 209–15

58. Kett, K., Rognum, T. O. and Brandtzaeg, P. (1987). Mucosal subclass distribution of immunoglobulin G-producing cells is different in ulcerative colitis and Crohn's disease of the colon. *Gastroenterology*, **93**, 919–24

59. MacDermott, R. P., Nash, G. S., Auer, I. O., Shlien, R., Lewis, B. S., Madassery, J. and Nahm, M. H. (1989). Alterations in serum immunoglobulin G subclasses in patients with ulcerative colitis and Crohn's disease. *Gastroenterology*, **96**, 764–8

60. Helgeland, L., Tysk, C., Färnrot, G., Kett, K., Norheim-Andersen, S. and Brandtzaeg, P. (1991). The IgG subclass distribution in serum and rectal mucosa of monozygotic twins with or without inflammatory bowel disease. *Gut* (Submitted)

61. Iizuka, M. (1990). IgG subclass-containing cells in the human large bowel of normal controls, non-IBD colitis, and ulcerative colitis. *Gastroenterol. Jpn.*, **25**, 24–31

62. Hamann, A., Jablonski-Westrich, D., Scholz, K. U., Duijvestijn, A., Butcher, E. C. and Thiele, H. G. (1988). Regulation of lymphocyte homing. I. Alterations in homing receptor expression and organ-specific endothelial venule binding of lymphocytes upon activation. *J. Immunol.*, **140**, 737–43

63. Duijvestijn, A. M., Schreiber, A. B. and Butcher, E. C. (1986). Interferon-γ regulates an antigen specific for endothelial cells involved in lymphocyte traffic. *Proc. Natl. Acad. Sci. USA*, **83**, 9114–8

64. Duijvestijn, A. and Hamann, A. (1989). Mechanisms and regulation of lymphocyte migration. *Immunol. Today*, **10**, 23–8

65. Bjerke, K. and Brandtzaeg, P. (1986). Immunoglobulin- and J chain-producing cells associated with lymphoid follicles in the human appendix, colon and ileum, including Peyer's patches. *Clin. Exp. Immunol.*, **64**, 432–41

66. Kilian, M., Mestecky, J. and Russell, M. W. (1988). Defense mechanisms involving Fc-dependent functions of immunoglobulin A and their subversion by bacterial immunoglobulin A proteases. *Microbiol. Rev.*, **52**(2), 296–303

67. Mestecky, J. and Russell, M. W. (1986). IgA subclasses. *Monogr. Allergy*, **19**, 277–301

68. Chao, L. P., Steele, J., Rodrigues, C., Lennard-Jones, J., Stanford, J. L., Spiliadis, C. and Rook, G. A. W. (1988). Specificity of antibodies secreted by hybridomas generated from activated B cells in the mesenteric lymph nodes of patients with inflammatory bowel disease. *Gut*, **29**, 35–40

69. Zinberg, J., Vecchi, M., Sakamaki, S. and Das, K. M. (1987). Intestinal tissue associated antigens in the pathogenesis of inflammatory bowel disease. In Järnerot, G. (ed.), *Inflammatory Bowel Disease*, pp. 67–76 (New York: Raven Press)

70. Hibi, T., Ohara, M., Toda, K., Hara, A., Ogata, H., Iwao, Y., Watanabe, N., Watanabe, M., Hamada, Y., Kobayashi, K., Aiso, S. and Tsuchiya, M. (1990). In vitro anticolon antibody production by mucosal or peripheral blood lymphocytes from patients with ulcerative colitis. *Gut*, **31**, 1371–6

71. Halstensen, T. S., Mollnes, T. E., Garred, P., Fausa, O. and Brandtzaeg, P. (1990). Epithelial deposition of immunoglobulin G1 and activated complement (C3b and terminal complement complex) in ulcerative colitis. *Gastroenterology*, **98**, 1264–71

72. Das, K. M., Sakamaki, S. and Vecchi, M. (1989). Ulcerative colitis: specific antibodies against a colonic epithelial Mr 40,000 protein. *Immunol. Invest.*, **18**, 459–72

73. Takahasi, F., Shah, H. S., Wise, L. S. and Das, K. M. (1990). Circulating antibodies against human colonic extract enriched with a 40 kDa protein in patients with ulcerative colitis. *Gut*, **31**, 1016–20

74. Halstensen, T. S., Mollnes, T. E., Garred, P., Fausa, O. and Brandtzaeg, P. (1991). Surface epithelium-related activation of complement differs in Crohn's disease and ulcerative colitis. *Gut* (in press)

75. Podolsky, D. K. (1987). Glycoproteins in inflammatory bowel disease. In Järnerot, G. (ed.), *Inflammatory Bowel Disease*, pp. 53–65 (New York: Raven Press)

3
Coeliac disease

E. SAVILAHTI

Coeliac disease (CD) develops in the susceptible person after digestion of cereals containing gluten, the major protein of wheat, rye, barley and oats. The harmfulness of the gluten of the four grains diminishes in the above order; the toxicity of oats in the development of coeliac disease is uncertain[1,2]. The ethanol-soluble fraction of gluten, gliadin, contains the CD-inducing factor. All electrophoretically distinct fractions (α, β, γ and ω) have been shown to cause intestinal damage in coeliac patients[3]. Several smaller peptides digested from α-gliadin, all having 25–127 amino acid residues, were found to be toxic to the jejunal biopsy specimens of coeliac patients *in vitro*[4]. The largest sequences in common in these five toxic peptides were four amino acids; the toxicity of such small peptides has not, however, been shown.

CLINICAL ASPECTS OF COELIAC DISEASE

Symptoms of CD are due to a morphological lesion of the jejunum and its functional consequences: malabsorption of various nutrients. In the typical infantile patient, chronic diarrhoea and malabsorption leading to growth failure develop a few months after the introduction of gluten-containing cereals to the diet. The presentation of coeliac disease later in childhood is quite variable; the gastrointestinal symptoms may be absent, and the disease may be monosymptomatic, presenting as growth failure, iron-deficiency anaemia, rickets or folic acid deficiency[5]. The unexpectedly high concurrence of CD with such immune disorders as insulin-dependent diabetes mellitus[6], IgA deficiency[7] and malignancy[8] suggests that an immune disturbance is present in CD. In adults, chronic diarrhoea leading to malabsorption and malnutrition are major symptoms of coeliac disease; however, it is possible for healthy individuals to have a typical coeliac jejunal lesion without any symptoms[9]. While the classical form of infantile CD has been known for a century, adult CD was identified as the same disease only due to the similarity in morphology of the jejunal lesion and its response to a gluten-free diet[10,11].

It is not definitely known whether the jejunal lesion always develops after contact with gluten in the susceptible person, who then may remain asymptomatic for a variable period of time; or whether the jejunal lesion develops at any age due to environmental factors in the susceptible person. Adenovirus 12 has been implicated as such a factor: its early protein (E1b) shares an amino acid sequence similar to that in α-gliadin[12] and significantly more patients than controls have increased antibody titres against this virus[13]. Antibodies to the particular E1B protein synthesized by the infected epithelial cells could not be found in the sera of coeliac patients in a later study[14], and a search for adenovirus DNA in duodenal biopsy samples of 26 coeliac patients was negative[15]. High numbers of asymptomatic adults have lesions in the jejunum typical of CD[9], but on the other hand, some coeliacs develop after the documentation of normal jejunal biopsy (e.g. taken because of CD in family members)[16,17]. The variation in intestinal damage is also demonstrated by patients with dermatitis herpetiformis. The majority of patients with dermatitis herpetiformis have, in addition to the blistering skin disease, villous atrophy of varying degree[18,19]. Both skin disease and intestinal lesion are, like CD, gluten-dependent, both diseases segregate in the same families[2] and the patients share the same association with HLA haplotypes[20].

THE HEREDITARY BASIS OF COELIAC DISEASE

The familial nature of CD has been demonstrated by the finding of a high frequency of CD, $\sim 10\%$, among asymptomatic family members[11,21]. The association of CD with human major histocompatibility complex (MHC) antigens was first detected for human leukocyte antigen (HLA) B8[22]. This association proved to be secondary to the association with Dw3 (DR3) antigen[23]. The alleles rendering susceptibility to CD were shown to be DR3 and DR7[24-26]. Both alleles are in linkage disequilibrium with DQw2[27], which was found in all 60 patients tested; however only one of the patients in that study did not have HLA-DR3 or DR7 alleles. Interestingly, the highest relative risk was accompanied by the genotype DR5/DR7 (20X)[28]. It was recently shown that DR3-negative coeliac patients who carry DR5/DR7 alleles share parts of the same genetic information as individuals with a DR3DQw2 haplotype. The heterodimer encoded by DQA1 and DQB1 genes may be the structure rendering susceptibility for CD. While in DR3 + patients DQA1 and DQB1 genes are expressed in *cis* position, the DR5/DR7 phenotype may encode structurally almost the same DQ-heterodimer in *trans* position[29]. In another study the DQA gene rendering susceptibility to CD was carried with the DR6 allele[30]. The disease susceptibility would thus be linked to a special structure in the molecule which functions as a receptor for peptides on the surface of cells, which express HLA class II molecules, as for example antigen-presenting cells. This structural specificity of DQ chains can be recognized by T cells[31]. These receptors are expressed on the surface of epithelial cells of the jejunum. The interaction of gliadin fractions and the structurally specific surface protein cannot alone, however, explain the pathogenesis of coeliac disease, since the same combination of DQ genes as found in 98.9% of coeliacs was found also in 25% of normal controls[29].

MORPHOLOGY

General morphology

By light microscopy the villi of the jejunum are absent or stunted[10,32]. The mucosa is not atrophic. The lengths of the crypts are increased[10,32], and, in addition to this increase in length, the circumference of the crypts is increased; thus the total mass of the crypts is increased to a greater extent than could be calculated from their lengths alone[33]. The reduction of surface epithelium in comparison to the mass of lamina propria has been demonstrated using several types of morphometric measurements[10,34,35]. When specimens were taken from proximal and distal small intestine, changes were always more severe in the proximal intestine; clinical symptoms were associated with the extent of mucosal damage[11]. Gluten-dependence of the villous lesion was demonstrated by Anderson[36], who showed that the mucosa of paediatric patients with CD reverted to normal during a gluten-free diet.

Surface epithelial cells

By light microscopy the epithelial cells in the specimens of patients with untreated CD are flattened, and their cytoplasm shows vacuolization[10,32]. The brush border and basement membrane are ill-defined[34]. Both in electron microscopy and enzyme analysis, surface epithelial cells of coeliacs are immature[37]; they have short, irregular microvilli; their mitochondria are degenerated and numerous lysosomal and lipid lakes are visible[38]. In the crypt epithelial cells the frequency of mitoses was more than two-fold higher than in normal intestine[32,37]. Morphometric estimation of the cell kinetics indicates that the crypt-cell production rate in untreated CD is more than 5 times higher than that observed in controls[33]. A similar increase is, however, seen in other types of disease with crypt hyperplastic villous atrophy, such as in severe cow's milk allergy[39] (Fig. 3.1).

Lamina propria

Cellular infiltrate

The volume of the lamina propria in the jejunal specimens of patients with untreated CD is 2-3 times greater than in normal intestine[34,35,40]. The density of plasma cells is greater in untreated CD according to several studies[10,34,41,42], while that of lymphocytes was either lower[34,41] or at the level of the controls (Table 3.1)[42]. Eosinophils are unevenly distributed, but still significantly more numerous[10,34,42]; there are more deposits of eosinophilic cationic protein extracellularly in specimens from patients with untreated CD[44]. The number of neutrophils is 20-fold higher[40], and the release of

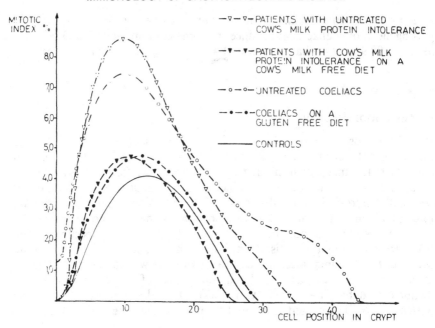

Figure 3.1 Mitotic index curves in the biopsy specimens from patients with CD, intestinal cow's milk allergy and villous atrophy and controls. (From ref. 39, with permission)

myeloperoxidase to the gut lumen is greater, but no myeloperoxidase deposits are seen in the lamina propria[44].

In the lamina propria the density of CD3 + cells is unchanged[46,47], while their absolute number expressed as cells per mm of muscularis mucosae is greater because of the larger volume of lamina propria[46]. While Selby *et al.*[48] found a slight increase in the proportion of CD8 + cells in the lamina propria, no change in CD4/CD8 ratio was seen in two other studies[46,47]. The number of T cells expressing activation markers in the lamina propria is higher[49]; this quantity of activated T lymphocytes being more pronounced among CD4 + cells[52]. The increase of activated T cells may give rise to the

Table 3.1 Inflammatory cells in the lamina propria

Increase in plasma cells[10,34,41,42]
Increase in mast cells[43]
Increase in eosinophils[10,34,42]
   increase in eosinophilic cationic protein[44]
Increase in neutrophils[40,44]
   quantity of myeloperoxidase is normal[44]
Increase in enterochromaffin cells[45]
Density of lymphocytes lower[34,41] or normal[42]
   the volume of lamina propria is 3 times higher than for normal intestine
   total number of lymphocytes is higher
CD4/CD8 ratio is not changed[46,47] or slightly decreased[48]
Activated T cells present[49]
TCR-γ/δ + cells increased[50] or unchanged[51]

observed increase of soluble interleukin-2 receptor in the serum of coeliac patients during a gluten-containing diet[53]. The density of γ/δ TCR bearing lymphocytes was about twice that observed in the normal intestine[50]; their density was not changed during a gluten-free diet or challenge. While Jenkins et al.[54] found more CD8+ cells in the lamina propria of patients with dermatitis herpetiformis than in that of coeliacs, we have found the proportion of CD4 and CD8 positive cells quite similar in the two diseases[55].

Immunoglobulin-producing cells

Several studies have indicated that the densities of immunoglobulin-containing cells in the lamina propria of patients with coeliac disease and dermatitis herpetiformis are significantly higher than in controls (Table 3.2). While the proportion of lamina propria is at the same time greater, the total number of Ig-containing cells calculated for a fixed length of mucosa is at least three times higher than in controls[62]. The higher number of IgA-containing cells may not be so pronounced in adult patients as in young coeliacs, though in our own study no difference was apparent between the numbers of IgA-containing cells of children with CD who were below and above the age of 2 years[61]. IgA-containing cells are mostly large mononuclear cells with granular cytoplasm, though in coeliac mucosa the proportion of small round cells is higher[65]. The cells were most densely concentrated below the surface epithelium[61,62]. The number of IgA2-subclass-producing cells is increased to a greater proportion (3.9 times that observed in controls) than that of IgA1-producing cells (1.7 × controls). Cells containing both subclasses were co-stained with J chain in a high percentage (89–98%) of both untreated and treated coeliacs, as well as in controls[66]. Stimulation of the IgA-producing system may be followed in some patients by the disappearance of IgA, the resulting IgA deficiency being permanent or transient[7]. IgA is also seen in the apical parts of epithelial cells and in the basement membrane, suggesting transportation. There is also striated staining between the epithelial cells[61,62]. By immunoelectron microscopy, dense IgA deposits were demonstrated in the basement membranes of the epithelial cells, and the transport routes between the epithelial cells can be seen[65,67]. The secretory component is localized in the epithelium, in the same sites as in conrols, though in the surface epithelial cells its staining was less[68]. No complement deposits were associated with the basement membrane deposition of IgA[65].

The density of IgM-containing cells was 2.5 times that of the controls[61] and the numbers in a fixed mucosal unit about 5 times[62]. The extracellular staining with anti-IgM serum is similar to that with anti-IgA, but weaker, and probably shows the secretion of IgM through epithelial cells and the basement membrane[61,62,65]. In proportion, the change in the numbers of IgG cells is most pronounced, more than 6 times that of controls; these cells still are much rarer than cells containing IgA or IgM, about 5% of the total number of Ig-containing cells[61,62]. In the mucosa of untreated coeliacs the proportion of cells containing the IgG2 subclass is higher than that of specimens from treated patients and patients with food allergy; the proportion

Table 3.2 Density of immunoglobulin-containing cells in the lamina propria of jejunal mucosa of jejunal biopsy specimens from patients with coeliac disease and dermatitis herpetiformis

Study	IgA	IgM	IgG	IgE	Relation IgA:IgM:IgG	Patients
56	Major Ig	Higher	Normal	NS		Adults
57	Lower or normal	Higher	Higher	Normal		Adults
58	Normal	Higher	Higher	NS	44:32:24 (calculated from Figure 1, ref. 58)	Adults
59	Lower	Higher	Higher	NS	37:38:18 (calculated from Figure 2, ref. 59)	Adults
60	Higher (×1.4)	Higher (×2)	Normal	NS	85:11:4	Untreated children
60	Normal	Normal	Normal	NS	88:8:4	Children on GFD
60	Higher (×1.4)	Higher (×3.1)	Normal	NS	84:14:2	Children after challenge
61	Higher (×2)	Higher (×2.5)	Higher (×1.7)	Slightly increased	73:22:5	Untreated children
62	Higher (×1.5)	Higher (×2.8)	Higher (×3.9)	Slightly increased	66:28:6	Untreated adults
63	Higher (×2.4 total number)	Higher (×3.5 total number)	Higher (×5.1 total number)	Slightly increased	71:24:5	Untreated adults with DH and villous atrophy
63	Higher (×1.4 total number)	Higher (×1.5 total number)	Normal	Normal	78:20:2	Adults with DH and normal villous structure
64	Normal	Normal	Normal	NS	83:13:5	Children on GFD

GFD-gluten free diet

of these cells in the normal intestine has not been determined, because of their scarcity[69].

The density of IgE-containing plasma cells has been found to be low according to direct staining methods[61,62,70]. In studies using more sensitive indirect methods the density of IgE-positive cells has been found to be much higher[71,72] and probably includes counts for IgE-positive mast cells[72]. *In vitro* production of IgE by coeliac biopsies was also very low, and not different from that of control specimens[73]. IgE does not play a role in the pathogenesis of jejunal damage in coeliac disease.

Investigators looking for IgD-containing cells have found only a few positive cells in the lamina propria[61,62].

In vitro *immunoglobulin production by jejunal biopsy specimens*

Results in the *in vitro* culture of jejunal biopsy specimens from coeliacs have also indicated a higher production of both IgA and IgM, when specimens are taken from untreated patients or treated patients even after a short gluten challenge[73-76]. When isolated intestinal lymphocytes were studied, the spontaneous secretion of both IgA and IgM by jejunal lymphocytes of untreated coeliacs was higher than that of the controls, culturing with peripheral autologous T lymphocytes further increased IgA and IgM production, in contrast to little or no change in cultures of cells from normal jejunum or jejunum from patients with treated coeliac disease[77]. The IgG production was not increased *in vitro*[73,76]. Affinity chromatographic methods suggested that about half of the IgA and IgM production after the short gluten challenge was specific for gliadin[75]. Lycke *et al.* isolated jejunal lymphocytes and estimated their ability to produce gliadin antibodies at a single cells level using the ELISPOT technique: they found increased numbers of gliadin–antibody-producing cells in specimens from untreated coeliac patients, more than 60% of the cells producing IgA antibodies; in the majority of patients IgM-producing cells were also found, while only three out of eight patients produced IgG antibodies[78].

Conclusions on Ig production

Evidently, the lamina propria of coeliac patients actively produces IgA and IgM antibodies; the majority of which are probably specific anti-gliadin antibodies. This process is rapidly normalized during a gluten-free diet[61] (Fig. 3.2) and the numbers of these and IgG-containing cells become quite normal after treatment for 1–2 years[64]. When the intestine is normalized, the *in vitro* challenge with gliadin could not increase the immunoglobulin production of the specimens[73,76] or isolated jejunal lymphocytes[77]. The more intense staining of basement membranes with anti-IgA sera may merely reflect its increased secretion through the diminished surface area. Further, IgA and IgM are associated with the secretory component and joining chain in the coeliac mucosa as in the normal intestine. The IgA response seems to be protective, an attempt to exclude gliadin peptides and later, with the developing mucosal damage, other intruding food and microbial antigens.

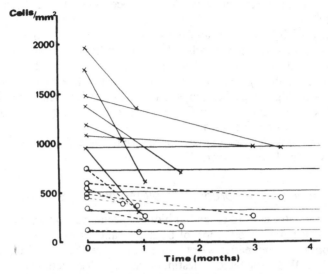

Figure 3.2 Follow-up results in seven patients treated with a gluten-free diet. × = IgA-containing cells of a patient, ○ = IgM-containing cells. Means ± SD for IgA- and IgM-containing cells in the controls are indicated. (From ref. 61, with permission)

Intraepithelial lymphocytes

The density of lymphocytes in the epithelium of CD patients with villous atrophy is significantly higher than in the normal intestine. In the normal epithelium, lymphocytes are located basally between the epithelial cells. In coeliac mucosa more lymphocytes are seen in the para- and supranuclear region of the epithelial cells[79,80]. Epithelial lymphocytes were also larger and there were more large (diameter > 9 μm) lymphoblastoid cells in the specimens of coeliacs than in control specimens[81]. The total number of lymphocytes when counted on a fixed length of muscularis mucosae is reduced on the surface; but when at the same time their number in enlarged crypts[33] is very much higher[82], the total number of lymphocytes on the given length of intestine is greater. In the crypts, the density of lymphocytes is approximately one-third of that in the surface[82]. The greater density of lymphocytes in the epithelium is not, however, specific for CD; it is seen in many types of small intestinal diseases with varying villous atrophy such as severe food allergy (particularly caused by cow's milk proteins)[83,84]. It has been proposed that a high mitotic index of lymphocytes would be specific for CD and DH[81,82], but Ferguson and Ziegler[85] found high frequency of mitosis also in specimens from patients with other jejunal disorders, the greater mitotic rate being associated with the higher density of lymphocytes. Most authors agree that the density of lymphocytes remains high in the epithelium even during a gluten-free diet[79,80,83,84] (Table 3.3).

Immunohistochemical analysis shows that only the α/β T-cell-receptor-positive cells react to gluten elimination and challenge (Fig. 3.3), while the increased

Table 3.3 Intraepithelial lymphocytes

	Normal intestine	Coeliac disease	Other causes of villus atrophy[79,80,83,84]
Density/100 epithelial cells	<40[79,80]	>40[79,80]	Higher or normal[79,80,83,84]
Total quantity		Higher[81]	Normal or higher
in the surface epithelium		Lower[81-82]	Normal or lower
in the crypts		Higher[81-82]	Higher
Morphology	Small lymphocytes[79-82]	Also larger mononuclear cells[81,82]	
Mitotic frequency	<0.5%[81,82]	>0.5%[81,82]	>0.5% (if density is higher)[85]
CD8 positive	>90%[46-48,86]	62-90%[46-48]	>90%[87,88]
CD4 positive	<10%[46-48,86]	<10%[46-48]	<10%
Interleukin-2 receptor positive	Absent[49,52]	Absent[49,52]	Absent[88]
TCR α/β positive	>90%[50,51,87]	50-80%[50,51,87]	>90%[87,88]
TCR γ/δ positive	<10%[50,51,87]	20-50%[50,51,87]	<10%[87,88]

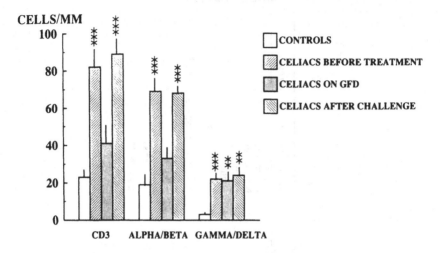

Figure 3.3 Mean numbers of lymphocytes/mm in the surface epithelium expressing surface antigens CD3, alpha/beta and gamma/delta for controls, patients with coeliac disease before treatment, during a gluten-free diet (GFD) and after a gluten challenge. SEM and the significance of the difference to the controls are shown (* $p < 0.05$, ** $p < 0.01$, *** $p < 0.001$). (From ref. 50, with permission)

number of $\gamma/\delta +$ cells remains unchanged[50]. In the normal intestine, the majority, over 80% of CD3+ intraepithelial T cells, are CD8+ suppressor/inducer T cells, and there are very few, if any, B cell or NK cells in the epithelium[86]. The density of CD3 + cells is much greater in active coeliac disease, and CD8 + cells predominate also in the coeliac epithelium[46,47]. T cells in the epithelium have not been found to bear activation markers[49,52]. Careful quantitation of intraepithelial T cells suggested that a considerable proportion of CD3 + cells did not bear either CD4 or CD8 antigen on their surface[46,47]. By double-staining methods the mean proportion of this CD3 +CD8 −CD4 population was 28%[89]. By studying the character of the T cell receptor (TCR) of IEL, it was shown that γ/δ-TCR-bearing cells are significantly higher in coeliac disease[50,51,87]. The proportion of $\gamma/\delta +$ cells varied during dietary treatment, being highest during gluten-free diet, about 35% of the number of CD3 + cells. During gluten-free diet the density of α/β TCR + cells was similar to that of controls in the surface epithelium, but the density of $\gamma/\delta +$ cells remained on the same, increased level as in untreated patients. During gluten challenge the density of α/β TCR + cells increased significantly, while the density of $\gamma/\delta +$ cells remained unchanged[50]. There is a constant, marked increase of the density of $\gamma/\delta +$ T cell in the epithelium of coeliacs, while the $\alpha/\beta +$ cells respond to gluten elimination and challenge. In specimens from patients with dermatitis herpetiformis (DH) a similar increase of $\gamma/\delta +$ cells has been found as in coeliacs[55], the proportion of $\gamma/\delta +$ cells being highest in DH patients having been on a gluten-free diet for many years and having normal jejunal morphology; it was 45% of that of CD3 + cells.

HLA antigen expression in epithelial cells

Major histocompatibility Class II molecules were shown to be present in the jejunal epithelium both in normal human intestine and in the intestine of patients with CD and DH[90]. In that study no difference was noted in the distribution of HLA-DR in normal or diseased jejunum. Later studies showed that in biopsies from coeliacs taken during a gluten-containing diet the staining is extended even to the bottom of crypts, and the epithelial cells are more heavily stained than cells in normal jejunum with anti-DR − monoclonal antibodies[72,91]. Installation of gluten to the jejunum of treated patients induced HLA-DR staining of crypt epithelial cells within an hour[92]. In the specimens of patients with treated CD the expression of HLA-DR on the epithelial cells is similar to that in normal intestine[72,92]. Although there is controversy on the expression of the DP and DQ molecules on the surface of epithelial cells in coeliac jejunum, in a recent study these antigens, too, could be shown in the same location as DR − antigen[93]. This would be expected, as the molecules are probably functionally similar. The presence of MHC Class II antigens may be important in transporting antigenic material from gut lumen to the basolateral surface of the epithelial cells to antigen-presenting cells in the lamina propria or to T cells in the epithelium. Whether they are antigen-presenting cells to T cells, leading directly to stimulation of a subgroup of T cells, is another possibility.

Progression of morphological change

In experiments with a single dose of gluten it has been shown that the accumulation of intraepithelial lymphocytes takes place within a few hours of the challenge with gluten[94]. Using graded amounts of gluten during challenge tests, Marsh found that the increase of intraepithelial lymphocytes was followed by crypt hyperplasia and increase in the total number of IE (both surface and crypt) lymphocytes, the villous atrophy being the last event in the development of the coeliac lesion in the intestine[95]. In the reports published on the progression of the CD in individuals, in five cases in the biopsy specimens taken before the diagnostic biopsy no changes could be found[17,96,97], while Marsh[16] found increased numbers of intraepithelial lymphocytes several years before the development of villous atrophy and crypt hyperplasia in two cases. In an asymptomatic father of a coeliac patient we have found higher than normal density of γ/δ TCR positive cells in an otherwise normal jejunal specimen; 2 years after this examination he developed symptomatic CD and villous atrophy with crypt hyperplasia of the jejunum[98]. Intermediate forms of gluten-induced jejunal damage are found in patients with DH: from total villous atrophy with crypt hyperplasia to a normal villous structure. The vast majority of DH patients show at least higher intraepithelial lymphocyte numbers[99], which is not fully normalized during a gluten-free diet. Even in cases with normal morphology, DH patients show activation of the local immunoglobulin-producing system: they have increased numbers of mucosal IgA cells[100] and secrete gliadin IgA and IgM antibodies to the jejunal fluid[101], and they have higher numbers of $\gamma/\delta +$ cells, particularly in the epithelium[55].

Morphology of the intestine of family members of coeliac patients

In addition to the asymptomatic cases found among family members of coeliac patients, others with grossly normal jejunal structure may show minor changes. Thirty-eight per cent of 52 first-degree relatives of patients with CD had higher numbers of intraepithelial lymphocytes; such numbers showed a highly significant association with HLA-DR3[102]. A similar frequency for a higher number of IE lymphocytes was found among 116 family members of 38 coeliac probands; this increase was not associated with HLA-DR3. An abnormally high density of $\gamma/\delta +$ cells in the epithelium was seen in 15% of these asymptomatic family members with grossly normal villous structure (Holm et al., in preparation).

Morphology of jejunal specimens of coeliacs when cultured in vitro

When specimens of mucosa from untreated coeliac patients are cultured in the absence of gluten, a remarkable improvement of the surface epithelial cells takes place within 24 h[103]. [³H] Thymidine incorporation shows that the mitotic activity of crypt cells was greatly increased in specimens of untreated coeliacs compared with controls; in specimens of the same patients after 6–15 weeks on a gluten-free diet the mitotic rate was intermediate[103]. This labelling could be further enhanced by cultivating the specimens in the presence of gluten[104]. Falchuk et al. demonstrated that the epithelial cells matured during in vitro culture, a maturation which was inhibited by adding gluten to the culture fluid[38]. However, gluten had no clear effect on the biopsy specimens of treated coeliac patients[38,105,106]. Such resistance to gluten of specimens from treated patients with coeliac disease strongly suggests that not all factors required for the development of jejunal damage in coeliac disease are present locally in the mucosa.

Supernatants of the culture medium of biopsy specimens from untreated coeliacs, when the specimens were cultured in the presence of α-gliadin, inhibited migration of leukocytes from normal persons[107]. This finding was corroborated by another group, who also reported that biopsies from treated patients did not secrete this migration-inhibition factor when cultured in the presence of gliadin[108].

SERUM ANTIBODIES SPECIFIC FOR COELIAC DISEASE

Antigliadin antibodies

Titres of antibodies to several food antigens have been found to be higher in the sera of patients with coeliac disease[5,109], but the most constant finding has been the strong reaction with gliadin. The use of enzyme-linked immunosorbent technique has simplified the determination of these antibodies in different immunoglobulin classes[110]. The increase in IgA-antigliadin–antibody titre is quite a sensitive marker of active coeliac disease[5,110-114], its specificity being higher than that of IgG antibodies. During a gluten challenge test over 90% of patients show either the IgA- or IgG-antigliadin response during the first 3 months of exposure, and the antibodies may appear before the development of jejunal damage; during continued gluten challenge in many patients there is decrease in the titre of gliadin antibody[112]. The development of this non-responsiveness may explain why some studies find a lower frequency of gliadin antibodies in adults than in children[113].

The origin and role of gliadin antibodies in the pathogenesis of coeliac disease is not clear. Together with the data on the production of antigliadin antibodies by the jejunal mucosa and on cells isolated from the mucosa (discussed above), one would expect them to be of mucosal origin. Gliadin antibody titres are normalized during a gluten-free diet, as are the numbers of immunoglobulin-producing cells in the jejunum. On average, more than half of the IgA antigliadin antibodies are polymeric[114], this relation being similar to that secreted by intestinal lamina propria cells[115]. Immunoblotting analysis showed that the antibodies from coeliacs react with the same epitopes of gliadin as those from persons having high gliadin antibodies, but not CD (as, for example, patients with Crohn's disease) and from rabbits immunized parenterally[116,117]. Still, the magnitude of the antibody response to gliadin is of quite another order compared to that for other food proteins. When we used the same monoclonal antibodies to titrate the IgA and IgG gliadin and β-lactoglobulin antibodies we found that the mean titres to gliadin were 100–1000 times higher than those to β-lactoglobulin[118]. The B cells of coeliacs respond to gliadin abnormally. This may not be due to primary abnormality of B cells, but secondary: for instance to the affinity of the surface receptors of antigen-presenting cells to gliadin, or to lack of specific suppressor T cells.

Reticulin and endomysial antibodies

Reticulin–antibody formation is another humoral response quite specific for CD. These antibodies react with reticulin fibres in several organs, both of human and rodent origin[119]. The IgG class antibody was more common in children with coeliac disease than that observed in adults[120]. Later it was shown that IgA-reticulin antibody test has a high specificity and sensitivity in paediatric patients with CD[121]. However, the variation between laboratories determining the test is great[5]. Attempts to show cross reactivity between reticulin and gliadin antibodies have repeatedly failed[119,120].

An antibody reacting with connective tissue around smooth muscle fibres of primate gastrointestinal tract (endomysial antibody) has been claimed to be specific for CD and DH[122]. By the detecting methods used, these reticulin and endomysium antibodies seem to be crossreactive: both antibodies can be absorbed with human liver homogenates, while rodent liver absorption eradicated staining in rodent tissues, but activity remained in the endomysium test performed on monkey oesophagus[123]. The origin of both reticulin and endomysial antibodies is unknown. The reticulin (or endomysial) antibody can fix in vitro to the reticulin fibres of human intestine[119,123], but not to the epithelial cells. The titres of both gliadin and reticulin antibody associate with the severity of the jejunal damage observed in patients with dermatitis herpetiformis[124]. Both reticulin and endomysial antibodies disappear during a gluten-free diet[5,120-123]. The role of these antibodies in the pathogenesis of jejunal damage is speculative: by fixing to the basement membranes of the epithelium they may play a part in the pathogenesis.

PATHOGENESIS OF COELIAC DISEASE

Morphology of the mucosal lesion in CD indicates that epithelial cells are lost from the surface rapidly. These surface epithelial cells are immature and young, but still show the morphology of dying cells. Compensatory mechanisms in the crypts are activated, but are not capable of replacing the rapidly destroyed epithelial cell mass. These events lead to villous atrophy and crypt hyperplasia.

We have presented some data concerning the vigorous immune reaction taking place in the mucosa of the patient with CD when taking gluten-containing food, and of some of its reflections in the systemic immune response. There are several possibilities which may kill or induce the death of the epithelial cells.

1. direct T cell cytotoxicity;
2. antibody-dependent T cell cytotoxicity – the fixation of gliadin to the epithelial cells and the presence of gliadin antibodies would activate this cytotoxicity;
3. lymphokine-programmed death of the epithelial cells;
4. autoimmune reaction of the basal membrane of the epithelial cells interacting with the nutrition or attachment of the epithelial cells.

Many details of the possible processes are known, but the pieces have not been put together. One of the basic events could be the connection with gliadin peptides and the CD-specific DQ heterodimer, which is expressed on the epithelial cells. Present knowledge indicates a fairly common structure for the heterodimer; there should be a more specialized structure with high affinity to the toxic gliadin peptides, if the combining of the special antigen receptor has a central role in the pathogenesis of CD and DH. Another hereditary factor is probably the presence of high numbers of γ/δ TCR-bearing cells in the epithelium. Too little is known about the functions of these cells to allow speculation upon their exact role. As indicated, several other types of inflammatory cells are present in much higher number in the lamina propria: this is probably due to secretion of lymphokines and interferon-γ by the lymphocytes participating in the immune reaction.

Acknowledgements

Financial support from the Sigrid Juselius foundation for the preparation of this manuscript is gratefully acknowledged.

COELIAC DISEASE

References

1. Dicke, W. K., Weijers, H. A. and van de Kamer, J. H. (1953). An investigation into the injurious constituents of wheat in connection with their action on patients with coeliac disease. *Acta Paediatr. (Uppsala)*, **42**, 34–42
2. Ciclitira, P. J. and Hall, M. A. (1990). Coeliac disease. *Bailliere's Clin. Gastroenterol.*, **4**, 43–61
3. Ciclitira, P. J., Evans, D. J., Fagg, N. K., Lennox, E. S. and Dowling, R. H. (1984). Clinical testing of gliadin fraction in coeliac disease. *Clin. Sci.*, **66**, 357–64
4. de Ritis, G., Auricchio, S., Jones, H. W., Lew, E. J., Bernardin, J. E. and Kasarda, D. D. (1988). *In vitro* (organ culture) studies of the toxicity of specific A-gliadin peptides in celiac disease. *Gastroenterology*, **94**, 41–9
5. Auricchio, A., Greco, L. and Troncone, R. (1988). Gluten-sensitive enteropathy in childhood. *Pediatr. Clin. N. Am.*, **35**, 157–87
6. Savilahti, E., Simell, O., Koskimies, S., Rilva, A. and Åkerblom, H. K. (1986). Celiac disease in insulin-dependent diabetes mellitus. *J. Pediatr.*, **108**, 690–3
7. Savilahti, E., Pelkonen, P., Verkasalo, M. and Koskimies, S. (1985). Selective deficiency of immunoglobulin A. *Klin. Pädiat.*, **197**, 336–40
8. Swinson, C. M., Slavin, G., Coles, E. C. and Booth, C. C. (1983). Coeliac disease and malignancy. *Lancet*, **1**, 111–15
9. Hed, J., Lieden, G., Ottosson, E., Ström, M., Walan, A., Groth, O., Sjögren, F. and Franzen, L. (1986). IgA anti-gliadin antibodies and jejunal mucosal lesions in healthy blood donors. *Lancet*, **2**, 215.
10. Rubin, C. E., Brandborg, L. L., Phelps, P. C. and Taylor, H. C. (1960). Studies of celiac disease. I. The apparent identical and specific nature of the duodenal and proximal jejunal lesions in celiac disease and idiopathic sprue. *Gastroenterology*, **38**, 28–49
11. MacDonald, W. C., Brandborg, L. L., Flick, A. L., Trier, J. S. and Rubin, C. E. (1964). Studies of celiac sprue. IV. The response of the whole length of the small bowel to a gluten-free diet. *Gastroenterology*, **47**, 573–89
12. Kagnoff, M. F., Raleigh, K. A., Hubert, J. J., Bernardin, J. E. and Kasarda, D. D. (1984). Possible role for a human adenovirus in the pathogenesis of celiac disease. *J. Exp. Med.*, **160**, 1544–57
13. Kagnoff, M. F., Paterson, Y. J., Kumar, P. J., Kasadra, D. D., Carnone, F. R., Unsworth, D. J. and Austin, R. K. (1987). Evidence for the role of a human intestinal adenovirus in the pathogenesis of coeliac disease. *Gut*, **28**, 995–1001
14. Howdle, P. D., Blair Zajdel, M. E., Smart, C. J., Tredjdosiewicz, L. K., Blair, G. E. and Losowsky, M. S. (1989). Lack of serological response to an E1B protein of adenovirus 12 in coeliac disease. *Scand. J. Gastroenterol.*, **24**, 282–6
15. Carter, M. J., Willococks, M. M., Mitchison, H. C., Record, C. O. and Madeley, C. R. (1989). Is a persistent adenovirus infection involved in coeliac disease? *Gut*, **30**, 1563–7
16. Marsh, M. N. (1989). Studies of intestinal lymphoid tissue. XIII. Immunopathology of the evolving celiac sprue lesion. *Path. Res. Pract.*, **185**, 774–7
17. Mäki, M., Holm, K., Koskimies, S., Hällström, O. and Visakorpi, J. K. (1991). Normal small bowel biopsy followed by coeliac disease. *Arch. Dis. Child.* (In press)
18. Fry, L., Keir, P., McMinn, R. H., Cowan, J. D. and Hoffbrand, A. V. (1967). Small-intestinal structure and function and haematological changes in dermatitis herpetiformis. *Lancet*, **2**, 729–33
19. Hall, R. P. (1987). The pathogenesis of dermatitis herpetiformis: Recent advances. *J. Am. Acad. Dermatol.*, **16**, 1129–44
20. Hall, R. P., Sanders, M. E., Duquesnoy, R. J., Katz, S. I. and Shaw, S. (1990). Alterations in HLA-DP and HLA-DQ antigen frequency in patients with dermatitis herpetiformis. *J. Invest. Dermatol.*, **93**, 501–5
21. Auricchio, S., Mazzacca, G., Tosi, R., Visakorpi, J., Mäki, M. and Polanco, I. (1988). Coeliac disease as a familial condition: identification of asymptomatic coeliac patients within family groups. *Gastroenterol. Int.*, **1**, 25–31
22. Falchuk, Z. M., Rogentine, G. N. and Strober, W. (1972). Predominance of histocompatibility antigen HL-A8 in patients with gluten-sensitive enteropathy. *J. Clin. Invest.*, **51**, 1602–5
23. Solheim, B. G., Ek, J., Thune, P. O., Baklien, K., Bratlie, A., Rankin, B., Thoresen, A. B. and Thorsby, E. (1976). HLA antigens in dermatitis herpetiformis and coeliac disease.

Tissue Antigens, **7**, 57–9
24. Demarchi, M., Carbonara, A., Ansaldi, N., Santini, B., Barbera, C., Borelli, I., Rossino, P. and Rendine, S. (1983). HLA-DR3 and DR7 in coeliac disease: immunogenetic and clinical aspects. *Gut*, **24**, 706–12
25. Mearin, M. L., Biemond, I., Pena, A. S., Polanco, I., Vazquez, C., Schreuder, G. T. M., Vries, R. R. P., de and Rood, J. J., van (1983). HLA-DR phenotypes in Spanish coeliac children: their contribution to the understanding of the genetics of the disease. *Gut*, **24**, 523–37
26. Verkasalo, M., Tiilikainen, A., Kuitunen, P., Savilahti, E. and Backman, A. (1983). HLA antigens and atrophy in children with coeliac disease. *Gut*, **24**, 306–10
27. Tosi, R., Vismara, D., Tanigaki, N., Ferrara, G. B., Cicimarra, F., Buffolano, W., Follo, D. and Auricchio, S. (1983). Evidence that celiac diseases is primarily associated with a DC locus allelic specificity. *Clin. Immunol. Immunopathol.*, **28**, 395–404
28. Trabace, S., Giunta, A., Rosso, M., Marzorati, D., Cascino, I., Tettamanti, A., Mazzilli, M. C. and Gandini, E. (1984). HLA-ABC and DR antigens in celiac children. *Vox. Sang.*, **46**, 102–6
29. Sollid, L. M., Markussen, G., Ek, J., Gjerde, H., Vartdal, F. and Thorsby, E. (1989). Evidence for a primary association of celiac disease to a particular HLA-DQ alpha/β heterodimer. *J. Exp. Med.*, **169**, 345–50
30. Koskimies, S., Lipsanen, V., Mäki, M. and Visakorpi, J. (1991). HLA and family studies. In Mearin, M. L. and Mulder, C. J. J. (eds), *Coeliac Disease, 40 years Glutenfree*. (Dordrecht: Kluwer), pp. 10–14
31. Lundin, K. A., Sollid, L. M., Qvigstad, E., Markussen, G., Gjertsen, A. A., Ek, J. and Thorsby, E. (1990). T lymphocyte recognition of a celiac disease-associated *cis*-or *trans*-encoded HLA-DQ α/β-heterodimer. *J. Immunol.*, **145**, 136–9
32. Shiner, M. and Doniach, I. (1960). Histopathologic studies in steatorrhea. *Gastroenterology*, **38**, 419–40
33. Wright, N., Watson, A., Morley, A., Appleton, D. and Marks, J. (1973). Cell kinetics in flat (avillous) mucosa of the human small intestine. *Gut*, **14**, 701–10
34. Kuitunen, P. (1966). Duodeno-jejunal histology in the malabsorption syndrome in infants. *Ann. Paediatr. Fenn.*, **12**, 101–32
35. Risdon, A. and Keeling, J. W. (1974). Quantitation of the histological changes found in small intestinal biopsy specimens from children with suspected coeliac disease. *Gut*, **15**, 9–18
36. Anderson, C. M. (1960). Histological changes in the duodenal mucosa in coeliac disease-reversibility during treatment with a gluten-free diet. *Arch. Dis. Child.*, **35**, 419–27
37. Padykula, H. A., Strauss, E. W., Ladman, A. J. and Gardner, E. H. (1961). A morphologic and histochemical analysis of the human jejunal epithelium in non tropical sprue. *Gastroenterology*, **40**, 735–65
38. Falchuk, Z. M., Gebbard, R. L., Sessons, C. and Strober, W. J. (1974). An *in vitro* model of gluten-sensitive enteropathy. *J. Clin. Invest.*, **53**, 487–500
39. Kosnai, I., Kuitunen, P., Savilahti, E., Rapola, J. and Kohegyi, J. (1980). Cell kinetics in the jejunal epithelium in malabsorption syndrome with cows' milk protein intolerance and in coeliac disease of childhood. *Gut*, **21**, 1041–6
40. Dhesi, I., Marsh, M. N., Kelly, C. and Crowe, P. (1984). Morphometric analysis of small intestinal mucosa. II. Determination of lamina propria volumes, plasma cell and neutrophil populations within control and coeliac disease mucosae. *Virchow's Arch. (Pathol. Anat.)*, **403**, 173–80
41. Holmes, G. K. T., Asquith, P., Stokes, P. L. and Cooke, W. T. (1974). Cellular infiltrate of jejunal biopsies in adult coeliac disease in relation to gluten withdrawal. *Gut*, **15**, 278–83
42. Lancaster-Smith, M., Kumar, P. J. and Dawson, A. M. (1975). The cellular infiltrate of the jejunum in adult coeliac disease and dermatitis herpetiformis following the reintroduction of dietary gluten. *Gut*, **16**, 683–8
43. Strobel, S. B., Busittil, A. and Ferguson, A. (1983). Human intestinal mucosal mast cells: expanded population in untreated coeliac disease. *Gut*, **24**, 222–7
44. Hällgren, R., Colombel, J. F., Dahl, R., Fredens, K., Kruse, A., Jacobsen, N. O., Venge, P. and Rambaud, J. C. (1989). Neutrophil and eosinophil involvement of the small bowel in patients with celiac disease and Crohn's disease: studies on the secretion rate and immunohistochemical localization of granulocyte granule constituents. *Am. J. Med.*, **86**, 56–64
45. Wheeler, E. E. and Challacombe, D. N. (1984). Quantification of enterochromaffin cells with serotonin immunoreactivity in the duodenal mucosa in coeliac disease. *Arch. Dis.*

Child., **59**, 523–7
46. Jenkins, D., Goodall, A. and Scott, B. B. (1986). T-lymphocyte populations in normal and coeliac small intestinal mucosa defined by monoclonal antibodies. *Gut*, **27**, 1330–7
47. Verkasalo, M., Arato, A., Savilahti, E., and Tainio, V.-M. (1990). Effect of diet and age on jejunal and circulating lymphocyte subsets in children with coeliac disease: persistence of CD4-8- intraepithelial T cells through treatment. *Gut*, **31**, 422–5
48. Selby, W. S., Janossy, G., Bofill, M. and Jewell, D. P. (1983). Lymphocyte subpopulations in the human small intestine. The findings in normal mucosa and in the mucosa of patients with adult coeliac disease. *Clin. Exp. Immunol.*, **52**, 219–28
49. Kelly, J., O'Farrelly, C., O'Mahony, C. and Weir, D. G. (1987). Immunoperoxidase demonstration of the cellular composition of the normal and coeliac small bowel. *Clin. Exp. Immunol.*, **68**, 177–88
50. Savilahti, E., Arato, A. and Verkasalo, M. (1990). Intestinal γ/δ receptor bearing T lymphocytes in celiac disease and inflammatory bowel diseases in children. Constant increase in celiac disease in the epithelium of celiac disease. *Pediatr. Res.*, **28**, 579–82
51. Halstensen, T. S., Scott, H. and Brandtzaeg, P. (1989). Intraepithelial T cells of the TcRγ/δ + CD8– and V $\delta 1/J\delta$ 1+ phenotypes are increased in coeliac disease. *Scand. J. Immunol.*, **30**, 665–72
52. Griffiths, C. E. M., Barrison, E. G., Leonar, J. N., Caun, K., Valdimarsson, H. and Fry, L. (1988). Preferential activation of CD4 T lymphocytes in the lamina propria of gluten-sensitive enteropathy. *Clin. Exp. Immunol.*, **73**, 280–3
53. Crabtree, J. E., Heatley, R. V., Juby, L. D., Howdle, P. D. and Losowsky, M. L. (1989). Serum interleukin-2-receptor in coeliac disease: response to treatment and gluten challenge. *Clin. Exp. Immunol.*, **77**, 345–54
54. Jenkins, D., Goodall, A. and Scott, B. (1989). T-cell and plasma cell populations in coeliac small intestinal mucosa in relation to dermatitis herpetiformis. *Gut*, **30**, 955–8
55. Savilahti, E., Arata, A., Reunala, T. and Verkasalo, M. (1991). Intestinal γ/δ receptor bearing T lymphocytes are increased in coeliac disease and dermatitis herpetiformis. In Mearin, M. L. and Mulder, C. J. J. (eds), *Coeliac Disease, 40 years Glutenfree.* (Dordrecht: Kluwer), pp. 73–80
56. Rubin, W., Fauci, A. S., Sleisenger, M. H. and Jeffries, G. H. (1965). Immunofluorescent studies in adult celiac disease. *J. Clin. Invest.*, **44**, 475–85
57. Douglas, A. P., Crabbe, P. A. and Hobbs, J. R. (1970). Immunochemical studies of the serum, intestinal secretions and intestinal mucosa in patients with adult celiac disease and other forms of the celiac syndrome. *Gastroenterology*, **59**, 414–25
58. Söltoft, J. (1970). Immunoglobulin-containing cells in non-tropical sprue. *Clin. Exp. Immunol.*, **6**, 413–20
59. Pettingale, K. W. (1971). Immunoglobulin-containing cells in the coeliac syndrome. *Gut*, **12**, 291–6
60. Jos, J., Rey, J. and Frezal, J. (1972). Etude immuno-histochimique de la muqueuse intestinale chez l'enfant. I. Les syndromes de malabsorption. *Arch. Franc. Pediatr.*, **29**, 681–98
61. Savilahti, E. (1972). Intestinal immunoglobulins in children with coeliac disease. *Gut*, **13**, 958–64
62. Baklien, K., Brandtzaeg, P. and Fausa, O. (1977). Immunoglobulins in jejunal mucosa and serum from patients with adult coeliac disease. *Scand. J. Gastroenterol.*, **12**, 149–59
63. Baklien, K., Fausa, O., Thune, P. O. and Gjone, E. (1977). Immunoglobulins in jejunal mucosa and serum from patients with dermatitis herpetiformis. *Scand. J. Gastroenterol.*, **12**, 161–8
64. Scott, H., Ek, J., Baklien, K. and Brandtzaeg, P. (1980). Immunoglobulin-producing cells in jejunal mucosa of children with coeliac disease on a gluten-free diet and after gluten challenge. *Scand. J. Gastroenterol.*, **15**, 81–8
65. Perkkiö, M., Savilahti, E. and Kuitunen, P. (1981). Semi-quantitative analysis of immunoglobulins and complement fractions 3 and 4 in the jejunal mucosa in coeliac disease and in food allergy in childhood. *Acta Pathol. Microbiol. Scand. (A)*, **89**, 343–50
66. Kett, K., Scott, H., Fausa, O. and Brandtzaeg, P. (1990). Secretory immunity in celiac disease: Cellular expression of immunoglobulin A subclass and joining chain. *Gastroenterology*, **99**, 386–92
67. Jos, J. and Labbe, F. (1976). Ultrastructural localization of IgA globulins in normal and coeliac intestinal mucosa using immunoenzymatic methods. *Biomedicine*, **24**, 425–34

68. Jos, J., Labbe, F., Geny, B. and Griscelli, C. (1979). Immunoelectron-microscopic localization of immunoglobulin A and secretory component in jejunal mucosa from children with coeliac disease. *Scand. J. Gastroenterol.*, **9**, 441–50

69. Rognum, T. O., Kett, K., Fausa, O., Bengtsson, U., Kilander, A., Scott, H., Gaarder, P. I. and Brandtzaeg, P. (1989). Raised number of jejunal IgG2-producing cells in untreated adult coeliac disease compared with food allergy. *Gut*, **30**, 1574–80

70. Wood, G. M., Howedle, P. D., Trejdosiewicz, L. K. and Losowsky, M. S. (1987). Jejunal plasma cells and in vitro immunoglobulin production in adult coeliac disease. *Clin. Exp. Immunol.*, **69**, 123–32

71. Scott, B. B., Goodall, A., Stephenson, P. and Jenkins, D. (1984). Small intestinal plasma cells in coeliac disease. *Gut*, **25**, 41–6

72. Arato, A., Savilahti, E., Tainio, V.-M., Verkasalo, M. and Klemola, T. (1987). HLA-DR expression, natural killer cells, and IgE containing cells in the jejunal mucosa of coeliac children. *Gut*, **28**, 988–94

73. Wood, G. M., Shires, S., Howdle, P. D. and Losowsky, M. S. (1986). Immunoglobulin production by coeliac biopsies in organ culture. *Gut*, **27**, 1151–60

74. Loeb, P. M., Strober, W., Falchuk, Z. M. and Laster, L. (1971). Incorporation of L-leucine14C into immunoglobulins by jejunal biopsies of patients with celiac sprue and other gastrointestinal disease. *J. Clin. Invest.*, **50**, 559–69

75. Falchuk, Z. M. and Strober, W. (1974). Gluten-sensitive enteropathy: synthesis of antigliadin antibody in vitro. *Gut*, **15**, 947–52

76. Fluge, G. and Aksnes, L. (1983). Quantification of immunoglobulins after organ culture of human duodenal mucosa. *J. Pediatr. Gastroenterol. Nutr.*, **2**, 62–70

77. Crabtree, J. E., Heatley, R. V. and Losowsky, M. L. (1989). Immunoglobulin secretion by isolated intestinal lymphocytes: spontaneous production and T-cell regulation in normal small intestine and in patients with coeliac disease. *Gut*, **30**, 347–54

78. Lycke, N., Kilander, A., Nilsson, L.-A., Tarkowski, A. and Werner, N. (1989). Production of antibodies to gliadin in intestinal mucosa of patients with coeliac disease: a study at the single cell level. *Gut*, **30**, 72–7

79. Ferguson, A. and Murray, D. (1971). Quantitation of intraepithelial lymphocytes in human jejunum. *Gut*, **12**, 988–94

80. Ferguson, A. (1977). Intraepithelial lymphocytes of the small intestine. *Gut*, **18**, 921–37

81. Marsh, M. N. (1980). Studies of intestinal lymphoid tissue. III. Quantitative analysis of epithelial lymphocytes in the small intestine of human control subjects and of patients with celiac sprue. *Gastroenterology*, **79**, 481–92

82. Marsh, M. N. (1989). Studies of intestinal lymphoid tissue. XV. Histopathologic features suggestive of cell-mediated reactivity in jejunal mucosae for patients with dermatitis herpetiformis. *Virchows Archiv. A, Pathol. Anat.*, **416**, 125–32

83. Mavromichalis, J., Brueton, M. J., McNeish, A. S. and Anderson, C. M. (1976). Evaluation of the intraepithelial lymphocyte count in the jejunum in childhood enteropathies. *Gut*, **17**, 600–3

84. Kuitunen, P., Kosnai, I. and Savilahti, E. (1982). Morphometric study of the jejunal mucosa in various childhood enteropathies with special reference to intraepithelial lymphocytes. *J. Ped. Gastroenterol. Nutr.*, **1**, 525–31

85. Ferguson, A. and Ziegler, K. (1986). Intraepithelial lymphocyte mitosis in a jejunal biopsy correlates with intraepithelial lymphocyte count, irrespective of diagnosis. *Gut*, **27**, 675–79

86. Selby, W. S., Janossy, G. and Jewell, D. P. (1981). Immunohistological characterisation of intraepithelial lymphocytes of the human gastrointestinal tract. *Gut*, **22**, 169–76

87. Spencer, J., Isaacson, P. G., Diss, T. C. and MacDonald, T. T. (1989). Expression of disulfide-linked and non-disulfide-linked forms of the T cell receptor γ/δ heterodimer in human intestinal intraepithelial lymphocytes. *Eur. J. Immunol.*, **19**, 1335–8

88. Cuenod, B., Brousse, N., Goulet, O., Potter, S. D., Mougenot, J.-F., Ricour, C., Guy-Grand, D. and Cerf-Bensussan, N. (1990). Classification of intractable diarrhea in infancy using clinical and immunohistological criteria. *Gastroenterology*, **99**, 1037–43

89. Spencer, J., MacDonald, T. T., Diss, T. C., Walker-Smith, J. A., Ciclitira, P. J. and Isaacson, P. G. (1989). Changes in intraepithelial lymphocyte subpopulations in coeliac disease and enteropathy associated T cell lymphoma (malignant histiocytosis of the intestine). *Gut*, **30**, 339–46

90. Scott, H., Brandtzaeg, P., Solheim, B. G. and Thorsby, E. (1981). Relations between

HLA-DR-like antigens and secretory component (SC) in jejunal epithelium of patients with coeliac disease or dermatitis herpetiformis. *Clin. Exp. Immunol.*, **44**, 233–8

91. Arnaud-Battandier, F., Cerf-Bensussan, N., Amsellem, R. and Schmitz, J. (1986). Increased HLA-DR expression by enterocytes in children with celiac disease. *Gastroenterology*, **91**, 1206–12

92. Ciclitira, P. J., Nelufer, J. M., Ellis, H. J. and Evans, D. J. (1986). The effect of gluten on HLA-DR in the small intestinal epithelium of patients with coeliac disease. *Clin. Exp. Immunol.*, **63**, 101–4

93. Marley, N. J., Macartney, J. C. and Ciclitira, P. J. (1987). HLA-DR, DP and DQ expression in the small intestine of patients with coeliac disease. *Clin. Exp. Immunol.*, **70**, 386–93

94. Shiner, M. and Shmerling, D. H. (1972). The immunopathology of coeliac disease. *Digestion*, **5**, 69–88

95. Marsh, M. N. (1989). The immunopathology of the small intestinal reaction in gluten-sensitivity. *Immunol. Invest.*, **18**, 509–31

96. Egan-Mitchell, B., Fottrell, P. F. and McNicholl, B. (1981). Early or pre-coeliac mucosa: development of gluten enteropathy. *Gut*, **22**, 65–9

97. Kuitunen, P., Savilahti, E. and Verkasalo, M. (1986). Late mucosal relapse in a boy with coeliac disease and cows' milk allergy. *Acta Pediatr. Scand.*, **75**, 340–2

98. Mäki, M., Holm, K., Collin, P. and Savilahti, E. (1991). Increase of γ/δ T cell receptor bearing lymphocytes in normal small bowel mucosa of a patient with latent coeliac disease. *Gut* (In press)

99. Fry, L., Seah, P. P., McMinn, R. M. and Hoffbrand, A. V. (1972). Lymphocytic infiltration of epithelium in diagnosis of gluten-sensitive enteropathy. *Br. Med. J.*, **3**, 371–4

100. Kosnai, I., Karpati, S., Savilahti, E., Verkasalo, M., Bucsky, P. and Török, E. (1986). Gluten challenge in children with dermatitis herpetiformis: a clinical, morphological and immunohistochemical study. *Gut*, **27**, 1464–70

101. O'Mahony, S., Vestey, J. P. and Ferguson, A. (1990). Similarities in intestinal humoral immunity in dermatitis herpetiformis without enteropathy and in coeliac disease. *Lancet*, **335**, 1487–90

102. Marsh, M. N., Bjarnason, I., Shaw, J., Ellis, A., Baker, R. and Peters, T. J. (1990). Studies of intestinal lymphoid tissue. XIV-HLA status, mucosal morphology, permeability and epithelial lymphocyte populations in first degree relatives of patients with coeliac disease. *Gut*, **31**, 32–6

103. Trier, J. S. and Browning, T. H. (1970). Epithelial-cell renewal in cultured duodenal biopsies in celiac sprue. *N. Engl. J. Med.*, **283**, 1245–50

104. Fluge, G. and Aksnes, L. (1981). Labelling indices after 3H-thymidine incorporation during organ culture of duodenal mucosa in coeliac disease. *Scand. J. Gastroenterol.*, **16**, 921–8

105. Jos, J., Lenoir, G., deRitis, G. and Rey, J. (1975). *In vitro* pathogenetic studies of coeliac disease. *Scand. J. Gastroenterol.*, **10**, 121–8

106. Fluge, G. and Aksnes, L. (1981). Morphological and morphometric assessment of human duodenal biopsies maintained in organ culture. *In vitro* influences of gluten in coeliac disease. *Scand. J. Gastroenterol.*, **16**, 555–67

107. Ferguson, A., MacDonald, T. T., McClure, J. P. and Holden, R. J. (1975). Cell-mediated immunity to gliadin within the small-intestinal mucosa in coeliac disease. *Lancet*, **1**, 895–97

108. Howdle, P. D., Bullen, A. W. and Losowsky, M. S. (1982). Cell-mediated immunity to gluten within the small intestinal mucosa in coeliac disease. *Gut*, **23**, 115–22

109. Carswell, F. and Ferguson, A. (1972). Food antibodies in serum – a screening test for coeliac disease. *Arch. Dis. Child.*, **47**, 594–6

110. Unsworth, D. J., Manuel, P. D., Walker-Smith, J. A., Campbell, C. A., Johnson, G. D. and Holborow, E. J. (1981). New immunofluorescent blood test for gluten sensitivity. *Arch. Dis. Child.*, **56**, 864–8

111. Savilahti, E., Viander, M., Perkkiö, M., Vainio, E., Kalimo, K., and Reunala, T. (1983). IgA antigliadin antibodies: a marker of mucosal damage in childhood coeliac disease. *Lancet*, **1**, 320–2

112. Bürgin-Wolff, A. and Lentze, M. J. (1990). Relation of antigliadin antibodies to gluten-sensitive enteropathy. B. Diagnostic significance of antibodies against gliadin in celiac disease in children. In Chorzelski, T. O., Beutner, E. H., Kumar, V. and Zalewski, T. K. (eds), *Serologic Diagnosis of Celiac Disease*. Boca Raton, FL: CRC Press), pp. 59–76

113. Scott, H., Fausa, O., Ek, J. and Brandtzaeg, P. (1984). Immune response patterns in coeliac disease. Serum antibodies to dietary antigens measured by an enzyme linked immunosorbent assay (ELISA). *Clin. Exp. Immunol.*, **57**, 25–32
114. Mascart-Lemone, F., Cadranel, S., Van den Broeck, J., Dive, C., Vaerman, J. P. and Duchateau, J. (1988). IgA immune response patterns to gliadin in serum. *Int. Arch. Allergy Appl. Immunol.*, **86**, 412–19
115. Kutteh, W. H., Prince, S. J. and Mestecky, J. (1982). Tissue origins of human polymeric and monomeric IgA. *J. Immunol.*, **128**, 990–5
116. Vainio, E. (1986). Immunoblotting analysis of antigliadin antibodies in the sera of patients with dermatitis herpetiformis and gluten-sensitive enteropathy. *Int. Arch. Allergy Appl. Immunol.*, **80**, 157–63
117. Skeritt, J. H., Johnson, R. B., Hetzel, P. A., la Broody, J. T., Shearman, D. J. C. and Davidson, G. P. (1987). Variation of serum and intestinal gluten antibody specificities in coeliac disease. *Clin. Exp. Immunol.*, **68**, 189–99
118. Rautonen, J., Rautonen, N. and Savilahti, E. (1991). Antibodies to gliadin in children with coeliac disease. *Acta Paediatr. Scand.* (In press)
119. Seah, P. P., Fry, L., Fossiter, M. A., Hoffbrand, A. V. and Holborow, E. J. (1971). Anti-reticulin antibodies in childhood coeliac disease. *Lancet*, **2**, 681–2
120. von Essen, R., Savilahti, E. and Pelkonen, P. (1972). Reticulin antibody in children with malabsorption. *Lancet*, **1**, 1157–9
121. Mäki, M., Hällström, O., Vesikari, T. and Visakorpi, J. K. (1984). Evaluation of a serum IgA-class reticulin antibody test for the detection of childhood celiac disease. *J. Pediatr.*, **105**, 901–5
122. Zalewski, T., Chorzelski, T. P., Kapuscinska, A., Radzikowski, T., Beutner, E. H., Karczewska, K., Czerwionka-Szarflarska, Kumar, V., Rossi, T. and Sulej, J. (1990). Significance of IgA-class endomysial antibodies in the diagnosis of celiac disease. In Chorzelski, T. O., Beutner, E. H., Kumar, V. and Zalewski, T. K. (eds), *Serologic̀ Diagnosis of Celiac Disease*. (Boca Raton, FL: CRC Press), pp. 88–104
123. Hällstrom, O. (1989). Comparison of IgA-class reticulin and endomysium antibodies in coeliac disease and dermatitis herpetiformis. *Gut*, **30**, 1225–32
124. Vainio, E., Kosnai, I., Hällström, O., Karpati, S., Mäki, M. and Reunala, T. (1986). Antigliadin and antireticulin antibodies in children with dermatitis herpetiformis. *J. Pediatr. Gastroenterol. Nutr.*, **5**, 735–9

4
Immunology of gastrointestinal food allergy in infancy and early childhood

J. A. WALKER-SMITH

Intolerance to various foods, especially the proteins of cows' milk, has been recognized in children for many years. Such food intolerance may be due to a variety of causes; for example, a congenital digestive enzyme defect such as sucrase–isomaltase deficiency, an acquired digestive enzyme defect such as lactase deficiency secondary to small intestinal mucosa damage, or the conditions may be immunological in origin.

Adverse reactions after food ingestion may be classified as follows:

1. Toxic effects, including those due to bacterial contamination and food additives.
2. Intolerance phenomena due to enzyme deficiencies, e.g. lactose intolerance as a sequel to lactase deficiency.
3. Allergic reactions.
4. Symptoms which resemble allergic reactions but which are not elicited by immunological phenomena. To this category belong symptoms caused by histamine releasers, e.g. strawberries, where histamine release is not the consequence of an immunological reaction.

The term 'food idiosyncrasy' has been used in the sense of a non-immunological abnormal response to food. There is, however, increasing evidence that dietary protein intolerance may be mediated by an allergic reaction or reactions affecting the gastrointestinal tract. It is those syndromes of dietary protein intolerance occurring in infancy and childhood that have an immunological pathogenesis which are the subject of this chapter.

DEFINITIONS

Gastrointestinal food allergies may be defined as clinical syndromes which are characterized by the onset of gastrointestinal symptoms following food ingestion where the underlying mechanism is an immunologically mediated reaction within the gastrointestinal tract.

A food-sensitive enteropathy is a disorder characterized by an abnormal small intestinal mucosa whilst having the offending food in the diet; the abnormality is reversed by an elimination diet only to recur once more on challenge with the relevant food. It may be permanent, as occurs in coeliac disease, and this disorder will not be discussed further here since it is covered elsewhere in this book. It may, however, be temporary, and such disorders are confined to infancy and early childhood and will be discussed in this chapter.

Food-induced colitis is a disorder where ingestion of food produces a colitis which is reversed by an elimination diet and which relapses on challenge.

CLINICAL SPECTRUM

Clinical intolerance to a variety of food proteins has been described. The most common are cows' milk, cereals, soy protein, eggs and fish; intolerance to tomatoes, oranges, bananas, meat, nuts and chocolates has been described[1]. There is no consistent association between a particular food and specific syndromes. In fact the clinical manifestations that may occur in cows' milk protein intolerance are large in number and diverse in nature, involving a range of organ pathology[2,3].

Broadly, gastrointestinal reactions to food in children with food allergy may be divided into those that manifest quickly, i.e. within minutes to an hour of food ingestion, and those in which the onset is slow, taking hours or days after food ingestion. Both types of reaction may occur individually or together in different children. Yet there are clear immunological differences between these groups. For example, it has been shown by Fallstrom et al.[4] that children with slow-onset reactions to cows' milk feedings have significantly elevated titres of IgG antibodies against both native and digested β-lactoglobulin, when compared with both controls and those children who develop symptoms quickly after milk ingestion. These children also tended to have higher levels of IgA antibody to both native and processed milk.

Seven out of nine children with quick-onset cows' milk allergy had significant IgE antibodies to cows' milk, yet these were not found in the slow-onset group.

However, elevated titres of IgE antibodies to cows' milk protein have been observed in some children with slow-onset reactions with enteropathy, although these findings are more typical of quick reactors. Such elevated titres can on occasion be found in milk-tolerant, atopic children.

AGE OF ONSET AND DURATION OF SYNDROMES

The incidence of gastrointestinal food allergy is greatest in the first months and years of life; it decreases with age. This is especially true for late-onset reactions to food with food-induced small intestinal mucosal damage[5]. Indeed there is no evidence that gastrointestinal syndromes of allergic origin do cause small intestinal mucosal damage in adult life or older children. These gastrointestinal food syndromes of early childhood appear to be temporary in duration, although it does seem possible – as in the case of cows' milk protein intolerance – that gastrointestinal syndromes may be replaced with the passage of time by syndromes involving other systems.

QUICK-ONSET SYNDROMES

These syndromes are usually easy to diagnose on historical grounds. The children often have an individual and family history of atopy, peripheral eosinophilia, elevated total serum IgE levels and positive RAST and skin-prick tests to specific foods.

When there is intolerance to a number of foods, diets involving the elimination of a number of foods may be impractical or ineffective on their own. However, the addition of disodium cromoglycate may be highly effective as in the group of children described by Syme[6]. Its therapeutic dose is empirical at present[7]; it is usually 100 mg twice daily. Curiously, if oral disodium cromoglycate alleviates symptoms these may not relapse when the drug is discontinued.

Little information is available concerning small intestinal mucosa in these quick-onset syndromes, as children with these disorders are not usually biopsied. Theoretically, from animal studies the small intestinal mucosa may be normal. These patients need to be distinguished from cases of eosinophilic gastroenteritis.

Eosinophilic gastroenteritis is a disorder characterized by gastrointestinal thickening with oedema and dense infiltration of eosinophils. It usually affects the gastric antrum and proximal small intestine[8]. It is usually a disorder of young adults but may occur in children[9]. Clinically it is characterized by protein-losing enteropathy and peripheral eosinophilia. IgE levels may be elevated and some patients have been reported to respond to a cows' milk-free diet. Although most are not responsive to diet manipulation, some patients respond to disodium cromoglycate but most will require steroids.

SLOW-ONSET SYNDROMES

Whereas quick-onset syndromes often present to allergy clinics, by contrast the slow-onset syndromes usually present as a gastrointestinal problem to paediatric or paediatric gastroenterology clinics. Such children may often have failure to thrive. In these cases there is often no clear history of food ingestion being related to the onset of symptoms.

Diagnosis may be difficult. Accurate diagnosis centres upon the following three groups of test:

1. Investigation of gastrointestinal structure, e.g. proximal small intestinal mucosal biopsy.
2. Investigation of gastrointestinal function, e.g. intestinal sugar permeability.
3. Investigation of immunological function:
    (a) systemic, e.g. specific antibody production;
    (b) gut-associated, e.g. studies of local antibody-producing cells.

Once these initial investigations have been performed, dietary elimination and challenge continue to have an important diagnostic role. This approach is of best value when such elimination and challenge is related to gastrointestinal structure and function, i.e. serial observations. At present there are no simple laboratory tests available for routine diagnostic screening of children with these slow-onset gastrointestinal symptoms. In individual patients cows' milk antibody estimation is not diagnostically useful.

In children such problems often overlap with gastrointestinal infection, thus making diagnosis difficult. Unless full microbiological study of the stools is done, i.e. stool electron microscopy for viruses, as well as stool bacterial culture, infection of the gastrointestinal tract can be easily overlooked. Food allergy and infection often coexist.

TRANSIENT FOOD-SENSITIVE ENTEROPATHIES

Changes in the structure of the small intestinal mucosa in response to the ingestion of particular foods provide clear objective evidence of food-sensitive disorders affecting the small intestinal mucosa. This approach of using serial small intestinal mucosal biopsies related to dietary elimination and challenge was first used for the diagnosis of coeliac disease in the Interlaken or ESPGAN Diagnostic Criteria. Coeliac disease is a state of permanent food-sensitivity, but there also exists a group of temporary food-sensitive enteropathies, presenting in infancy. Indeed, a number of foods apart from gluten have now been shown to produce food-sensitive enteropathies in infancy. These include cows' milk protein, soy protein, eggs, chicken, ground rice and fish.

PATHOLOGY

Most information available concerns cows' milk-sensitive enteropathy and is based upon small intestinal mucosal biopsy. What evidence there is for other food-sensitive enteropathies suggests that the pathology is essentially similar. The characteristic feature is small intestinal mucosal damage of variable extent and severity[10-12]. The lesion is often patchy[13]. Within one biopsy there may be a wide range of morphological appearances from normal to severe abnormality. Indeed, a single normal small intestinal mucosal biopsy does not exclude this diagnosis. Ideally a double-port small-intestinal biopsy capsule should be used to ensure as wide a sampling as possible[14].

The changes which will be described are non-specific and can be established to be induced by cows' milk only by means of serial small-intestinal biopsies taken first at the time of initial diagnosis on a cows' milk-containing diet; second after clinical remission on a cows' milk-free diet and thirdly after a clinical relapse after a return to a cows' milk-containing diet, i.e. a cows' milk challenge. Despite their non-specific nature, when these biopsy changes are found in children with the typical clinical features, i.e. chronic diarrhoea and failure to thrive and other causes such as giardiasis have been excluded, their presence is an indication for a therapeutic trial of a cows' milk-free diet. When there is a rapid clinical response to such a diet, from a practical viewpoint, the diagnosis of cows' milk-sensitive enteropathy has been established. However, from a strictly scientific viewpoint the diagnosis can be said to have been established only when this is followed by a clinical and histological relapse following cows' milk challenge.

The histological changes found in cows' milk-sensitive enteropathy are indistinguishable from those found in post-enteritis enteropathy. As the two disorders overlap it may not be possible to distinguish them without an early cows' milk challenge. This in practice may not be practical, as it may not be seen to be a helpful aid to management, and early cows' milk challenge carries the risk of a severe relapse.

The classical lesion found in the small intestinal mucosa is crypt hyperplastic villous atrophy of variable severity (Fig. 4.1). It is usually less severe than that found in coeliac disease. A flat mucosa is quite uncommon, and nowadays the lesion is usually less severe. This decline in severity of the mucosal lesion in cows' milk-sensitive enteropathy has been well documented in Finland[15] It probably relates chiefly to the development of less sensitizing cows' milk formulae and also earlier diagnosis.

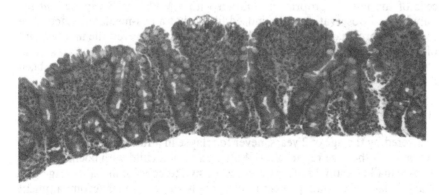

Figure 4.1 Severe partial villous atrophy on biopsy of small intestine of an infant with cows' milk-sensitive enteropathy showing crypt hyperplastic villous atrophy

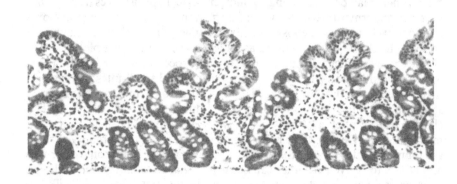

Figure 4.2 Mild partial villous atrophy on biopsy of small intestine of an infant with cows' milk-sensitive enteropathy with shortening of villi and normal crypt length, i.e. normoplastic villous atrophy

The mucosa is characteristically thin[16]. Whilst there is some lengthening of the crypts the most characteristic feature is shortening of the villi (crypt normoplastic villous atrophy) (Fig. 4.2). The epithelial abnormality is less severe than in coeliac disease. However, functional damage to the enterocyte is usually present with depression of disaccharidase activity especially lactase[17].

There may be an elevation of the intraepithelial lymphocyte count but not usually to the levels found in coeliac disease[18]. Recently it has been found that gamma/delta T cells are increased in the intraepithelial lymphocyte population of patients with coeliac disease[19]. It has been suggested that this change is specific for coeliac disease[20]. However, when 15 abnormal small intestinal biopsies were looked at from children with cows' milk-sensitive enteropathy/post-enteritis syndrome, two had increased levels of intraepithelial T cells and gamma/delta intraepithelial lymphocytes, i.e. findings indistinguishable from coeliac disease[21].

There is increased expression of the markers of T cell activation on the T cells of the lamina propria in children with CMPSE/PES (Spencer *et al.*, unpublished observation). It is indeed likely that a cell-mediated reaction in the lamina propria is the basis of the abnormality. However, the involvement of IgE in the immunological response of the lamina propria to cows' milk challenge in children with cows' milk-sensitive enteropathy has been described[22,23].

After a relatively short period on a cows' milk-free diet all these changes either heal completely, or significantly improve on a cows' milk-free diet.

Unlike coeliac disease these disorders are temporary and have usually recovered by the age of 2 years, never to relapse in adult life. One remarkable exception is the case reported by Watt *et al.*[24] of a child with coeliac disease whose small intestinal mucosa was responsive to cows' milk till the age of 7 years. In fact cows' milk protein intolerance is an occasional accompaniment of coeliac disease at the time of presentation, but rapidly disappears as the child responds to a gluten-free diet.

PATHOGENESIS

In order to explore the pathogenetic role of allergic reactions in gastrointestinal allergy, Type I, Type III and Type IV reactions have been induced in experimental animals. Type I or reaginic allergic reaction may be produced in a rat which has been immunized and then challenged with an intravenous dose of antigen[25]. The effect of such an immediate allergic reaction is the development within 5 or 10 min of microscopic oedema, mucus secretion, and increased blood flow. Histologically, the mucosa may be entirely normal or merely show some oedema of the lamina propria and small subepithelial blebs.

In a study of intraluminal antigen challenge of actively or passively immunized pigs to produce a Type III or immune complex allergic reaction, a massive influx of polymorphs to the mucosa was shown but without morphological damage[26]. In a similar model in rabbits, deposition of immune complexes in the gut wall was shown, but an enteropathy did not develop[27].

A variety of Type IV, local cell-mediated reactions in the mucosa have been produced in animals including graft-versus-host disease, rejection of transplanted allografts of intestine, and parasite infections in the T cell-depleted host[28–30]. These models show that the earliest changes in these cell-mediated reactions are infiltration of lymphocytes into the lamina propria and the epithelium. The crypts lengthen (i.e. become hypertrophied) and crypt cell production rate is increased. Villi are shortened. These changes are mediated by lymphokines secreted by activated T cells. Thus, there is a compelling morphological incidence in these animal studies to suggest that cell-mediated immunity may produce small intestinal enteropathy.

Similar evidence is now available in human fetal small intestinal mucosa by fetal gut organ culture (see Chapter 8).

So it could be hypothesized in gastrointestinal food allergy, where there is a cell-mediated reaction, that lymphocytes in the small intestinal mucosa lamina propria, which have been sensitized to dietary antigen, interact with food antigens that enter the mucosa from the gut lumen. This leads to activation of T lymphocytes leading to crypt hypertrophy and reduction in villous height. Whether an IgE-mediated reaction plays any part, such as triggering the reaction, remains unclear.

Abnormalities of the small intestinal mucosa have been reported in children suffering temporary intolerance to cows' milk protein, soy protein, gluten, eggs, chicken, ground rice and fish. The evidence that the enteropathy is directly related to ingestion of a particular food is based upon serial small intestinal biopsy studies related to dietary elimination and challenge. The enteropathy is not usually as severe as that seen in coeliac disease, although a flat mucosa may occasionally be seen.

In some cases the children appear to develop food intolerance after an acute episode of gastroenteritis. The underlying causes of these temporary food intolerances of infancy probably relate to a transient sensitization of the child to dietary antigens, which may be a result of a breach of the mucosal barrier. The precise mechanisms which cause the enteropathy are unclear, although the application of the Gell and Coombs classification of hypersensitivity reaction provides a basis for investigation as described above. For the reactions to occur the offending food antigen must enter the mucosa in appropriate amounts to cause sensitization. There are two hypotheses regarding this process: one suggests sensitization caused from an overstimulation of the immune system by excess antigen entry, the other proposes a minimal entry of antigen sufficient to stimulate a reaginic response, which in turn leads to increased antigen entry leading to mucosal damage. In the experimental animal it has been shown that intestinal anaphylaxis can lead to increased uptake of intestinal luminal antigens[31]. Both hypotheses may be correct.

Post-enteritis food-sensitive enteropathies may result from excess local food antigen entry in susceptible individuals following gut damage induced by viral or bacterial pathogens. An hypothesis relating acute gastroenteritis and cows' milk sensitive enteropathy is illustrated in Fig. 4.3.

It is known from the observations of Gruskay and Cook[32] that excess antigen absorption (in their studies egg albumin) occurs in infants with acute gastroenteritis. This has been well documented in animal studies of viral enteritis[33]. Clinical studies have also shown increased entry of both small molecular weight sugars in acute gastroenteritis[34], and a larger molecular weight protein, horseradish peroxidase, in post-enteritis food-sensitive enteropathies as observed using organ culture[35].

So there are probably two syndromes, a primary disorder of immunological origin and a secondary disorder, a sequel of mucosal damage. Abnormal handling of dietary antigens across the intestinal mucosa probably occurs in infants with gastrointestinal food allergy. This may be related to a temporary immunodeficiency state such as transient IgA deficiency[36], or to non-specific small intestinal mucosal damage from any cause permitting excess antigen

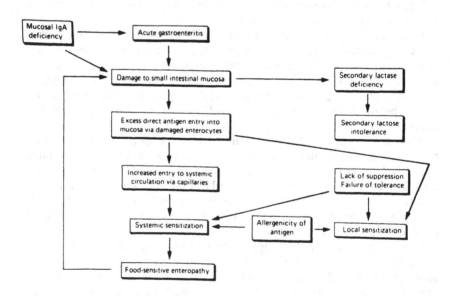

Figure 4.3 Hypothesis: relationship between gastroenteritis and lactose intolerance with cows' milk-sensitive enteropathy

entry as referred to above. There is indeed clinical evidence that acute enteritis may be followed not only by lactose intolerance but by more persistent and longer-lasting cows' milk-sensitive enteropathy[37,38].

In the experimental animal, increased protein antigen uptake occurs when the mucosa is damaged by parasitic infection[25]. The pathogenic role of circulating antibodies to cows' milk remains to be established. Lippard *et al.*[39] showed that at whatever age a child first begins to drink cows' milk, cows' milk antigen and then cows' milk antibody can be detected in the child's blood. Delire *et al.*[40] have found that all neonates fed on cows' milk have in their blood immune complexes containing cows' milk protein antigens, and IgG antibodies of maternal origin. Despite these findings, only a few children go on to develop cows' milk protein intolerance. How such a state of clinical intolerance develops is unknown. Even the presence of a high level of serum anti-milk antibodies is not necessarily associated with damage, e.g. there is a high incidence of elevated titres of cows' milk antibodies in children with both coeliac disease and kwashiorkor[41] yet, as a rule, these children improve clinically on a cows' milk-containing diet.

As stated earlier the local reaction in the small intestine may be mediated via one of the allergic reactions as classified by Gell and Coombs[42], namely Type I, Type III and Type IV.

The importance of Type I reaction in the gut would be in allowing increased amounts of antigen to cross the mucosa by causing capillary dilatation and increased permeability, allowing large amounts of antigen into the systemic circulation to initiate secondary immunization. If this antigen meets tissue fixed IgE on mast cells then a Type I reaction would occur, e.g. in the skin (rash), in the gut (diarrhoea) and in bronchial mucosa (wheeze). Thus the very variable clinical reactions encountered can be accounted for by differences in antigen reaching IgE on mast cells in different sites in the body.

Involvement of systemic immunity, and the local immune system, could explain the transient nature of the illness. The illness could disappear after a period on a milk-free diet when the small intestinal mucosa local immune system was mature enough to prevent much antigen getting through. The role of cell-mediated immunity would come into play in the case of those children who mounted a cell-mediated reaction in the small intestinal mucosa and so an enteropathy.

The allergenicity or antigenicity of the cows' milk formula may be of critical importance in pathogenesis.

Manuel *et al.*[43] showed a remarkable difference in the incidence of delayed recovery between infants fed with different formulae immediately after an acute attack of gastroenteritis. Old formula Pregestimil (high osmolality and based on a casein hydrolysate) and A1 110 (based on casein) and standard SMA (an adapted formula) were compared for infants aged under 6 months. It is likely that delayed recovery in these circumstances is related to cows' milk-sensitive enteropathy; 26% of infants fed with the casein formula A1 110 developed delayed recovery compared with only 5% with Pregestimil and the very low figure of 2.5% with SMA. This latter figure may have been by chance unusually low. Nevertheless, when these milks were tested in an animal model (guinea pigs) then similar results were found; A1 110 was sensitizing, Pregestimil not sensitizing at all and SMA sensitized significantly less often[13,44].

Thus, adapted feeding formulae appear to be much less sensitizing than the older infant feeding formula still routinely used in much of the developing world. This is consistent with the decline in the severity of cows' milk-sensitive enteropathy in societies where such milks are now universally used. Thus the allergenicity of the milk formula fed at the time of an acute attack of gastroenteritis may be a central factor in the development of cows' milk-sensitive enteropathy. However, other as yet unidentified factors must also play a part.

GENETIC FACTORS

Boys and girls appear to be equally affected. Although an atopic family history is often very common, no definite genetic factor has been identified. Kuitunen et al.[10] have shown an HLA status identical to that of the community. However, Swarbrick et al.[45] have shown, in animals, a genetic variation in the control of antigen absorption by the gut. If this is so in humans, certain individuals may be more predisposed to develop dietary protein intolerance than are others.

FOOD-SENSITIVE COLITIS

Rubin[46] described rectal loss of fresh blood which responded to cows' milk withdrawal. Gryboski[47] described eight children with cows' milk colitis diagnosed by response to cows' milk elimination. The main clinical features were explosive bloody diarrhoea, shock, pallor and colitis. The diagnosis was based upon evaluation of sigmoidoscopic appearances and rectal biopsy. No pathogens were isolated. The advent of safe colonoscopy and multiple mucosal biopsy, even in early infancy, has clearly established food-sensitive or allergic colitis as an important case of chronic blood diarrhoea in infancy. Colonoscopically there is patchy erythema of the mucosa and petechiae, and there may be aphthoid ulceration. Histopathologically, oedema and infiltration with eosinophils have been reported, although others describe a histopathological appearance not dissimilar to ulcerative colitis with an inflammatory infiltrate; however, both changes disappear on a cows' milk-free diet, only to reoccur on early challenge. Similar appearances are seen in Crohn's disease, Behçet's disease, amoebiasis and chronic granulomatous disease. Even breast-fed infants whose mothers drink much cows' milk may develop cows' milk colitis. β-Lactoglobulin has been demonstrated in the breast milk of lactating mothers, although the amounts are very small.

This disorder needs to be distinguished from ulcerative colitis and Crohn's colitis. However, ulcerative colitis has been observed to remit in a group of five children when on a milk-free diet, all having both symptomatic and histological relapse after milk was reintroduced; such treatment is not curative. It has also been suggested that ulcerative proctitis may at times be caused by local IgE-mediated reaction to cows' milk protein. Thus, a response to cows' milk elimination may not accurately discriminate between these disorders and true cows' milk-sensitive colitis. The diagnosis rests upon endoscopy and the histopathology demonstrated by mucosal biopsy and the subsequent clinical course. In food-sensitive colitis there may be a dense infiltration of eosinophils in the mucosa, and the lesion resolves on food elimination *pari passu* with clinical remission.

There is an association with atopy, and serum IgE may be elevated in some cases. Olives et al.[48] have studied the relationship between cows' milk colitis and cows' milk-sensitive enteropathy. Twenty-nine children with cows' milk-sensitive enteropathy were studied. In only 7% was severe colitis observed both endoscopically and histologically, but in 86% a microscopic colitis was demonstrated. However, it is clear that the large and small intestines are not always affected at the same time, and the selectivity of organ damage remains unexplained.

CONCLUSION

It is now clearly established that a variety of foods, but particularly cows' milk, may be associated with food allergy causing structural and functional damage to the intestinal mucosa both large and small. Such disorders appear to be temporary and are a feature of early childhood.

TREATMENT

Therapy is the temporary elimination of the offending food. In children with intolerance to cows' milk protein, a cows' milk protein hydralysate, either casein or whey, is recommended.

References

1. Bleumink, E. (1974). Allergies and toxic protein in food. In Hekkens, W. Th. J. M. and Pena, A. S. (eds), *Coeliac Disease*. Leyden: Stenfert Kroese, p. 46
2. Bahna, S. L. and Heiner, D. C. (1980). *Allergies to Milk*. New York: Grune & Stratton.
3. Hill, D. J., Firer, M. A., Shelton, M. J. and Hosking, C. S. (1986). Manifestations of milk allergy in infancy: clinical and immunologic findings. *J. Paediatr.*, 109, 270–6
4. Fallstrom, S. P., Ahlstedt, S., Carlsson, B., Lonnerdal, S. and Hanson, L. A. (1986). Serum antibodies against native, processed and digested cows' milk protein intolerance. *Clin. Allergy*, 16, 417–23
5. Dannaeus, A. and Johansson, S. G. O. (1979). A follow-up study of infants with adverse reactions to cows' milk. *Acta Paediat. Scand.*, 68, 377–83
6. Syme, J. (1979). Investigation and treatment of multiple intestinal food allergy in childhood. In Pepys, J. and Edwards, A. M. (eds), *The Mast Cell: Its Role in Health and Disease*. Tunbridge Wells: Pitman Medical, pp. 438–42
7. Kocoshis, S. and Gryboski, J. D. (1979). Use of cromolyn in combined gastrointestinal allergy. *J. Am. Med. Assoc.*, 242, 1169–73

8. Marshak, R. H., Lindner, A., Maklansky, D. and Gelt, A. (1981). Eosinophilic gastroenteritis. *J. Am. Med. Assoc.*, **245**, 1677–80
9. Katz, A. J., Goldman, H. and Grand, R. J. (1977). Gastric mucosal biopsy in eosinophilic (allergic) gastroenteritis. *Gastroenterology*, **73**, 705
10. Kuitunen, P., Visakorpi, J. K., Savilahti, E. and Pelkonen, P. (1975). Malabsorption syndrome with cows' milk intolerance clinical findings and course in 54 cases. *Arch. Dis. Childh.*, **50**, 351
11. Fontaine, J. L. and Navarro, J. Small intestinal biopsy in cows' milk protein allergy in infancy. *Arch. Dis. Childh.*, **50**, 357
12. Walker-Smith, J. A. (1975). Cows' milk protein intolerance, transient food intolerance of infancy. *Arch. Dis. Childh.*, **50**, 347
13. Manuel, P. D., Walker-Smith, J. A. and France, N. E. (1979). Patchy enteropathy. *Gut*, **20**, 211
14. Kilby, A. (1976). Paediatric small intestinal biopsy capsule with two ports. *Gut*, **17**, 158
15. Verkasalo, M., Kuitunen, P., Savilahti, E. and Tiilikainen, A. (1981). Changing pattern of cows' milk intolerance. *Acta Paediatr. Scand.*, **70**, 289–295
16. Maluenda, C., Phillips, A. D., Briddon, A. and Walker-Smith, J. A. (1984). Quantitative analysis of small intestinal mucosa in cows' milk sensitive enteropathy. *J. Paediatr. Gastroenterol. Nutr.*, **3**, 349–57
17. Walker-Smith, J. A., Kilby, A. and France, N. E. (1978). Reinvestigation of children previously diagnosed as coeliac disease. In McNicholl, N., McCarthy, C. F. and Fottrell, P. B. (eds), *Perspectives in Coeliac Disease*. Lancaster: MTP Press, p. 267
18. Phillips, A. D., Rice, S. J., France, N. E. and Walker-Smith, J. A. (1979). Small intestinal lymphocyte levels in cows' milk protein intolerance. *Gut*, **20**, 509
19. Spencer, J., Isaacson, P. G., Diss, T. C. and MacDonald, T. T. (1989). Expression of disulfide-linked and non-disulfide linked forms of the T cell receptor γ/δ heterodimer in human intestinal intraepithelial lymphocyte. *Eur. J. Immunol.*, **19**, 1335–8
20. Walker-Smith, J. A., Guandalini, S., Schmitz, J., Shmerling, D. H. and Visakorpi, J. K. (1990). Revised criteria for diagnosis of coeliac disease. *Arch. Dis. Child.*, **65**, 909–11
21. Spencer, J., Isaacson, P. G., MacDonald, T. T., Thomas, A. J. and Walker-Smith, J. A. (1991). Gamma/Delta T cells and the diagnosis of coeliac disease. *Clin. Exp. Immunol.*, **85**, 109–13
22. Shiner, M., Ballard, J. and Smith, M. E. (1975). The small intestinal mucosa in cows' milk allergy. *Lancet*, **1**, 136
23. Kilby, A., Walker-Smith, J. A. and Wood, C. B. S. (1976). Small intestinal mucosa in cows' milk allergy. *Lancet*, **1**, 53
24. Watt, J., Pincott, J. R. and Harries, J. T. (1983). Combined cow's milk protein and gluten-induced enteropathy: common or rare. *Gut*, **24**, 165–70
25. Bloch, K. J., Bloch, K. B., Sterns, M. and Walker, W. A. (1979). Intestinal uptake of macromolecules VI. Uptake of protein antigen *in vivo* in normal rats and rats infested with *Nippostrongyloides* and *Brasiliensis* or subject to mild systemic anaphylaxis. *Gastroenterology*, **77**, 1039
26. Bellamy, J. E. C. and Nielsen, N. O. (1974). Immune-mediated emigration of neutrophils into the lumen of the small intestine. *Infect. Immunol.*, **9**, 615
27. Accinni, L., Brentjens, J. R., Albini, E. O., O'Connell, D. W., Pawlowski, I. B. and Andres, G. A. (1978). Deposition of circulating antigen–antibody complex in the gastrointestinal tract of rabbits with chronic serum sickness. *Am. J. Dig. Dis.*, **23**, 1098
28. MacDonald, T. T. and Ferguson, A. (1976). Hypersensitivity reactions in the small intestine. 2. Effects of allograft rejection on mucosal architecture and lymphoid cell infiltrate. *Gut*, **17**, 81
29. MacDonald, T. T. and Ferguson, A. (1977). Hypersensitivity reactions in the small intestine. 3. The effects of allograft rejection and of graft-versus-host disease on epithelial cell kinetics. *Cell Tissue Kinet.*, **10**, 301
30. Ferguson, A. and MacDonald, T. T. (1978). Effects of local delayed hypersensitivity on the small intestine. *Immunology of the Gut*. Ciba Foundation Symposium 46. Amsterdam: Elsevier, North Holland, p. 35
31. Walker, W. A., Wu, M. and Isselbacher, K. J. (1975). Intestinal uptake of macromolecules. III. Studies on the mechanism by which immunization interferes with antigen uptake. *J. Immunol.*, **115** (3), 854–61
32. Gruskay, F. L. and Cook, R. E. (1955). The gastrointestinal absorption of unaltered protein in normal infants and in infants recovering from diarrhoea. *Paediatrics*, **16**, 763
33. Keljo, D. F., Butler, D. G. and Hamilton, J. R. (1985). Altered jejunal permeability to

macromolecules during viral enteritis in the piglet. *Gastroenterology*, **88**, 998–1004

34. Ford, R. P. K., Menzies, I. S., Phillips, A. D., Walker-Smith, J. A. and Turner, M. W. (1985). Intestinal sugar permeability: relationship to diarrhoeal disease and small bowel morphology. *J. Paediatr. Gastroenterol. Nutr.*, **4**, 568–75

35. Jackson, D., Walker-Smith, J. A. and Phillips, A. D. (1983). Macromolecular absorption by histologically normal and abnormal small intestine mucosa in childhood: an *in vitro* study using organ culture. *J. Paediatr. Gastroenterol. Nutr.*, **3**, 235–40

36. Taylor, B., Norman, A. P., Orgel, H. A., Stokes, C. R., Turner, M. W. and Soothill, J. (1973). Transient IgA deficiency and pathogenesis of infantile atopy. *Lancet*, **2**, 111

37. Harrison, B. M., Kilby, A., Walker-Smith, J. A., France, N. E. and Wood, C. B. S. (1976). Cows' milk protein intolerance: a possible association with gastroenteritis lactose intolerance and IgA deficiency. *Br. Med. J.*, **1**, 1501–4

38. Walker-Smith, J. A. (1982). Cows' milk intolerance as a cause of postenteritis diarrhoea. *J. Paediatr. Gastroenterol. Nutr.*, **1**, 163–75

39. Lippard, V. W., Schloss, O. M. and Johnson, P. A. (1936). Immune reactions induced in infants by intestinal absorption of incompletely digested cow's milk proteins. *Am. J. Dis. Childh.*, **51**, 562

40. Delire, M., Cambiaso, C. L. and Masson, P. L. (1978). Circulatory immune complexes in infants fed on cows' milk. *Nature (Lond.)*, **272**, 632

41. Chandra, R. K. (1976). Immunological consequences of malnutrition including fetal growth retardation. In *Food and Immunology*, Swedish Nutrition Foundation Symposium XIII. Stockholm: Almqvist & Wiksell.

42. Gell, P. G. H. and Coombs, R. R. A. (1968). Classification of allergic reactions responsible for hypersensitivity and disease. In Gell, P. G. H. and Coombs, R. R. A. (eds), *Clinical Aspects of Immunology*. Oxford and Edinburgh: Blackwell, p. 575

43. Manuel, P. D. and Walker-Smith, J. A. (1981). A comparison of three infant feeding formulae for the prevention of delayed recovery after infantile gastroenteritis. *Acta Paediatr. Belg.*, **34**, 13–20

44. McLaughlan, P., Anderson, K. J. and Coombs, R. R. A. (1981). An oral screening procedure to determine the sensitizing capacity of infant feeding formulae. *Clin. Allergy*, **11**, 311

45. Swarbrick, E. T., Stokes, L. K. and Soothill, J. (1979). The absorption of antigens after immunisation and the simultaneous induction of specific tolerance. *Gut*, **20**, 121–5

46. Rubin, M. I. (1940). Allergic intestinal bleeding in the newborn: a clinical syndrome. *Am. J. Med. Sci.*, **200**, 385–92

47. Gryboski, J. D. (1967). Gastrointestinal milk allergy in infants. *Paediatrics*, **40**, 354–62

48. Olives, J. P., LeTallec, C., Bloom, E., Agnese, P., Familiades, J. and Ghisolfi, J. (1988). Colitis and cows' milk protein sensitive enteropathy. *Paediatr. Res.*, **24**, 412

5
Immunology of intractable diarrhoea

B. CUENOD and N. CERF-BENSUSSAN

Intractable diarrhoea can be defined as a severe syndrome of diarrhoea persisting over 1 month in spite of digestive rest and intravenous feeding. It is a rare syndrome, mainly observed in children. Miscellaneous causes have been identified. The aim of this chapter is to review immunological disorders responsible for intractable diarrhoea in children. The possible role of autoimmunity will be considered first, then the association of intractable diarrhoea and immunodeficiencies.

INTRACTABLE DIARRHOEA AND AUTOIMMUNITY

Several observations[1-15] summarized in Table 5.1, have led to the concept of autoimmune enteropathy. In the patients described, enteropathy was ascribable neither to a dietary antigen nor to an infectious agent, and was associated with extradigestive symptoms known to be autoimmune, with circulating enterocyte autoantibodies and/or with intestinal mononuclear cell activation. Several features of this syndrome deserve to be emphasized.

Clinical features

1. Outset of the disease is usually early during the first 2 years of life. Several neonatal cases of poor prognosis have been reported (Table 5.1).
2. The vast predominance of boys, as well as the familial history in several male patients, suggest that some cases may be X-linked inherited. Two reports are particularly significant; one by Ellis et al. of two male cousins born from two sisters[4]; the second by Powell et al. of a family with 17 boys with various autoimmune disorders associated in eight cases with a severe protracted diarrhoea[5].

Table 5.1 Autoimmune enteropathy

References	Sex	Familial history	Age of onset	Associated diseases	Gut autoantibody	Other autoantibody	Histology[a]	Outcome[b]
McCarthy et al. (1978)	M	+	14 years	IgA deficiency	+	none	TVA Crypt hyperplasia	CP = +
Unsworth et al. (1982); Walker-Smith et al. (1982)	M		15 months	0	+	Pancreatic islets Nucleus Smooth muscle	TVA Crypt hyperplasia LP infiltration	St/C = 0 CP = ± CSA = 0
Ellis et al. (1982)	M	+	2 weeks	Glomerulopathy Nephritis	+	Renal tubule Red blood cells	TVA	C/CP = 0; death
Ellis et al. (1982)	M	+	1 day	Dermatitis Diabetes Haemolytic anemia	Not tested	Immune complexes	P2 = cryptites LP infiltration	Death
Powell et al. (1982)	M	+	7 months	Diabetes Haemolytic anemia Infections	Not tested	Not tested	Severe VA ↑ mitoses LP infiltration	St = 0; death
Martini et al. (1983)	M	+	2 years	Glomerulopathy	+	Renal tubule Basement membrane Nucleus Immune complexes	TVA LP infiltration	St/CP = clinical + but no histological + St/CP = 0; death
Savilahti et al. (1985)	F	−	3 years	Diabetes Arthritis Pericarditis	Low titres	Nucleus	TVA ↓ mitotic rate	
Savage et al. (1985)	M	+	4 months	Hypothyroidism Thrombopenia	+	Thyroid Pancreatic islets Nucleus smooth muscle	STVA	P1: St/CP/Aza = 0; death P2: spontaneous +
Mirakian et al. (1986), 12 cases	M = 8 7/12, F = 4	M −	1–20 months	Diabetes = 3/12 Alopecia = 2/12 Hypothyroidism 2/12 Thrombopenia 2/12	+ High titres 4/12 Low titres 8/12	Pancreatic islets Nucleus Microsomes Thyroglobulin Smooth muscle Mitochondria Parietal cells	Partial VA = 7/12 STVA = 3/12 Normal 1/12? LP infiltration Cryptites = 3/7	St ± Aza = +(8/12)

76

Table 5.1 (Cont.)

References	Sex	Familial history	Age of onset	Associated diseases	Gut autoantibody	Other autoantibody	Histology[a]	Outcome[b]
Kanof et al. (1987)	F	0	1 day	0	Not tested	Not tested	Severe VA ↑ mitoses Cryptites LP infiltration Fibrosis Colonic lesions	St = 0; death
Catassi et al. (1988)	M		13 years	Variable Hypogamma-globulinaemia	+	Microsomes	TVA Crypt hyperplasia	Death
Bernstein et al. (1988)	M	–	22 months	0	–	–	TVA Crypt hyperplasia LP infiltration	CSA = recovery
Mitton et al. (1989)	M		7 months	0	+	Microsomes Renal brush border	TVA Crypt hyperplasia Inflammation Crypt abscesses in colon	St = 0; death
Cuenod et al. (1990), 7 cases	M = 7	1/7	1–8 months	Thrombopenia and haemolytic anemia = 1/7 Polyarthritis and Sjögren = 1/7 Diabetes = 1/7 IgG2, IgG4 deficiency = 1/7	Not tested	Thrombocytes Red blood cells Nucleus	Severe to TVA ↑ or normal mitoses LP infiltration Cryptites = 3/7 Colonic lesions = 3/7	1: spontaneous + 3: CP/Aza/St/Ig = + 3: CP/CSA + St/anti-lymphocyte Ig = 0; death

[a] TVA = total villous atrophy; LP = lamina propria; VA = villous atrophy; STVA = subtotal villous atrophy.
[b] + = improvement; ± = limited improvement; 0 = no effect of treatment; CP = cyclophosphamide; St = steroids; CSA = cyclosporine A; Aza = azathioprine.

77

3. Although the absence of immunodeficiency has been included in the definition of autoimmune enteropathy, this point should probably be reconsidered[17]. Thus Powell et al. have noted an abnormal sensitivity to viral infections in their patients, although there was no characterized immunodeficiency[5]. Moreover, three patients with either IgA deficiency[1], common variable hypogammaglobulinaemia[12], or IgG2 and IgG4 deficiency[15], all conditions predisposing to autoimmune diseases, presented a syndrome identical to other patients. Finally, it is tempting to speculate that the neonatal onset of several autoimmune diseases in some patients reflects a profound defect of immune regulations.

4. Diarrhoea is usually characterized as secretory. Its intensity is variable. In our series, three patients with a faecal output over 150 ml/kg per day also had intermittent blood and mucus discharges. These severe clinical symptoms were associated with the most severe and extensive histological lesions and were of poor prognosis[15].

Histological features

Severe or subtotal villous atrophy is usual, and associated with intestinal mononuclear cell infiltration. Intestinal mononuclear cell infiltration contributes to differentiate autoimmune enteropathy from other cases of intractable diarrhoea, possibly related to an inherited defect of enterocytic differentiation[15,16].

Mitotic rate is variable. Low mitotic rate has been observed[7]. Yet, in most cases, severe to total villus atrophy (TVA) was associated with crypt hyperplasia (Table 5.1). The latter histological picture can initially lead one to suspect coeliac disease. However, in coeliac disease TVA is associated with a striking increase in the number of intraepithelial lymphocytes (IEL)[18] and a more moderate T cell infiltration of the superficial lamina propria (Kutlu et al., submitted). In contrast, T cell infiltration in autoimmune enteropathy predominates in lamina propria with no or a moderate increase of IEL[15]. Recent immunohistochemical studies have also demonstrated an increase in the subset of IEL expressing a T cell receptor (TCR) of the $\gamma\delta$ type in coeliac disease[19,20]. This is not observed in autoimmune enteropathy, where the T cell increase is restricted to the TCR $\alpha\beta+$ subset[15,17].

In some patients, TVA is associated with destructive lesions of the crypts. In the latter cases, similar colonic and rectal lesions are often associated[10,11,14,15]. In one of our patients ulcerative gastritis and oesophagitis were also present[15]. All reported patients presenting such severe lesions have died in spite of all therapeutic attempts, including heavy immunosuppression in three of our patients (Table 5.1).

Pathogenic hypotheses

Clinical and biological data support the hypothesis of an autoimmune process. Yet the immune mechanisms possibly involved in the pathogenesis of intestinal damage are not defined. The deleterious effect of enterocyte autoantibodies detected in the serum of most tested patients was first suspected[1-4,7-10,12,14,17]. In one study a high titre of autoantibodies fixing complement was associated with the most severe histological lesions[10]. Yet *in situ* detection of autoantibodies observed in one patient[1] was absent in another[7]. Moreover, a precise kinetic study performed in one patient showed that appearance of autoantibodies had followed that of intestinal lesions[2]. Treatment by cyclophosphamide induced disappearance of autoantibodies but only minimal histological and clinical improvement[3]. Finally, autoantibodies were not detected in all patients (Table 5.1) and on the contrary were observed at low titres in other enteropathies[10]. Altogether, these data suggest that autoantibodies may appear secondary to gut epithelial lesions and are more likely to play an aggravating than a primary role in epithelial damage.

Recently, the possible role of intestinal T cells activated by an autoimmune process has been propounded[15]. Indeed, studies of murine models of graft-versus-host disease[21,22], as well as of human fetal organ cultures[23], have demonstrated that excessive activation of intestinal T cells can lead to villous atrophy associated or not with crypt destruction. The primary role of T lymphocytes using the TCR $\alpha\beta$ in the pathogenesis of autoimmune diseases has been demonstrated in several animal models and is strongly suspected in humans (reviewed in ref. 24). The mechanisms by which T cells can induce epithelial damage are unclear. T cells may act directly against epithelial cells by exerting a cytotoxic activity or through a lymphokine secretion. They could also recruit and activate macrophages and/or favour the production of autoantibodies. In the future, the study of the intestinal T cell repertoire may help to demonstrate the presence of a clone of autoreactive T cells.

Management and prognosis

Although spontaneous recovery has been reported, prognosis of autoimmune enteropathy is globally severe (Table 5.1). Total parenteral nutrition is required for prolonged periods. Because of the clues in favour of an autoimmune disease, or of the associated autoimmune disorders, various immunosuppressive treatments have been attempted. Steroids, azathioprine, cyclophosphamide and more recently cyclosporin A have induced durable improvement and even recovery in several patients[17] (Table 5.1). Yet other patients have only been minimally or transitorily improved by heavy immunosuppressive regimens, including in three of our patients, cyclophosphamide, cyclosporin A and steroids and antilymphocytic immunoglobulins. Altogether, the various reports suggest that a neonatal onset, a diarrhoea exceeding 150 ml/kg per day, extensive crypt destruction, associated lesions of colon and/or of the upper digestive tract, severe renal involvement and perhaps high titres of circulating enterocyte autoantibodies are criteria of bad prognosis, associated with a poor response to immunosuppressive treatment and with a fatal outcome.

INTRACTABLE DIARRHOEA AND IMMUNODEFICIENCIES

Diarrhoea is common in patients with immunodeficiencies (ID) either primary or acquired. Only primary ID will be considered here, as severe acquired immunodeficiency syndrome (AIDS) is discussed in another chapter. Severity and frequency of digestive symptoms depend on the nature and intensity of the immune defect.

Primary humoral deficiencies

Characteristics of the main primary B cell ID are summarized in Table 5.2 (for review see ref. 25).

Isolated IgA deficiency, the most frequent primary ID (prevalence: 1/600 in Europe) is rarely associated with diarrhoea, probably because of the compensatory hyperplasia of intestinal IgM and IgG plasma cells. Protracted diarrhoea might be more frequent in cases of associated IgG2 and/or IgG4 deficiency[26] but is mainly observed in global humoral ID (Table 5.2)[25,27,30]. Thus, before treatment with intravenous immunoglobulins, approximately 30% of patients with agammaglobulinaemia had protracted diarrhoea.

Protracted diarrhoea in B cell ID has been ascribed to prolonged infestation by *Giardia*, less frequently to microbial overgrowth. A high prevalence of coeliac disease has been reported in IgA deficiency[32]. Finally, as discussed above, rare cases of autoimmune intractable diarrhoea have been observed in patients with IgA ID, IgG2 and IgG4 ID, and in common variable hypogammaglobulinaemia, all conditions predisposing to autoimmune diseases[25].

In patients with severe humoral ID, substitutive treatment by intravenous immunoglobulins[33] has markedly decreased the frequency of both digestive and extradigestive symptoms. One patient with IgG2 and IgG4 deficiency and autoimmune enteropathy was also markedly improved by immuno-globulins[15]. Immunoglobulins are given every 3–4 weeks at an approximate dose of 200 mg/kg. Residual levels of IgG over 5 g/L are necessary to ensure protection in patients with complete absence of immunoglobulins. This treatment is, however, counterindicated in isolated IgA ID because of the high risk of inducing anti-IgA autoantibodies. In cases of associated IgG deficiency, immunoglobulins can be given while regularly checking for anti-IgA autoantibodies. Their detection should lead to the use of immunoglobulin preparations deprived of IgA.

Primary cellular immunodeficiencies

Primary T cell deficiencies are related to an inborn defect of T cell differentiation which leads either to an absence of mature T cells (severe combined immunodeficiencies = SCID) or to their defective functions (combined immunodeficiencies = CID)[25,34]. Main T cell defects responsible for protracted or untractable diarrhoea are listed in Table 5.3.

Table 5.2 Main primary B cell immunodeficiencies

	Clinical consequences	Defect	Origin	Others
1. Global defects				
(a) X-linked agamma-globulinaemia	ORL and pulmonary bacterial infections Diarrhoea Arthritis (mycoplasma) Infections by enteroviruses	Blockage at pre-B cell stage Absence of mature B cells and Ig	Localized in Xq21.3q23	Antenatal diagnosis possible
(b) Hyper-IgM with defective isotypic switch[25]	Idem Bacterial meningitis	Switch defect, probably extrinsic	(1) X-linked (Xq27) (2) Autosomal recessive (3) Related to fetal rubella	
(c) Common variable hypogamma-globulinaemia (CVH)[28]	ORL and pulmonary infections Diarrhoea Autoimmune diseases Cancers	?	Linked to MHC Class III[28] Class II[29 a]	
2. IgA deficiency	Rarely symptomatic diarrhoea Autoimmune diseases Cancers	?	Idem to CVH[28 a]	
3. IgG isotype deficiencies[31 a]	Idem to CVH	?		

[a] CVH, IgA deficiency and Ig isotype deficiencies may be related diseases as suggested by genetical linkage to the same regions of MHC, and by the fact that they may be observed in the same family and successively in the same patient.

Table 5.3 Main T cell immunodeficiencies

	Inheritance	Mechanisms	Criteria useful for diagnosis
1. Severe combined ID[25]			
(a) Reticular dysgenesis	Autosomal recessive[a]	Unknown defect of granulocyte + lymphocyte precursor	Alymphocytosis + agranulocytosis
(b) Alymphocytosis	Autosomal recessive[a]	Unknown defect of the precursor for B and T cells	Absence of T and B cells
(c) Deficiency in T cell precursors	1-X-linked: + + (Xq11-q13)[a,b] 2-autosomal recessive ±[a]	Unknown defect of the T cell precursor	Absence of T cells, presence of B and NK cells
(d) Adenoside deaminase (ADA) deficiency	Autosomal recessive[a,b]	Accumulation of purine metabolites leading to lymphocyte death	Undetectable ADA activity in red blood cells
2. Combined ID			
(a) Defective HLA class II expression[39]	Autosomal recessive[a]	Defective antigen presentation to T cells	Class II B cells, macrophages and activated T cells
(b) Defective CD3-TCR expression[40,41]	?	Defective antigen recognition by T cells	Low CD3 expression
(c) Defective signal transduction[42]	?	Defective coupling of CD3 with signal transducers	See ref. 42
(d) ID with nanism and short limbs	?	?	
(e) Deficiency in purine nucleoside phosphorylase[25]	Autosomal recessive[a]	Idem ADA deficiency	Undetectable enzymatic activity in red blood cells
3. Di George's syndrome[25]	Embryopathy Defective migration of 3rd and 4th pharyngeal pouches	More or less severe thymic hypoplasia	Associated malformations (hypoparathyroidia, cardiopathy, dysmorphy)

[a] Possible antenatal diagnosis.
[b] Possible detection of parents at risk.

Severe combined immunodeficiencies

In SCID patients, diarrhoea is present in approximately 70% of cases. It appears early after birth together with prominent extradigestive symptoms, particularly lower respiratory tract infections[25,35].

The mechanisms of the secretory diarrhoea, which leads to profound malnutrition and cachexia when the immunological defect is not corrected, are not entirely understood.

1. Intestinal infections by microorganisms with an intracellular cycle (*Salmonella*, mycobacteriae, candida, viruses, particularly cytomegalovirus and adenoviruses) can be demonstrated in some patients.
2. Profuse diarrhoea associated with exudative enteropathy has been observed in a few patients with graft-versus-host disease following unirradiated blood transfusions or maternal transmission of mature T cells via the placenta[35].
3. In some patients, diarrhoea persists in spite of effective intestinal decontamination, total parenteral nutrition and in the absence of demonstrable pathogens until bone marrow transplantation has allowed complete immunological recovery. This recalls observations in AIDS where detectable pathogens can be identified in only 50% of patients with diarrhoea. In AIDS patients without intestinal pathogens, low-grade villous atrophy, hyporegeneration, and decreased activity of brush-border enzymes were observed[36]. Together with experimental data[37], it may suggest that intestinal T cells play a direct role in the maintenance of normal mucosal architecture[36].

Diagnosis of SCID relies on simple immunological tests: enumeration of lymphocytes, intradermal reaction with PHA. Other tests are necessary to differentiate the various defects responsible for SCID (Table 5.3).

Prognosis depends on early diagnosis which allows early isolation in a sterile environment.

Treatment consists in bone marrow transplantation which brings normal lymphoid precursors. Chances of recovery are 90% in cases of HLA-compatible grafts and 60% in partially HLA-mismatched grafts[38]. Antenatal diagnosis is possible, as well as, for some diseases, detection of parents at risk[25,39].

Combined immunodeficiencies

Several CID related to T cell dysfunctions have been described recently[25,34,40-43]. These defects compatible with a survival of several years are responsible for severe viral infections, intractable diarrhoea and autoimmune diseases.

Defective expression of HLA class II molecules is the best characterized disease[40]. In this disease, mainly observed in North African children, HLA Class II genes are normal but cannot be expressed. It has been shown that a DNA binding protein called RF-X fails to bind to a promoter of HLA Class II genes called the X-box[36].

Absence of HLA Class II antigens on antigen-presenting-cells leads to the defective activation of T cells unable to recognize antigens. This defect can be demonstrated by the lack of *in vitro* or *in vivo* (intradermal reaction) responses of T cells to antigens and the lack of specific antibodies.

Intractable diarrhoea is observed in over 70% of patients, and can be the first symptom. Identified pathogens are similar to those found in SCID patients. In addition, profuse diarrhoea related to cryptosporidiae has been observed in several patients, associated in one case with sclerosing cholangitis.

Diagnosis is made on the absence of HLA Class II molecules on monocytes, B cells and activated T cells.

Treatment relies on bone marrow transplantation which is more difficult to perform than in SCID because the presence of T cells requires prior chemotherapy[38].

Other identified defects hampering T cell activation are summarized in Table 5.3. The frequency and severity of diarrhoea in these patients is variable and depends on the severity of the immunodeficiency.

CONCLUSION

The frequent association of intractable diarrhoea with immunological disorders underlines the importance of the gut-associated lymphoid tissue (GALT). On one hand, 30% of severe B cell ID and most severe T cell ID result in protracted or intractable diarrhoea, underlining the role of GALT in the protection of the mucosa and the body. On the other hand, abnormal activation of GALT can lead to severe mucosal damage and intractable diarrhoea. This emphasizes the importance of as yet poorly defined regulatory mechanisms able to prevent excessive activation of GALT by the numerous intraluminal antigenic stimuli.

These observations indicate that thorough immunological investigations are required in children with intractable diarrhoea.

References

1. McCarthy, D. M., Katz, S. I., Gazze, L., Waldmann, T. A., Nelson, D. L. and Strober, W. (1978). Selective IgA deficiency associated with total villous atrophy of the small intestine and an organ-specific anti-epithelial cell antibody. *J. Immunol.*, **120**, 932–8
2. Walker-Smith, J. A., Unsworth, D. J., Hutchins, P., Phillips, A. D. and Holborrow, E. J. (1982). Autoantibodies against gut epithelium in child with small-intestinal enteropathy. *Lancet*, **1**, 566–7
3. Unsworth, J., Hutchins, P., Mitchell, J., Philipps, A., Hindocha, P., Holborow, J. and Walker-Smith, J. (1982). Flat small intestinal mucosa and autoantibodies against the gut epithelium. *J. Pediatr. Gastroenterol. Nutr.*, **1**, 503–13
4. Ellis, D., Fischer, S. E., Smith, W. I. and Jaffe, R. (1982). Familial occurrence of renal and intestinal disease associated with tissue autoantibodies. *Am. J. Dis. Child.*, **136**, 323–6
5. Powell, B. R., Buist, N. R. M. and Stenzel, P. (1982). An X-linked syndrome of diarrhoea, polyendocrinopathy, and fatal infection in infancy. *J. Pediatr.*, **100**, 731–7
6. Martini, A., Scotta, M. S., Notarangelo, L. D., Maggiore, G., Guarnaccia, S. and De Giacomo, C. (1983). Membranous glomerulopathy and chronic small-intestinal enteropathy associated with autoantibodies directed against renal tubular basement membrane and the cytoplasma of intestinal epithelial cells. *Acta Paediatr. Scand.*, **72**, 931–4

7. Savilahti, E., Pelkonen, P., Holmberg, C., Perkkio, M. and Unsworth, J. (1985). Fatal unresponsive villous atrophy of the jejunum, connective tissue disease and diabetes in a girl with intestinal epithelial cell antibody. *Acta Paediatr. Scand.*, **74**, 472–6

8. Savage, M. O., Mirakian, R., Wozniak, E. R., Jenkins, H. R., Malone, M., Phillips, A. D., Milla, P. J., Bottazzo, G. F. and Harries, J. T. (1985). Specific autoantibodies to gut epithelium in two infants with severe protracted diarrhoea. *J. Pediatr. Gastroenterol. Nutr.*, **4**, 187–95

9. Unsworth, D. J. and Walker-Smith, J. A. (1985). Autoimmunity in diarrhoeal disease. *J. Pediatr. Gastroenterol. Nutr.*, **4**, 375–80

10. Mirakian, R., Richardson, A., Milla, P. J., Walker-Smith, J. A., Unsworth, J., Savage, M. O. and Bottazzo, G. F. (1986). Protracted diarrhoea of infancy: evidence in support of an autoimmune variant. *Br. Med. J.*, **293**, 1132–6

11. Kanof, M. E., Rance, N. E., Hamilton, S. T., Luk, G. D. and Lake, A. M. (1987). Congenital diarrhoea with intestinal inflammation and epithelial immaturity. *J. Pediatr. Gastroenterol. Nutr.*, **6**, 141–6

12. Catassi, C., Mirakian, R., Natalini, G., Sbarbati, A., Cinti, S., Coppa, G. V. and Giorgi, P. L. (1988). Unresponsive enteropathy associated with circulating enterocyte autoantibodies in a boy with common variable hypogammaglobulinemia and type I diabetes. *J. Pediatr. Gastroenterol. Nutr.*, **7**, 608–13

13. Bernstein, E. F. and Whitington, P. F. (1988). Successful treatment of atypical sprue in an infant with cyclosporine. *Gastroenterology*, **95**, 199–204

14. Mitton, S. G., Mirakion, R., Larcher, Dillon, M. J. and Walker-Smith, J. A. (1989). Enteropathy and renal involvement in an infant with evidence of widespread autoimmune disturbance. *J. Pediatr. Gastroenterol. Nutr.*, **8**, 397–400

15. Cuenod, B., Brousse, N., Goulet, O., De Potter, S., Mougenot, J. F., Ricour, C., Guy-Grand, D. and Cerf-Bensussan, N. (1990). Classification of intractable diarrhoea in infancy using clinical and immunohistological criteria. *Gastroenterology*, **99**, 1037–43

16. Davidson, G. P., Cutz, E., Hamilton, J. R. and Gall, D. G. (1978). Familial enteropathy: a syndrome of protracted diarrhoea from birth, failure to thrive, and hypoplastic villus atrophy. *Gastroenterology*, **75**, 783–90

17. Walker-Smith, J. A. (1991). Coeliac disease and autoimmune enteropathy. In Mearin, M. and Mulder, C. J. J. (eds), *Coeliac Disease: 40 years Glutenfree*, Dordrecht: Kluwer, pp. 131–6

18. Ferguson, A. (1977). Intraepithelial lymphocytes of the small intestine. *Gut*, **18**, 921–37

19. Halstensen, T. S., Scott, H. and Brantzaeg, P. (1989). Intraepithelial T cells of the TcRγ/δ + CD8- and Vδ1/φδ1 + phenotypes are increased in coeliac disease. *Scand. J. Immunol.*, **30**, 665–72

20. Spencer, J., Isaacson, P. G., Diss, T. C. and MacDonald, T. T. (1989). Expression of disulfide-linked and non disulfide-linked forms of the T cell receptor γ/δ heterodimer in human intestinal intraepithelial lymphocytes. *Eur. J. Immunol.*, **19**, 1335–8

21. MacDonald, T. T. and Ferguson, A. (1977). Hypersensitivity reactions in the small intestine 3-Effects of allograft rejection and graft-versus-host-disease on epithelial cell kinetics. *Cell Tissue Kinet.*, **10**, 301

22. Guy-Grand, D. and Vassalli, P. (1986). Gut injury in mouse graft-versus-host reaction. Study of its occurrence and mechanisms. *J. Clin. Invest.*, **77**, 1584–95

23. MacDonald, T. T. and Spencer, J. (1988). Evidence that activated cells play a role in the pathogenesis of enteropathy in humans. *J. Exp. Med.*, **167**, 1341–9

24. Kumar, V., Kono, D. H., Urban, J. L. and Hood, L. (1989). The T-cell repertoire and autoimmune diseases. *Ann. Rev. Immunol.*, **7**, 657–82

25. Cooper, M. D. and Butler, J. L. (1989). Primary immunodeficiency diseases. In Paul, W. E. (ed.), *Fundamental Immunology*. New York: Raven Press, pp. 1033–57

26. Oxelius, V. A., Laurell, A. B., Lindquist, B., Golebiowska, H., Axelson, V., Björkander, J. and Hanson, L. A. (1981). IgG subclasses in selective IgA deficiency. *N. Engl. J. Med.*, **304**, 1476–77

27. Geha, R. S., Hyslop, N., Alami, S., Farah, F., Schneeberger, E. E. and Rosen, F. S. (1979). Hyperimmunoglobulin M immunodeficiency (dysgammaglobulinemia). *J. Clin. Invest.*, **64**, 385–91

28. Cunningham-Rundles, C. (1989). Clinical and immunological analyses of 103 patients with common variable immunodeficiency. *J. Clin. Immunol.*, **9**, 22–3

29. French, M. and Dawkins, R. L. (1990). Central MHC genes, IgA deficiency and autoimmune

disease. *Immunol. Today*, **11**, 271–4
30. Olerup, O., Smith, C. I. E. and Hammarström, C. (1990). Different aminoacids at position 57 of the HLA DQβ chain associated with susceptibility and resistance to IgA deficiency. *Nature*, **347**, 289–90
31. Bremard-Oury, C., Aucouturier, P., Le Deist, F., Debré, M., Preud'homme, L. and Griscelli, C. (1986). The spectrum of IgG2 deficiencies. In Vossen, J. and Griscelli, C. (eds), *Progress in Immunodeficiency Research and Therapy*. Amsterdam: Excerpta Medica, vol. II, pp. 235–9
32. Cooper, B. T., Holmes, G. K. T. and Cooke, W. T. (1978). Coeliac disease and immunological disorders. *Br. Med. J.*, **537**, 5391
33. Stiehm, R. E., Ashida, E., Kwang, S. K., Winston, D. J., Haas, A. and Gale, R. P. (1987). Intravenous immunoglobulins as therapeutic agents. *Ann. Intern. Med.*, **107**, 307–82
34. Fischer, A. (1990). Primary immunodeficiencies. *Curr. Opinion Immunol.*, **2**, 439–44
35. Bremard-Oury, C., Durandy, A., Fischer, A., Le Deist, F. and Griscelli, C. (1984). A review of 58 patients with severe combined immunodeficiency. In Griscelli, C. and Vossen, J. (eds), *Progress in Immunodeficiency Research and Therapy*. Amsterdam: Elsevier, vol. 1, pp. 425–6
36. Ullrich, R., Zeitz, M., Heise, W., L'age, M., Höffken, G. and Riecken, E. O. (1989). Small intestinal structure and function in patients infected with human immunodeficiency virus (HIV): evidence for HIV-induced enteropathy. *Ann. Intern. Med.*, **111**, 15–21
37. Cummins, A. G., Labrooy, J. H. and Shearman, D. J. C. (1989). The effect of cyclosporin A in delaying maturation of the small intestine during weaning in rats. *Clin. Exp. Immunol.*, **75**, 451–6
38. Fischer, A., Griscelli, C., Friedriech, W. *et al.* (1986). Bone marrow transplantation of immunodeficiencies and osteopetrosis. A European survey 1968–1987. *Lancet*, **2**, 1080–3
39. De Sainte Basile, G. and Fischer, A. (1991). X-linked immunodeficiencies. Clues to genes involved in T- and B-cell differentiation. *Immunol. Today* (in press)
40. Griscelli, C., Lisowska-Grospierre, B. and Mach, B. (1989). Combined immunodeficiency with defective expression in MHC class II genes. *Immunodeficiency Rev.*, **1**, 135–54
41. Alarcon, B., Regueiro, J. R., Arnaiz-Villena, A. and Terhorst, C. (1988). Familial defect in the surface expression of the T-cell receptor–CD3 complex. *N. Engl. J. Med.*, **319**, 1203–9
42. Le Deist, F., Thoenes, G., Corado, J., Lisowska-Grospierre, B. and Fischer, A. (1991). Immunodeficiency with low expression of the T cell receptor/CD3 complex. Effect on T lymphocyte activation. *Eur. J. Immunol.* (In press)
43. Chatila, T., Wong, R., Young, M., Miller, R., Terhorst, C. and Geha, R. S. (1989). An immunodeficiency characterized by defective signal transduction in T lymphocytes. *N. Engl. J. Med.*, **320**, 696–702

6

Immunology of intestinal transplantation in humans and animals

N. BROUSSE, S. SARNACKI, D. CANIONI and N. CERF-BENSUSSAN

Small intestinal transplantation would represent the best definitive treatment for patients who have short bowel syndrome following pathological conditions such as necrotizing enterocolitis or midgut volvulus. These patients are indeed dependent on long-term parenteral nutrition, which is associated with complications such as liver impairment and infections[1].

Small intestinal transplantation (SIT) in humans is, however, not currently available as a standard surgical procedure. Despite the use of immunosuppressive drugs which have allowed control of graft rejection in animal models, rejection remains a major problem in clinical small intestinal transplantation[2]. Furthermore, the large amount of lymphoid tissue associated to the gut may suggest a possible risk of graft-versus-host (GVH) disease following intestinal transplantation.

This chapter considers first the use of experimental models to understand the mechanisms involved in intestinal graft rejection and to define treatments able to prevent this process. Second, the main clinical, histological and immunological data provided by the study of several intestinal allografts in humans will be described.

INTESTINAL TRANSPLANTATION IN ANIMALS

Experimental models

During the early 1960s, numerous investigations documented the technical feasibility of small bowel transplantation. In 1959, Lillehei was the first to describe a technique for functional orthotopic small bowel transplantation in the dog[3]. Then, heterotopic models involving transplantation of small intestinal segment in the neck or the abdomen in dogs and pigs have been described[4-8].

Experimental models of SIT were also developed in rats in order to control differences in donor and recipient MHC haplotypes and to facilitate immunological studies. The graft has been reimplanted either in heterotopic position with vena cava drainage[9] or in orthotopic position with portal venous drainage[10]. This orthotopic model was shown to prolong significantly the survival of the grafts as compared to that observed with the systemic venous outflow procedure[10,11]. The role of portal venous drainage in the better tolerance of allografts remains unclear.

Study of graft rejection

Histological study

The histological pattern of allograft rejection has been well described in rats either in fully allogeneic strain combinations or in a unidirectional host-versus-graft reaction. Whatever the strain combination studied, three phases of rejection have been described[12-14]. First, at an early stage, there was a moderate mononuclear infiltrate in the lamina propria (LP) around and under the crypts. Some crypts appeared to be mildly elongated with an increased number of mitoses. In small scattered foci, sloughing of crypt epithelium and isolated gland necrosis were already detectable. Madara *et al.* also reported early focal injury of endothelial cells of post-capillary venules in Peyer's patches (PP)[13]. In a second stage, lamina propria was distended by a dense infiltrate consisting predominantly of mononuclear cells. The number of necrotic crypts increased and villous atrophy varied from moderate to subtotal. The endpoint of graft rejection (Fig. 6.1) associated polymorphic

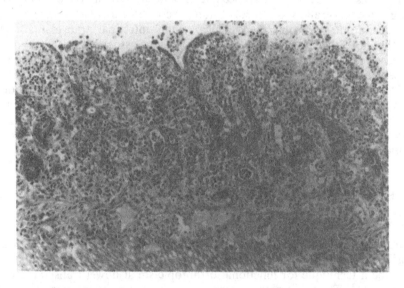

Figure 6.1 Small intestinal transplantation alone in the DA-PVG rat strain combination: acute graft rejection on day 6: mucosal atrophy and mononuclear cell infiltration with extensive crypt necrosis

infiltration with a predominance of polymorphonuclear cells, subtotal or total villous atrophy and extensive gland destruction resulting in some places in the disappearance of all epithelial structures and/or perforation of the intestinal wall. Mesenteric lymph nodes of the allografts contained a dense polymorphic infiltrate and the nodal architecture was destroyed.

The histological features thus suggest that the primary targets for rejection are most likely endothelial cells and crypt epithelial cells. Structural and functional impairment of villous epithelium appear as secondary to crypt injury.

Immunohistological study

Immunohistochemical studies have allowed study of traffic of allogeneic cells into the graft and aided definition of the phenotype of cells rejecting the graft.

Recipient cells identified by monoclonal antibodies specific for recipient MHC antigens were first seen in donor PP on postcapillary venules, 30 min following revascularization of the graft. By day 1, recipient cells had totally invaded T areas of PP. They were dividing and bore the IL2 receptor. Appearance of recipient cells in the lamina propria (LP) was delayed and started only on day 3 simultaneously with the appearance of first histological changes. These results indicate that priming of recipient cells against donor antigens occur in PP. Priming of intestinal T cells in PP was also shown to be the first step during the normal intestinal immune response. It seems likely that some factors – as yet unidentified – endowed lymphocytes stimulated in the microenvironment of PP with the ability to migrate into the intestinal mucosa. The fact that intestine is grafted together with these specialized lymphoid organs may contribute towards explaining the difficulties encountered in preventing intestinal graft rejection. On day 5–6, when epithelial lesions of rejection were patent, LP became massively infiltrated by CD8 + lymphocytes and by activated macrophages ED2 +, CD4 + and Ia +. Surprisingly, CD8 + lymphocytes infiltrating the graft were mainly CD5 – TCR $\alpha\beta$ –, suggesting that a large number of these lymphocytes may be non-specific NK cells probably recruited together with macrophages by a small number of allogeneic specific T cells. Abnormal expression of Class II MHC antigens, observed on crypt epithelium from day 3, reflected the increased secretion of IFN-γ by activated T cells infiltrating the graft[15].

Control of allograft rejection

Immunosuppression. Temporary control of rejection has been accomplished in dogs by better histocompatibility antigens matching and immunosuppressive therapy such as azathioprine (Imuran), prednisone and antilymphocyte globulin (ALG)[4-7]. In a canine model of orthotopic transplantation, daily intramuscular administration of cyclosporin A could prevent or delay rejection[15]. In pigs, prevention of rejection was obtained with cyclosporin A given parenterally[8]. Cyclosporin A has also proven to be remarkably effective in preventing rejection of small bowel grafts in different strain combinations of rats[16-19]. In some strain combinations the daily administration of cyclosporin A during the first week was sufficient to obtain indefinite survival of the graft[16,19]. Recently, new drugs have been tested for SIT in the rat model. Starzl et al. reported a significant prolongation of small bowel graft survival with short-term FK 506 immunosuppressive therapy in a strain combination where cyclosporin had been shown to be ineffective[20]. Other new immunosuppressive agents such as 15-deoxyspergualin (DSG) and rapamicin have been also used successfully in experimental small bowel transplantations[21,22]. However, as will be seen below, the very good efficiency of immunosuppressive drugs observed in animal models cannot be taken as entirely predictive of their efficiency in clinical small bowel transplantation. Thus, the poor efficiency of immunosuppressive drugs such as cyclosporin A in clinical transplantation, as well as the severe complications related to heavy non-specific immunosuppressive regimens, have led to the development of other more specific means to prevent rejection.

Pretreatment of the graft. Stangl et al. have attempted to reduce graft antigenicity by treating the donor 24 h prior to SIT with OX-42, a monoclonal antibody specific for dendritic cells and macrophages, and 14-4-4-S, a monoclonal antibody reacting with rat Class II antigen[23]. They have obtained a short but significant prolongation of the recipient's survival.

Pretreatment of the recipient. Pretreatment of the recipient with donor-specific blood transfusion (DST) has been shown to prolong significantly kidney allograft survival both in experimental[24] and clinical transplantation[25]. Thus the induction of graft tolerance by DST was also tested in small bowel transplantation. However, Martinelli et al.[26], and more recently de Bruin et al.[27], showed in a rat model that preconditioning with DST ameliorates GVH disease, but had no beneficial effect on the survival of small bowel allografts.

Pretransplant injection of donor strain spleen cells into the portal system of the recipient has also been reported in order to induce specific unresponsiveness of the host. However, although this method seemed to be effective in inducing tolerance of kidney[28] or heart graft[29], it did not promote long-term survival of small bowel graft without immunosuppression[30].

The mechanisms underlying specific unresponsiveness to donor alloantigens remain poorly understood: suppressor cells[31], soluble suppressor factor[28], anti-idiotypic antibodies[32] or clonal deletion of cytotoxic T cells[33] have been suggested. More recent data favoured a mechanism of anergy where allogeneic T cells remain present but are unable to mount an *in vivo* immunological response harmful to the graft[34].

Liver-induced tolerance. We have recently developed a rat model of double liver and intestinal transplantation which promoted long-term survival of small bowel graft without immunosuppression. The experiment was performed in an allogeneic DA to PVG combination where liver-induced tolerance has been well described for other organs. Rats received a heterotopic small bowel transplantation 17 days after an orthotopic liver graft. All animals with SIT alone had massive intestinal graft rejection between post-operative days 7 and 9. In contrast, survival of the graft in the double transplantation group was over 150 days.

Different mechanisms have been proposed to explain the liver-induced tolerance: clonal deletion of alloreactive T cells, suppressor cells, soluble suppressor factors such as soluble Class I MHC antigen[35]. However, the cellular basis of transplantation tolerance induced by liver grafting remains not fully elucidated.

In the double transplantation model, long-term survival of small bowel grafts was achieved in spite of strong mononuclear cell infiltrate (Fig. 6.2) of recipient origin in the LP which reached a peak 2 months after small bowel grafting and thereafter partially disappeared. The intensity of this infiltration on POD 70 contrasted with minor epithelial damage and favoured a mechanism of anergy which remains to be demonstrated by further studies (Fig. 6.3).

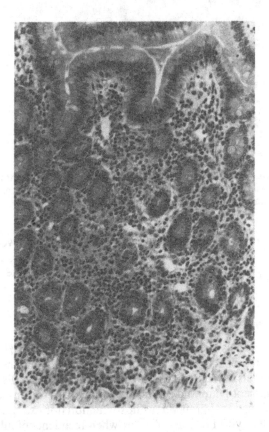

Figure 6.2 Combined liver/small bowel transplantation in the DA-PVG rat strain combination: minor histological lesions observed on day 15: mucosal mononuclear cell infiltration associated with scattered foci of crypt necrosis (arrow)

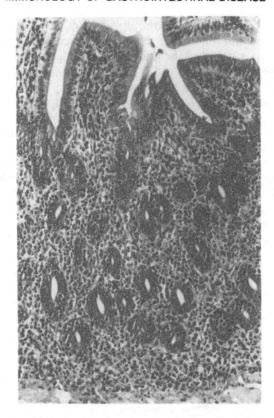

Figure 6.3 Combined liver/small bowel transplantation in the DA-PVG rat strain combination: minor histological lesions observed on day 70: persistence of an intense mucosal mononuclear cell infiltration contrasting with sparse isolated epithelial cell necrosis

Contrasting with these results, Starzl et al.[36] did not achieve tolerance of SIT in a cluster procedure where oesophagus, stomach, duodenopancreas and colon were grafted together with liver and small intestine.

Study of graft-versus-host (GVH) disease

In experimental models, clinical and histological signs of GVH disease were never observed in recipients of fully allogeneic grafts without immunosuppression. In the latter animals we have indeed observed that donor cells disappeared rapidly from recipient lymphoid organs (personal observation). GVH disease was seen in unidirectional graft versus host reaction (for example Lewis graft in a F1 Lew × BN hybrid recipient)[9,37] or when recipients of fully allogeneic grafts received an immunosuppressive treatment such as cyclosporin A[38] (which probably prolongs survival of donor cells in recipient lymphoid organs). Simultaneous host-versus-graft and graft-versus-host reactions were observed following Class II MHC incompatible small bowel transplantation[39]. The majority of the cells infiltrating the recipient's lymph nodes and spleen were of donor origin but failed to express Class II MHC antigens. The authors suggested that the GVH disease observed in this model was mediated by Class II MHC negative donor T lymphocytes which could not be recognized and eliminated by the recipient.

Pretreatment of the donor with ALG[40], irradiation[41], depletion of T-cell subsets[42], removal of mesenteric lymph nodes[43] and, more recently, administration of FK 506[44], permitted prevention of GVH disease in unidirectional models.

INTESTINAL TRANSPLANTATION IN HUMANS

Clinical results

Clinical results of intestinal fully HLA mismatched allografts in humans are summarized in Table 6.1. In spite of powerful immunosuppressive drugs, including antilymphocytic immunoglobulins, OKT3 monoclonal antibody and cyclosporin A – which prevented rejection effectively in animal models – most recent attempts of SIT alone have failed because of severe uncontrolled rejection[2,45]. In several other patients, failure was related to complications of immunosuppression which were often lethal. Thus, only two out of the 16 patients with SIT alone have a functional graft 2 years after transplantation[2,46,47]. These poor results contrast with the recent success of nine small bowel/liver transplantations[48,49] (and unpublished data), which suggests that in humans, as observed in our rat model, the liver may favour the tolerance of intestinal allografts. This result corroborates other recent observations in humans showing improved survival of kidney and pancreas allografts following liver transplantation. Four other small bowel/liver transplantations in a cluster procedure have been unsuccessful[50,51]. In the two patients who tolerated the graft, massive immunosuppression permitted control of graft rejection but occurrence of B cell lymphoproliferative syndrome induced by Epstein-Barr virus was responsible for a fatal outcome[50,51].

Because of the large amount of lymphoid tissue grafted together with the intestine in immunosuppressed recipients, GVH disease was expected to be a possible complication of human intestinal allografts. Although lymphocytes of donor origin could be detected in the peripheral blood of recipients during the first postoperative weeks[49], GVH disease has not been, as yet, a prominent problem in human HLA-mismatched intestinal transplantation. In one adult patient[48] who developed a skin rash on postoperative day 10, skin biopsy and detection of circulating T cells of donor origin have authenticated a mild GVH disease. In our experience clinical or biological extraintestinal signs of GVH were never observed. However in two children, systematic biopsies of the recipient colon on post-operative day 10 revealed scattered necrotic glands surrounded by a T cell infiltrate suggestive of mild intestinal GVH disease (Fig. 6.4). Similar but much more extensive lesions were observed at autopsy in an adult patient who died on postoperative day 21 of candida sepsis. In this patient the very poor nutritional status, together with massive

Table 6.1 Small intestinal transplantation in humans since introduction of cyclosporin A

Centre/ year	Intervention	Recipient age	Graft survival (days)	Outcome	Graft function	Ref.
Pittsburgh						
1983	Cluster	6.5 years	1	Haemorrhage*		51
1988	Cluster	3 years	192	LPD*		51
1990	SIT	Adult	>200	Still alive	?	49
1990	Liver/SIT	Adult	>200	Still alive	?	49
1990	Liver/SIT	Adult	>200	Still alive	?	49
1990	Liver/SIT	Infant	?	Still alive	?	PC
1990	Liver/SIT	Infant	?	Still alive	?	PC
1990	Liver/SIT	Infant	?	Still alive	?	PC
Toronto						
1985	SIT	26 years	12	CyA toxicity Encephalopathy Hypotension*		45
Paris						
1986	SIT	45 years	17	Sepsis*	0	PC
1987	SIT	9 months	1	Graft necrosis		2
1987	SIT	9 years	206	Visceral failure*	30%	2
1988	SIT	6 years	>500	Chronic rejection	50%	2
1988	SIT	3 years	60	Rejection, infection	50%	2
1989	SIT	5 months	>2 years	Still alive	100%	2
1989	SIT	9 months	25	Rejection	0	2
1989	SIT	4 years	200	Rejection	80%	PC
1990	SIT	20 months	1	Collapsus*	0	PC
1990	SIT	9 months	25	Rejection	0	PC
Chicago						
1987	SIT		10	Rejection		PC
1987	Cluster	17 months	4	Haemorrhage*		50
1988	Cluster	9 months	90	LPD*		50
Kiel						
1987	SIT	3 years	12	Rejection		46
1989	SIT	42 years	>2 years	Still alive	100%	46
Innsbruck						
1990	Cluster	45 years	1 year	Neoplasma Recurrence	?	PC
Ontario						
1988	SIT	8 years	15	Sepsis, rejection		47
1988	Liver/SIT	41 years	>2 years		100%	47, 48
1989	Liver/SIT	?	?	LPD*		PC
1989	Liver/SIT	?	2 years		?	PC
1990	Liver/SIT	?	>200		?	PC

*Died.

LPD, lymphoproliferative disease; SIT, small intestinal transplantation; PC, personal communication.

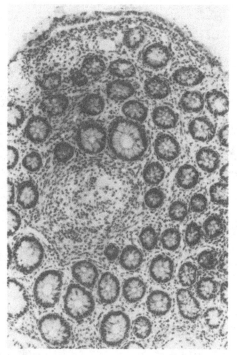

Figure 6.4 Graft-versus-host disease at day 10: scattered lesions of crypt necrosis in systematic colonic biopsy

immunosuppressive treatment, may have induced a profound T cell deficiency favouring occurrence of more severe intestinal GVH disease.

Histological and immunohistochemical signs of rejection

In our patients[52], as well as in the case reported by Hansman et al.[53], intestinal biopsies could be easily and repeatedly performed in the lower segment of the graft through the enterostomy. These biopsies have allowed precise description of the epithelial changes induced by the rejection process in humans, and enabled definition of early criteria of rejection useful to guide immunosuppressive treatment.

Acute rejection

More or less severe episodes of acute histological rejection have been observed in all our patients between postoperative day 8 and 75.

The first changes, detected only by immunohistochemistry (Fig. 6.5), included: (1) appearance of CD3+ cells in the deep mucosa beneath the crypts, some of which were activated as indicated by their expression of the p55 chain of the IL-2 receptor (CD25); (2) appearance of HLA-DR antigens

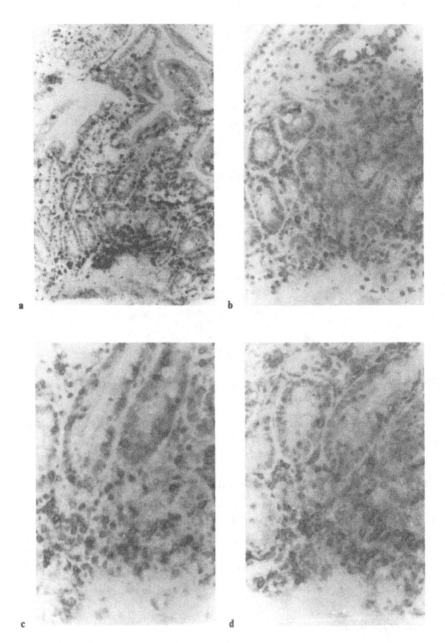

Figure 6.5 Early immunohistochemical changes suggestive of human graft rejection appearing at day 30 before histological lesions: a cluster of CD3+ cells is visible beneath the crypts (a), some of which are expressing IL-2R (CD25) (b). Increased numbers of CD8+ cells (c) and CD4+ cells (d) around the crypts

on crypt enterocytes reflecting the increased secretion of IFN-γ by activated T cells[54]; (3) decrease in the number of Ki67 + proliferating cells in the crypts. In one case the use of quinacrine, marker of the Y-chromosome, allowed confirmation that activated T cells were of recipient origin.

Focal necrosis of crypt enterocytes and oedema of villi, detected 2–5 days later, were the first histological lesions of rejection. When an appropriate early treatment of acute rejection was performed, a rapid and efficient control of the rejection process could be obtained with a marked decrease in the numbers of lamina propria CD3 + lymphocytes observed within a few days, followed by the reappearance of Ki67 + crypt enterocytes and the progressive disappearance of CD25 + cells. Lastly HLA-DR antigen expression also disappeared on crypt enterocytes.

In the absence of efficient immunosuppressive treatment, infiltration of lamina propria by activated T cells and CD68 macrophages increased rapidly. Concomitantly, crypt necrosis became extensive and associated with blunting of villi and sloughing of surface epithelium. Polymorphonuclear cells accumulated in the mucosal vessels, then extruded into the lamina propria and into the crypt lumen. In the most severe cases, mucosal epithelial structures were almost totally destroyed and replaced by an infiltrate of activated macrophages and polymorphonuclear cells (Fig. 6.6).

Hansman[53,55] proposed two markers useful for early detection of rejection: one is the decreased activity of brush border alkaline phosphatase: in our experience, the first histological lesions were limited to the crypts. Changes in alkaline phosphatase activity were more delayed. The second criterion was the appearance of numerous CD68 + (KiM6 + KiM7 +) macrophages in the submucosa. Yet in our paediatric experience submucosa was either absent or very small, which prevented the use of this marker.

Chronic rejection

Chronic rejection has been observed in only one of our patients[52]. It progressively appeared around the seventh month following several episodes of mild acute rejection. It was characterized (Fig. 6.7) by total villous atrophy with severe dystrophy of surface epithelium, fibrosis of mucosa, submucosa and muscular layers, endarteritis of submucosal vessels, infiltration of epithelium, lamina propria, submucosa and muscular layers by lymphocytes, mainly CD8 +, and macrophages. The presence of some CD25 + mononuclear cells and the strong epithelial expression of HLA-DR antigens reflected the persistent activation of graft infiltrating T cells. Although crypts were irregularly spaced there was no evidence of recent crypt necrosis. The intense staining of crypt enterocytes by Ki67 antibody and the unusual presence of Ki67 + surface enterocytes suggested an increase in epithelial cell renewal. On the 18th month post-transplantation the graft had become totally fibrous and was removed.

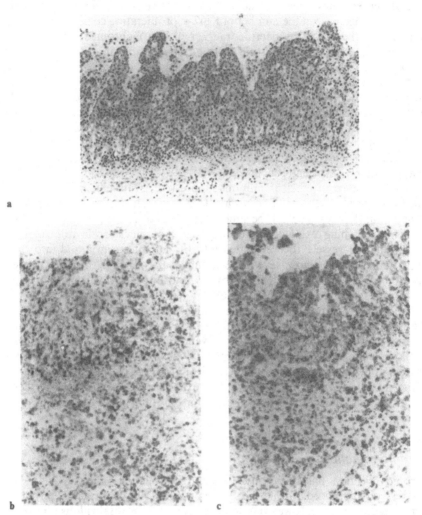

Figure 6.6 Acute rejection. Explantation at day 60. Histological lesions (**a**) showing epithelial damage and increased number of mononuclear cells. Immunohistochemical techniques revealed an increased number of CD3 + (**b**) and CD68 + (KiM7) cells (**c**) in the mucosa and submucosa.

PATHOGENESIS OF LESIONS IN INTESTINAL ALLOGRAFT REJECTION

The mechanisms by which T lymphocytes, sensitized in PP and reactivated in the intestinal mucosa by allogeneic histocompatibility antigens (expressed on macrophages, epithelial cells and endothelium), induce epithelial lesions of rejection have not been thoroughly studied[56]. However, conclusions can be drawn, based on data obtained in other types of grafts or in experimental models of T-cell induced intestinal damage[57] such as GVH disease[58-60].

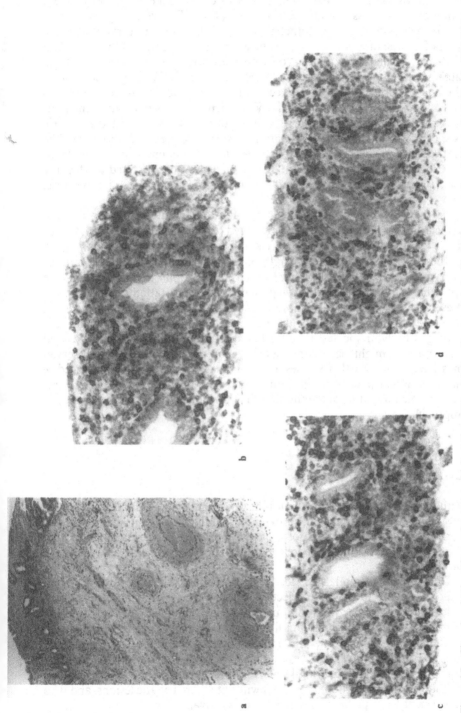

Figure 6.7 Chronic rejection 10 months post-transplantation. Mucosal atrophy associated with dense mucosal and submucosal fibrosis (7a). CD3+ (7b), CD8+ (7c) and CD68+ (7d) cells are increased

In acute rejection, early destruction of crypt epithelial cells might be mediated by direct cytotoxicity of T cells, or could be mediated by cytotoxic lymphokines such as tumour necrosis factor (TNF). By secreting lymphokines, T cells can also modify endothelial cells and thus favour entrance into the graft of a large number of non-specific effectors. TNF released by T cells can also activate macrophages and polymorphonuclears able in turn to release factors activating T cells, cytotoxic mediators (e.g. TNF, superoxide ions) or chemoattractants. The latter cells certainly play a major role in the late phases of acute rejection. In rats the phenotype of lymphocytes infiltrating the graft suggested the presence of a large number of non-MHC-restricted cytotoxic NK cells. However, such cells were rare in human rejected allografts. The cascade of non-specific events which amplify the immune reaction triggered by allogeneic T cells explains the major difficulties encountered to stop the rejection process once started, and emphasizes the importance of prevention, and of early detection of rejection.

In the single case of chronic rejection observed in humans[2,52], the association of villous atrophy and increased mitotic rate recalled observations made in various experimental models of T cell-induced epithelial damage[61]. In these models, the role of a lymphokine able to stimulate directly mitoses in crypts was suggested. Because of the severe dystrophic lesions of the surface epithelium and the marked intraepithelial T cell infiltration observed in the present case, it seems to us more likely that accelerated epithelial renewal occurred secondarily to compensate accelerated loss of surface epithelial cells damaged by lymphocytes. Finally, TNF secreted both by lymphocytes and macrophages might have contributed to the development of the observed massive fibrosis. Further studies allowing analysis of molecules produced *in situ* at different phases of rejection should help to identify the mechanisms responsible for epithelial lesions, and thus perhaps to design new therapeutic approaches.

CONCLUSION

Although animal models of small intestinal transplantation have been very promising, SIT in humans has proven very difficult to achieve and requires a particularly heavy immunosuppressive regimen responsible for severe iatrogenic complications. Therefore, SIT is not yet available as a standard procedure.

Data in animal models suggest that the gut-associated lymphoid system may contribute to promote rejection by favouring sensitization of T cells able to home into the intestinal mucosa of the graft.

Limited experimental and clinical data suggest that combined transplantation of the small intestine with the liver from the same donor may markedly improve graft survival. However, the data remained too sparse to draw conclusions. In addition, the risks of liver transplantation limit the indications of double transplantation in patients without severe hepatic lesions, and who can benefit from parenteral nutrition for survival.

Better understanding of the mechanisms involved in intestinal graft rejection and in immunological tolerance should help to design new therapies more adapted to clinical SIT than those currently available.

References

1. Grosfeld, J. L., Rescorla, F. J. and West, K. W. (1986). Short bowel syndrome in infancy and childhood. Analysis of survival in 60 patients. *Am. J. Surg.*, **151**, 41–6
2. Goulet, O., Révillon, Y., Jan, D., Brousse, N., De Potter, S., Cerf-Bensussan, N., Rambaud, C., Buisson, C., Pellerin, D., Mougenot, J. F., Fischer, A. and Ricour, C. (1990). Small bowel transplantation in children. *Transplant. Proc.*, **22**, 2499–500
3. Lillehei, R. C., Goott, B. and Miller, F. A. (1959). The physiological response of the small bowel of the dog to ischemia including prolongated in vitro preservation of the small bowel with successful replacement and survival. *Ann. Surg.*, **150**, 543–60
4. Preston, F. W., Macalad, F., Wachowski, T. J., Randolph, D. A. and Apostol, J. V. (1966). Survival of homografts of the intestine with and without immunsuppression. *Surgery*, **60**, 1203–10
5. Hardy, M. A., Quint, J. and Stale, D. (1970). Effect of antilymphocyte serum and other immunosuppressive agents on canine jejunal allografts. *Ann. Surg.*, **171**, 51–60
6. Taylor, R. M. R., Watson, J. W., Walker, F. C. and Watson, A. J. (1966). Prolongation of survival of jejunal homografts in dogs treated with azathioprine (Imuran). *Br. J. Surg.*, **53**, 134–8
7. Ruiz, J. O., Uchida, H., Schultz, L. S. and Lillehei, R. C. (1972). Problems in absorption and immunosuppression after entire intestinal transplantation. *Am. J. Surg.*, **123**, 297–303
8. Ricour, C., Revillon, Y., Arnaud-Battandier, F., Ghnassia, D., Weyne, P., Lauffenburger, A., Jos, J., Fontaine, J. L., Gallix, P. and Vaiman, M. (1984). Successful small bowel allografts in piglets using cyclosporine. *Transplant. Proc.*, **15**, 3019–26
9. Monchick, G. J. and Russell, P. S. (1971). Transplantation of small bowel in the rat: technical and immunological considerations. *Surgery*, **70**, 693–702
10. Schraut, W. H., Abraham, V. S. and Lee, K. K. (1985). Portal versus caval venous drainage for small bowel allografts. *Surgery*, **98**, 579–86
11. Schraut, W. H., Rosemurgy, A. S. and Ridell, R. M. (1983). Prolongation of intestinal allograft survival without immunosuppressive drug therapy. *J. Surg. Res.*, **34**, 597–607
12. Rosemurgy, A. S. and Schraut, W. H. (1986). Small bowel allografts. Sequence of histologic changes in acute and chronic rejection. *Am. J. Surg.*, **151**, 470–5
13. Madara, J. L. and Kirkman, R. L. (1985). Structural and functional evolution of jejunal allograft rejection in rats and the amelioration effects of cyclosporin therapy. *J. Clin. Invest.*, **75**, 502–12
14. Mosnier, J. F., Brousse, N., Calise, D., Muzeau, F., Gallix, P., Ricour, C. and Cerf-Bensussan, N. (1990). Etude des cellules immunitaires dans un modèle d'allotransplantation intestinale Lewis DA chez le rat avec cyclosporine. *Gastroenterol. Clin. Biol.*, **14** (2bis), A94
15. Reznick, R. K., Craddock, G. N., Langer, B., Gilas, T. and Cullen, J. B. (1982). Structure and function of small bowel allografts in the dog: immunosuppression with cyclosporin A. *Can. J. Surg.*, **25**, 51–5
16. Kirkman, R. L., Lear, P. A., Madara, J. L. and Tilney, N. L. (1984). Small intestine transplantation in the rat – immunology and function. *Surgery*, **96**, 280–6
17. Harmel, R. P. and Stanley, J. M. (1986). Improved survival after allogeneic small intestinal transplantation in the rat using cyclosporine immunosuppression. *J. Pediatr. Surg.*, **21**, 214–17
18. Preissner, W. Ch., Gundlach, M., Deltz, E. and Thiede, A. (1986). Allogeneic small bowel transplantation in the rat: immunosuppression by CsA and tolerance mechanism. *Transplant. Proc.*, **18**, 1427–8
19. Watson, A. J. M., Lear, P. A., Montgomery, A. *et al.* (1988). Water, electrolyte, glucose and glycine absorption in rat small intestinal transplant. *Gastroenterology*, **94**, 863–9
20. Lee, K. K. W., Stangl, S., Todo, S., Langrehr, J. M., Starzl, T. E. and Schraut, W. H. (1990). Successful orthotopic small bowel transplantation with short-term FK 506 immunosuppressive therapy. *Transplant. Proc.*, **22**, 78–9
21. Iga, C., Okajima, Y., Tadeka, Y. and Tezuka, K. (1990). Prolongated survival of small intestinal allografts in the rat with cyclosporine A, FK 506, and 15-deoxyspergualin. *Transplant. Proc.*, **22**, 1658

22. Stepkowski, S. M., Chen, H., Daloze, P. and Kahan, B. D. (1991). Rapamycin, a potent immunosuppressive drug for vascularized heart, kidney, and small bowel transplantation in the rat. *Transplantation*, **51**, 22–31

23. Stangl, M. J., Lee, K. K. W., Moynihan, H. L. and Schraut, W. H. (1990). Graft pretreatment with monoclonal antibodies prior to small bowel transplantation. *Transplant. Proc.*, **22**, 2483–4

24. Armstrong, H. E., Bolton, E. M., McMillian, I., Spencer, S. C. and Bradley, J. A. (1987). Prolongated survival of actively enhanced rat renal allografts despite accelerated cellular infiltration and rapid induction of both class I and class II MHC antigens. *J. Exp. Med.*, **164**, 891–907

25. Opelz, G., Sengar, D. P. S., Mickey, M. R. and Terasaki, P. I. (1973). Effect of blood transfusions on subsequent kidney transplants. *Transplant. Proc.*, **5**, 253

26. Martinelli, G. P., Knight, R. K., Kaplan, S., Racelis, D., Dikman, S. H. and Schanzer, H. (1989). Small bowel transplantation in the rat: effect of pretransplant blood transfusion and cyclosporine on host survival. *Transplantation*, **45**, 1021–6

27. de Bruin, R. W. F., Heineman, E., Meijssen, M. A. C., Jeekel, H. and Marquet, R. L. (1990). Small bowel transplantations in rats: the effect of pretransplant donor-specific blood transfusions on various segments of small bowel grafts. *Transplantation*, **50**, 928–30

28. Yoshimura, N., Matsui, S., Hamashima, T., Lee, C. J., Ohsaka, Y. and Oka, T. (1990). The effect of perioperative portal venous inoculation with donor lymphocytes on renal allograft survival in the rat. I. Specific prolongation of donor grafts and suppressor factor in the serum. *Transplantation*, **49**, 167–71

29. Rao, V. K., Burris, D. E., Gruel, S. M., Sollinger, H. W. and Burlingham, W. J. (1988). Evidence that donor spleen cells administered through the portal vein prolong the survival of cardiac allografts in rats. *Transplantation*, **45**, 1145–6

30. Wolf, Y. G., Dunaway, D. J. and Harmel, R. P. (1990). Small bowel transplantation following portal venous injection of donor strain spleen cells. *Transplant. Proc.*, **22**, 2493–4

31. Singh, S. K., Marquet, R. L., de Bruin, R. W. F., Westbroeck, D. L. and Jeekel, J. (1987). The role of suppressor cells in the blood transfusion phenomenon. *Transplant. Proc.*, **19**, 1442–4

32. Phelan, D. L., Rodey, G. E. and Anderson, C. B. (1989). The development and specificity of antiidiotypic antibodies in renal transplant recipients receiving single-donor blood transfusions. *Transplantation*, **48**, 57–60

33. van Twuyver, E., Kast, W. M., Mooijaart, R. D. J., Melief, C. J. M. and de Waal, L. P. (1989). Transfusion-induced skin allograft tolerance across an H-2 class I mismatch is caused by a clonal deletion of donor-specific cytotoxic T-lymphocyte precursors within the allograft. *Transplant. Proc.*, **21**, 1169–70

34. Dallman, M., Shiho, O., Page, T. H., Wood, K. J. and Morris, P. J. (1991). Peripheral tolerance to alloantigen results from altered regulation of the interleukin 2 pathway. *J. Exp. Med.*, **173**, 79–87

35. Kamada, N. (1985). The immunology of experimental liver transplantation in the rat. *Immunology*, **55**, 369–89

36. Murase, N., Demetris, A. J., Kim, D. G., Todo, S., Fung, J. J. and Starzl, T. E. (1990). Rejection of multivisceral allografts in rats: A sequential analysis with comparison to isolated orthotopic small-bowel and liver grafts. *Surgery*, **1108**, 880–9

37. Pomposelli, F., Maki, T., DeMichele, S. J., Kioyoizumi, T., Gaber, L., Balogh, K. and Monaco, A. P. (1985). Induction of graft-versus-host disease by small intestinal allotransplantation in rats. *Transplantation*, **40**, 343–7

38. Diflo, T., Maki, T., Balogh, K. and Monaco, A. P. (1989). Graft-versus-host disease in fully allogeneic small bowel transplantation in rats. *Transplantation*, **47**, 7–11

39. Lück, R., Klempnauer, J. and Steiniger, B. (1991). Simultaneous occurrence of graft-versus-host and host-versus-graft reactions after allogeneic MHC class II disparate small bowel transplantation in immunocompetent rats. *Transplant. Proc.*, **23**, 677–8

40. Schaffer, D., Maki, T., DeMichele, S. J., Karlstad, M. D., Bistrian, R. R., Balogh, K. and Monaco, A. P. (1988). Studies in small bowel transplantation: prevention of graft-versus-host disease with preservation of allograft function by donor pretreatment with antilymphocyte serum. *Transplantation*, **45**, 262–9

41. Lee, K. K. W. and Schraut, W. H. (1985). In vitro allograft irradiation prevents graft-versus-host disease in small bowel transplantation. *J. Surg. Res.*, **38**, 364–72

42. Schaffer, D., Simpson, M. A., Milford, E. L., Gottschalk, R., Maki, T. and Monaco, A. P. (1991). Donor pretreatment with monoclonal antibody for prevention of graft-versus-host disease following small bowel transplantation: effect of depletion of T-cell subsets. *Transplant. Proc.*, **23**, 679–81

43. Pirenne, J., Lardinois, F., D'Silva, M., Fridman, V., Boniver, J., Mahieu, P., Degiovanni, G. and Jacquet, N. (1990). Relevance of mesenteric lymph nodes to graft-versus-host disease following small bowel transplantation. *Transplantation*, **50**, 711–14

44. Hoffman, A. L., Makowka, X. C., Banner, B., Cramer, D. V., Pascualone, A., Todo, S. and Starzl, T. E. (1990). The effect of FK 506 on small intestine allotransplantation in the rat. *Transplant. Proc.*, **22**, 76–7

45. Cohen, Z., Silverman, R. E. and Wassez, S. G. (1986). Small intestinal transplantation using cyclosporine. Report of a case. *Transplantation*, **42**, 613

46. Deltz, E., Schroeder, P., Gundlach, M., Hansmann, M. L. and Leimenstoll, G. (1990). Successful clinical small-bowel transplantation. *Transplant. Proc.*, **22**, 2501

47. Grant, D., Wall, W., Zhong, R., Mimeault, R., Sutherland, F., Ghent, C. and Duff, J. (1990). Experimental clinical intestinal transplantation: initial experience of a Canadian centre. *Transplant. Proc.*, **22**, 2497–8

48. Grant, D., Wall, W., Mimeault, R., Zhong, R., Ghent, C., Garcia, B., Stiller, C. and Duff, J. (1990). Successful small-bowel/liver transplantation. *Lancet*, **335**, 181–4

49. Iwaki, Y., Starzl, T. E., Yagihashi, A., Taniwali, S., Abu-Elmagd, K., Tzakis, A., Fung, J. and Todo, S. (1991). Replacement of donor lymphoid tissue in small-bowel transplants. *Lancet*, **337**, 818–19

50. Williams, J. W., Sankary, H. N., Foster, P. F., Lowe, J. and Goldman, G. M. (1989). Splanchnic transplantation. An approach to the infant dependent on parenteral nutrition who develops irreversible liver disease. *J. Am. Med. Assoc.*, **261**, 1458–62

51. Starzl, T. E., Rowe, M. I., Todo, S., Jaffé, R., Tzakis, A., Hoffman, A. L., Esquivel, C., Porter, K. A., Venkataramanan, R., Makowka, L. and Duquesnoy, R. (1989). Transplantation of multiple abdominal viscera. *J. Am. Med. Assoc.*, **261**, 1449–57

52. Brousse, N., Canioni, D., Rambaud, C., Jarry, A., Guy-Grand, D., Goulet, O., Révillon, Y., Ricour, C. and Cerf-Bensussan, N. (1990). Intestinal transplantation in children: contribution of immunohistochemistry. *Transplant. Proc.*, **22**, 2495–6

53. Hansman, M. L., Deltz, E., Gundlach, M., Schroeder, P. and Radzun, H. J. (1989). Small bowel transplantation in a child. Morphologic, immunohistochemical, and clinical results. *Am. J. Clin. Pathol.*, **92**, 686–92

54. Cerf-Bensussan, N., Quaroni, A. and Kurnick, K. T. (1984). Intraepithelial lymphocytes modulate Ia expression by intestinal epithelial cells. *J. Immunol.*, **132**, 2244–52

55. Hansman, M. L., Hell, K., Gundlach, M., Deltz, E. and Schroeder, P. (1990). Immunohistochemical investigation of biopsies in a successful small bowel transplantation. *Transplant. Proc.*, **22**, 2502–3

56. Cerf-Bensussan, N., Brousse, N., Jarry, A., Goulet, O., Révillon, Y., Ricour, C. and Guy-Grand, D. (1990). Role of in vivo activated T cells in the mechanisms of villous atrophy in humans: study of allograft rejection. *Digestion*, **46**, 297–301

57. MacDonald, T. T. and Spencer, J. (1988). Evidence that activated mucosal T cells play a role in the pathogenesis of enteropathy in human small intestine. *J. Exp. Med.*, **167**, 1341–9

58. Mowat, A. and Ferguson, A. (1982). Intraepithelial lymphocyte count and crypt hyperplasia measure the mucosal component of the graft-versus-host reaction in mouse small intestine. *Gastroenterology*, **83**, 417–23

59. Guy-Grand, D. and Vassali, P. (1986). Gut injury in mouse graft-versus-host reaction. Study of its occurrence and mechanisms. *J. Clin. Invest.*, **77**, 1584–95

60. MacDonald, T. T. and Ferguson, A. (1977). Hypersensitivity reactions in small intestine. III. The effect of allograft rejection and of graft-versus-host disease on epithelial cell kinetics. *Cell Tissue Kinet.*, **10**, 301–12

61. Ferreira, R. D. C., Forsyth, L. E., Richman, P. I., Wells, C., Spencer, J. and MacDonald, T. T. (1990). Changes in the rate of crypt epithelial proliferation and mucosal morphology induced by a T-cell-mediated response in human small intestine. *Gastroenterology*, **98**, 1255–63

7
Intestinal graft-versus-host disease

A. McI. MOWAT

INTRODUCTION

The enteropathy caused by acute graft-versus-host (GVH) disease is an important clinical problem in patients receiving allogeneic bone marrow transplants (BMT), and intestinal damage is also an invariable feature of most animal models of GVH disease. The pattern of pathology in intestinal GVH disease also reproduces a variety of other, naturally occurring enteropathies. Thus, a knowledge of the pathophysiology of intestinal GVH disease is important both for improving the management of BMT patients and for understanding the immunopathogenesis of many other intestinal diseases. This chapter will review the pathogenesis of intestinal GVH disease, placing particular emphasis on the relationship between individual aspects of mucosal pathology and specific immune effector mechanisms.

BACKGROUND AND OCCURRENCE

GVH disease is the systemic immunological disorder which occurs after transfer of immunocompetent T lymphocytes into a genetically disparate, immunoincompetent host. The earliest description of GVH disease comes from the classical experiments performed by Medawar and colleagues, in which the majority of newborn mice given allogeneic lymphocytes developed a wasting disease characterized by weight loss, skin lesions and diarrhoea[1,2]. Similar features can be induced in a large number of different animal models, but the most important clinical form of GVH disease occurs after allogeneic BMT in humans. In this case the disorder is severe, as recipients are either inherently immunodeficient, or have been conditioned by high-dose irradiation and/or chemotherapy. This GVH disease is caused by contaminating T lymphocytes present in the BM. More rarely, mild GVH disease can occur in immunodeficient individuals given blood transfusions[3], while immunosuppressed recipients of small intestinal allografts are at considerable risk of GVH disease due to the large numbers of T lymphocytes within the transplanted bowel[4,5].

CLINICAL FEATURES OF GVH DISEASE

GVH disease occurs in a large proportion of patients receiving bone marrow (BM) from unrelated donors, and minor forms of the disease are not infrequent even when full HLA-matching has been performed[6,7]. In the earliest studies, GVH disease was almost universal and for many years it was the principal cause of mortality and morbidity in most BMT programmes[8-10]. More recently the severity and incidence of GVH disease have been reduced due to more effective immunosuppression of the recipient by cyclosporin A (CsA) and to regimes which purge the donor marrow of mature T lymphocytes. However, GVH disease is likely to remain an important clinical problem. Up to 70% of allogeneic BMT recipients still develop GVH disease in the face of improved therapy[11], while removal of T lymphocytes from the marrow is now known to be associated with an increased risk of graft failure[12-14]. In addition, the increasing use of intestinal allografts will provide an additional source of GVH disease.

Clinical GVH disease occurs in two forms: acute and chronic. These syndromes are defined according to their time of onset, acute GVH disease beginning within 100 days of BMT and chronic GVH disease occurring after this time. Despite the arbitrary nature of this division, the two diseases are quite distinct, often occurring independently in different patients, causing differing pathological syndromes and apparently involving distinct immunological mechanisms. Chronic GVH disease is a poorly understood disorder, causing immunological abnormalities and a generalized connective tissue disease-like syndrome. As intestinal disease is an infrequent consequence of chronic GVH disease (see below), this review will concentrate on acute GVH disease.

Acute GVH disease ranges from a mild inflammatory condition to a widespread, life-threatening disease. It is associated with damage to lymphoid tissues and other target organs. The bone marrow and immune system are always affected by acute GVH disease and the resulting immunological abnormalities have a profound influence on the outcome of the disease. Virtually every component of the immune system can be affected, with functional defects in B lymphocytes, accessory cells and all subsets of T lymphocytes having been described[15-19]. These abnormalities reflect direct attack on immunocytes themselves, as well as destruction of the lymphoid organs and thymus[20]. The immunological defects predispose the patient to secondary infections which are one of the most important features of the disease.

The infectious consequences of acute GVH disease are further predisposed to by the damage which disrupts the integrity of non-lymphoid tissues. Despite its systemic nature, the pathogenic immune response affects a rather limited number of tissues (Table 7.1). The majority of individuals with acute GVH disease have evidence of skin disease, while a smaller but variable proportion

Table 7.1 Tissue distribution of pathology in acute GVH disease

Lymphohaemopoietic
Bone marrow
Lymphoid organs

Non-lymphoid
Skin
Intestine
Liver

Pancreas
Salivary glands
?Lung

develop intestinal and liver pathology. Exocrine tissues such as the pancreas and salivary glands are also affected in some cases, but there is little convincing evidence that damage extends to other organs. Although pulmonary abnormalities have been described[21-23], the lung is not generally accepted to be a target of acute GVH disease as it is difficult to discriminate between primary consequences of GVH disease and secondary effects of irradiation, chemotherapy or infection.

The reasons underlying the restricted pattern of tissue pathology are unknown. Although it has been suggested that GVH disease damages only organs whose epithelia are capable of enhanced expression of Class II MHC antigens[24], many such tissues (e.g. kidney) are not involved in GVH disease. It seems more likely that the enhanced Class II MHC expression which occurs is merely a non-specific consequence of an ongoing local immune response. Epithelia are the principal target of acute GVH disease, with epidermal dyskeratosis and necrosis being the characteristic features of cutaneous GVH disease[25-28], while GVH disease in the liver produces bile duct lesions similar to those found in primary biliary cirrhosis[29,30]. Epithelial damage also characterizes the intestinal pathology of acute GVH disease, and this shares many features of the pathology in other epithelial tissues. Thus, the following discussion of the immunopathogenesis of intestinal GVH disease should be seen as relevant to the tissue pathology in other target organs.

INTESTINAL GVH DISEASE

As we have noted, intestinal pathology is a characteristic feature of acute GVH disease in all species examined, including humans. Most work on human intestinal GVH disease is necessarily descriptive, while detailed studies of immunopathogenesis have mainly been performed in experimental animals, particularly rodents. The clinicopathological features of intestinal GVH disease have been amply reviewed[7-9,31-34] and the principal purpose of this review is to present a synthesis of the immunological mechanisms responsible for the intestinal damage. In each section we will discuss clinical and experimental information together, but where appropriate will indicate how these might differ.

Occurrence

Diarrhoea was one of the most characteristic features of the runting disease described in the early studies of allospecific tolerance in neonatal mice, and it soon became apparent that intestinal damage played an important part in the animals' deterioration[1,2]. Subsequent work which began to define the immunological basis of experimental GVH disease confirmed the high frequency of diarrhoea[35,36], and this sign was rapidly noted in the earliest studies of patients given allogeneic BMT. Clinical intestinal GVH disease usually appears 3–6 weeks after BMT[7] but its exact incidence is difficult to estimate, as intestinal biopsies are not performed routinely in many centres and clinically obvious disease is likely to represent only the most severe end of the spectrum of pathology[34]. However, most studies suggest that before purging of marrow T cells was initiated, up to 30% of recipients of allogeneic BMT developed clinically apparent intestinal GVH disease[10,33,34], and it is widely accepted that clinical criteria greatly underestimate the true occurrence of the condition.

Intestinal pathology appears to be an invariant feature of GVH disease in experimental animals, even in models which have few other signs of tissue damage or immunological dysfunction. Thus, the intestine may be particularly susceptible to the effector mechanisms of GVH disease.

Clinical consequences of intestinal GVH disease

The main clinical features of severe intestinal GVH disease are diarrhoea, malabsorption and protein-losing enteropathy. These have profound metabolic consequences for affected individuals. Diarrhoea is the commonest sign and clinical GVH disease often leads to profuse, watery, sometimes bloody diarrhoea[7]. A variety of mechanisms could be responsible for this feature (Table 7.2). The most obvious is destruction of mature enterocytes, with resultant defects in digestion and absorption of sugars[37,38] leading to osmotic water loss. Secondly, small intestinal damage in acute GVH disease is associated with the appearance of immature or abnormal enterocytes on the villus (see below). Both these abnormalities will interfere with the transport of ions and water across the enterocyte and, if severe, are likely to produce a cholerogenic type of diarrhoea. In a similar way, colonic damage may alter

Table 7.2 Possible mechanisms for diarrhoea in intestinal GVH reaction

---

Small intestine

Disaccharidase deficiency in epithelium due to enterocyte damage → luminal sugars + osmotic water loss

Increased proportion of immature enterocytes → enzyme deficiency + abnormal water transport

Protein + water exudation through hyperpermeable epithelium

Large intestine

Damage to colonic enterocytes → water reabsorption

---

water reabsorption in the large intestine. Finally, diarrhoea and fluid loss may be secondary to protein-losing enteropathy (see below).

Epithelial transport functions are severely disrupted by GVH disease, with evidence of increased leakage of serum proteins into the gut and resulting hypoproteinaemia[36,39,40]. In addition, animal studies show that there is enhanced uptake of luminal material through the damaged mucosa, including sugars, proteins and bacterial endotoxin[41,42]. In addition to their obvious metabolic effects, these transport abnormalities may have pathological implications for the patient. The increased uptake of food proteins may predispose the individual to a harmful immunological hypersensitivity response[43,44], while the higher levels of circulating endotoxin have been associated with release of inflammatory mediators such as tumour necrosis factor-α (TNF-α) and other acute-phase proteins[45].

Malabsorption of essential nutrients occurs due to deficiencies in brush-border enzymes (see below) and to the loss of absorptive surface area secondary to villus atrophy. Patients with stomach lesions due to GVH disease are at risk of further metabolic complications due to persistent vomiting and fluid loss.

Distribution of intestinal GVH disease

Acute GVH disease can affect the entire gastrointestinal tract, but the mouth and small and large intestines show the most frequent and most severe damage (Fig. 7.1). GVH disease in the squamous epithelium of the oral cavity is analogous to that occurring in the skin, and buccal biopsy provides a useful means of diagnosing and assessing GVH disease in humans. Of the gastrointestinal tract proper, the oesophagus is rarely affected by acute GVH disease, while gastric GVH disease is an uncommon, if clinically important, feature[7,32]. Because of the lack of appropriate clinical material it is difficult to assess the relative severity and incidence of GVH disease in different regions of the human large and small bowel. It has been reported that the colon and ileum are most seriously affected[9], and certainly rectal biopsy has become widely used as a diagnostic procedure[7,32,46]. However, a recent study suggests that although rectal damage occurs in over 50% of patients with intestinal GVH disease, virtually all these patients also had small intestinal pathology, and the remaining patients had damage which was confined to the small bowel[32]. The distribution of intestinal GVH disease in experimental animals is also controversial, although the small intestine is usually affected to some extent. An early report that the ileum was most severely affected in murine GVH disease[47] was not confirmed by later workers[36]. Recent studies in mice have suggested that the colon is particularly susceptible to GVH disease, with the ileum showing the next highest incidence and the stomach exhibiting little or no pathology[48]. These discrepancies may reflect the techniques used to identify the intestinal damage, and it is important to note that, in our experience, accurate morphometry is often required to reveal small intestinal injury.

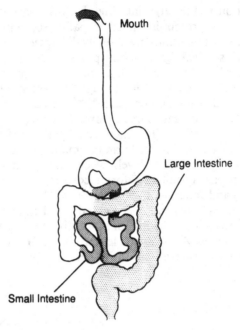

Figure 7.1 Distribution of intestinal damage in acute GVH disease. The small and large intestine are worst affected

NATURE OF THE INTESTINAL PATHOLOGY

The gross pathology of clinical GVH disease has been reviewed extensively elsewhere[7–10,32,33] and in this review we will concentrate on individual aspects of cellular pathology and on pathogenic processes.

Evolution of epithelial pathology

Severe intestinal inflammation, with macroscopic ulceration of the ileum and colon, associated with focal degeneration of the crypts were noted in early work on murine GVH disease[2,49]. Later, more detailed studies found small intestinal dilatation and bloody exudates, together with villus atrophy, crypt necrosis and increased extrusion of necrotic cells from the villus tip[36,47,50,51]. Small intestinal GVH disease in humans produces similar features, with mucosal thickening preceding ulceration, crypt abcesses and mucosal denudation (Fig. 7.2)[7–9,32]. Colonic GVH disease is associated with an analogous pattern of pathology[48,52].

Dividing crypt cells appear to be the principal targets of intestinal GVH disease. Although the most characteristic features of established disease are focal necrosis and degeneration of individual crypts, the earliest experimental studies also found crypt lengthening and increased mitotic activity[36,47,50,53]. More detailed work in animals shows clearly that stimulation of crypt cell

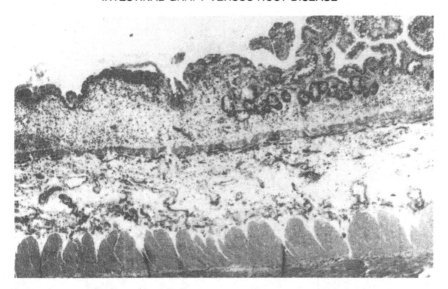

Figure 7.2 Appearance of established small intestinal damage in a patient with severe acute GVH disease after allogeneic BMT. There is a spectrum of damage ranging from mild villus atrophy, to complete necrosis in areas denuded of surface epithelium and crypts (H and E, ×37)

proliferation is the first detectable mucosal lesion[53-57]. This occurs within the first few days of GVH disease and precedes the onset of villus atrophy by several days (Fig. 7.3). In other models, crypt hyperplasia may be the only feature of intestinal GVH disease[54,56,58,59].

The increased mitotic activity of crypt cells is accompanied by other effects on the differentiation of enterocytes (Table 7.3), including an increased rate of exit of cells from the crypts and more rapid migration up the villus[38,50]. This reflects greater upward pressure from the enlarged crypt cell population and an absolute increase in the number of villus enterocytes (unpublished observations). As a result, the villus has a decreased proportion of cells with mature enzyme function, and jejunal lactase and aminopeptidase activities do not develop until much higher up the villus than normal[38]. These defects are balanced partly by the fact that the rate of differentiation of new enterocytes is also enhanced[38] and the activity of some brush-border enzymes may actually be increased[37]. This effect on differentiation is further evidenced by enhanced expression of Class II MHC molecules on villus enterocytes and the aberrant appearance of these molecules on crypt cells[60,61]. In humans this may be the only indication of intestinal GVH disease, and it affects the entire gastrointestinal tract[46,61,62]. Most Class II MHC expression is restricted to the basolateral surface of enterocytes, with HLA-DR expression being more prominent than HLA-DP, and there is virtually no HLA-DQ expression[62].

In severe intestinal GVH disease these early alterations in epithelial cell proliferation and differentiation are followed by a more destructive phase of pathology, typified by the appearance of villus atrophy (Fig. 7.4). Once again, crypt cells appear to bear the brunt of the immunological attack, and mature

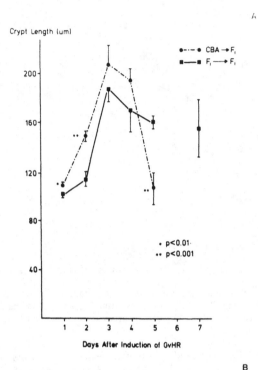

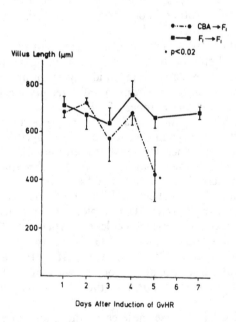

Figure 7.3 Development of crypt hypertrophy (**A**) and villus atrophy (**B**) during a destructive GVH reaction in irradiated mice. A large increase in crypt length, which is accompanied by markedly increased mitotic activity, occurs very quickly and before villus damage is seen

112

Table 7.3 Effects of GVH reaction on behaviour of intestinal crypt cells

Increased proliferation rate
Enhanced migration on to villus
More rapid differentiation of enzymes
Induction of expression of Class II MHC molecules
Ultimately, suppression of proliferation + apoptosis→necrosis

villus enterocytes are relatively spared, even in the presence of severe villus atrophy (unpublished observations). As the disease progresses, increasing numbers of apoptotic bodies can be seen in the crypts (Fig. 7.5)[27,28], while the terminal phase is characterized by the crypt abcesses and necrosis which are typically reported in human studies[47,50,51,27]. At this time necrosis of villus enterocytes can also be observed, and these end-stage events may partly reflect the superimposed effects of ischaemia and/or infection.

It should be noted that, although villus atrophy is the outstanding feature of severe GVH disease, it occurs in the absence of damage to the villus enterocytes themselves. In animals the appearance of villus atrophy requires a particularly intense period of crypt hyperplasia, which reaches its peak shortly before villus atrophy can be demonstrated (Fig. 7.3). One possible explanation for this could be that intense crypt hyperplasia creates a hyperdynamic, unstable mucosa, which cannot maintain the column of mature enterocytes necessary for intact villus architecture. An alternative possibility is suggested by animal experiments, which show that the appearance of villus atrophy is frequently accompanied by a sudden cessation in crypt cell mitotic activity (Fig. 7.3). Thus, villus atrophy may reflect immunological injury to crypt cells which prevents maintenance of epithelial renewal and integrity.

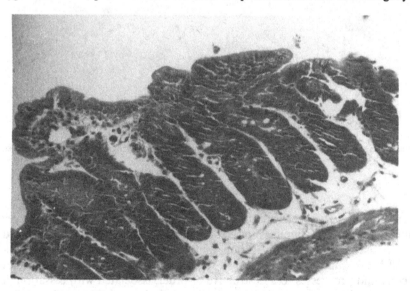

Figure 7.4 Destructive enteropathy in murine GVH reaction. Many crypts remain long and hyperplastic, but there is also necrosis of individual enterocytes and severe villus atrophy. The mucosa is devoid of lymphoid cells (HPE ×200)

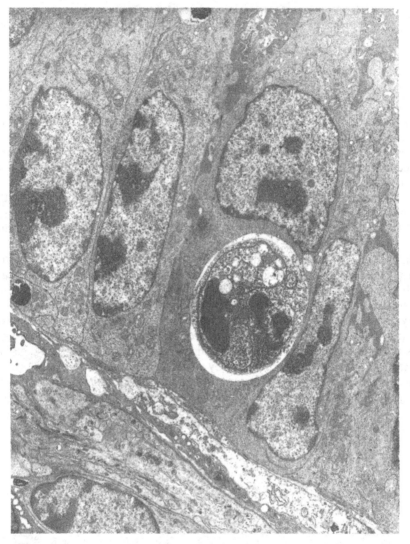

Figure 7.5 Apoptic body in a jejunal crypt during the terminal stages of acute GVH disease in mice ($\times 3960$)

In summary, crypt cells are the principal targets of intestinal GVH disease. Initially, the immune stimulus produces a proliferative enteropathy characterized by increased crypt cell proliferation, migration and differentiation, but with no effects on mature enterocytes. In severe cases this early phase intensifies rapidly and progresses to a destructive disorder associated with cessation of crypt cell mitotic activity and crypt necrosis. Only at this stage does villus atrophy appear, and this is paralleled by apoptosis of crypt stem cells rather than destruction of villus enterocytes themselves.

Effects of intestinal GVH disease on non-absorptive elements of the mucosa

There are few studies of the effects of GVH disease on the non-absorptive cells of the epithelium, but goblet cell hyperplasia is often seen, presumably reflecting the local inflammatory response. Destruction of enteroendocrine cells has also been noted in both experimental and clinical GVH disease (Table 7.4)[7]. Acute GVH disease also damages many components of the extracellular matrix and underlying tissues which are involved in maintaining the integrity of the intestine, including the epithelial basement membrane, which disintegrates as villus atrophy develops (unpublished observations). Swelling of the intestinal vascular endothelium has also been noted in irradiated mice with severe GVH reaction[27], and haemorrhagic exudates are present during the terminal stages of intestinal GVH disease[47,63]. We have recently found that mice dying of GVH disease have evidence of segmental ischaemia (unpublished observations), and it seems likely that destruction or occlusion of the local blood supply contributes to the failure of intestinal function.

Effects of GVH disease on intestinal lymphoid cells and immune function

Lamina propria

The effects of GVH disease on the systemic immune system are reflected in alterations in intestinal lymphoid cell populations. As with the epithelial pathology, the effects on mucosal lymphoid cells occur in two phases. Initial studies in experimental animals emphasized that severe GVH disease leads to depletion of mucosal lymphoid cells (Fig. 7.4)[2,47,64,65] and a similar phenomenon is found in humans with acute GVH disease[8,9]. This depletion of the local immune system can eventually produce marked reductions in the numbers of plasma cells in the lamina propria[66]. In contrast, the early phase of GVH disease is associated with infiltration of the mucosa by lymphoblasts[36,63]. These infiltrating cells are predominantly T lymphocytes of donor origin which accumulate close to the crypts, and their presence correlates with the severity of the mucosal damage[67,68]. Both CD4+ and CD8+ T cells are present in the infiltrate, but there is some evidence that

Table 7.4 Depletion of enteroendocrine cells during acute GVH disease in mice

	Enteroendocrine cells		Crypt hyperplasia	Villus atrophy
	Villus	Crypt		
Controls	+ +	+ + +	−	−
Day 14 GVH disease	±	+	+ + +	+ +
Day 21 GVH disease	+	+/+ +	+ +	+ + +

The number of enteroendocrine cells (determined by immunoperoxidase detection of chromogranin) both in the villus and crypt epithelium decreases as villus atrophy occurs

clinical intestinal GVH disease correlates with an excess of CD4+ T cells in the lamina propria[62].

Epithelium

One component of the lymphocytic infiltration of the gut in GVH disease is an increased density of intraepithelial lymphocytes (IEL). An increased IEL count is one of the earliest detectable signs of intestinal GVH disease in experimental animals (Fig. 7.6A), and it rises in parallel with other proliferative features of GVH reaction, such as crypt hyperplasia[54,55]. As villus atrophy develops there is a parallel loss of IEL (Fig. 7.6B)[54,55,58]. Studies in mice indicate that the infiltrating IEL include donor-derived T cells, as well as radioresistant lymphocytes of host origin. Most of these IEL retain the unusual CD8+ phenotype which characterizes this population under normal circumstances[68]. In clinical GVH disease, the excess of CD8+ IEL remains in the rectum and small bowel[62,69], although one recent report has suggested there may be a relative increase in the proportion of CD4+ IEL in crypt epithelium[62]. Interestingly, animal studies indicate that GVH disease produces an increase in the subset of IEL which express the $\alpha\beta$ form of the T cell receptor and express a heterodimeric CD8 molecule (Table 7.5)[70]. These latter cells appear to represent the progeny of donor-derived CD8+ T lymphoblasts which infiltrate the lamina propria after activation in the Peyer's patches and migration via the thoracic duct[67,68,71]. As IEL may produce a range of cytokines in GVH disease (see below), the presence of activated donor T cells in this site may have important consequences for the mucosal pathology.

Other lymphoid cells

The altered populations of mucosal lymphocytes are accompanied by changes in other lymphoid cells. Depletion of Ia$^+$ macrophages and dendritic cells has been reported in murine GVH disease[68] and is a possible factor in producing dysfunction of the intestinal immune system (see below).

Table 7.5 Effects of GVH disease on subsets of intraepithelial lymphocytes in mice

Marker	Percentage IEL positive	
	Control	GVH disease
CD4+	13	10
CD3+	75	80
CD3+ $\alpha\beta$TcR+	32	43
CD8α+	60	70
CD8α+ $\alpha\beta$TcR+	18	27
CD8α+ CD8β+	18	28

There is an increased proportion of T cells expressing the $\alpha\beta$ T cell receptor, together with increased numbers of CD8+ cells which express the $\alpha-\beta$ heterodimeric form of the CD8 molecule

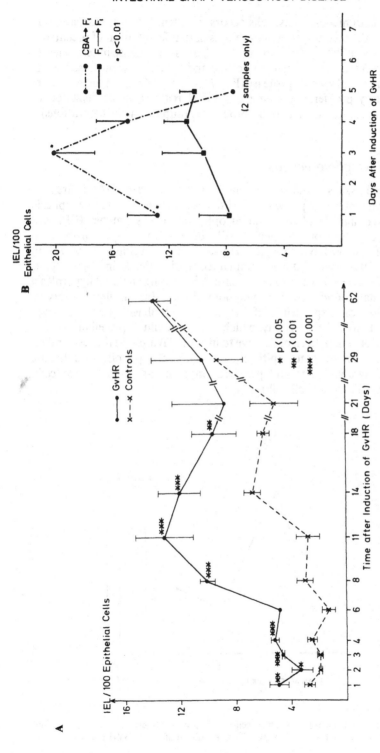

Figure 7.6 Behaviour of intraepithelial lymphocyte populations in different forms of intestinal GVH reaction. IEL counts increase rapidly in both proliferative (**A**) and destructive (**B**) enteropathy. However, the IEL counts remain increased for some time in the proliferative GVH reaction in unirradiated (CBA × BALB/c)F₁ mice, while IEL disappear rapidly as GVH reaction progresses in irradiated F₁ hosts given CBA donor cells (**B**)

Hyperplasia of mucosal mast cells occurs in rodent GVH disease, and this may reflect both recruitment of mature cells and differentiation of precursors within the mucosa[54,67,68,72,73]. In parallel, there is an increase in serum levels of interleukin-3 (IL-3)[74], while the intestine and serum show increased levels of mucosal mast cell specific protease (Fig. 7.7)[72,73,75]. These changes parallel the other, early proliferative changes of GVH reaction while depletion of MMC may occur as villus atrophy progresses (unpublished observations).

Organized lymphoid tissues

The organized tissues of the gut-associated lymphoid tissue (GALT) are also involved in the intestinal phase of GVH disease and show a similar biphasic pattern of damage. Depletion and atrophy of Peyer's patches (PP) is a characteristic feature of late, acute GVH disease and may contribute to depletion of mucosal lymphocytes. However, the development of PP in isografts of fetal small intestine implanted under the kidney capsule is accelerated in mice with early GVH disease[58], indicating an initial hyperplasia similar to that found in other lymphoid tissues. In parallel, the crypts supplying the dome epithelium of PP share the biphasic pattern of crypt hyperplasia, followed by atrophy, which occurs in villus epithelium[76].

In conclusion, the pattern of damage to intestinal lymphoid tissues parallels that found in the associated epithelium with an early period of infiltration by donor T lymphoblasts and proliferation of non-specific effector cells, followed by depletion of all cell types.

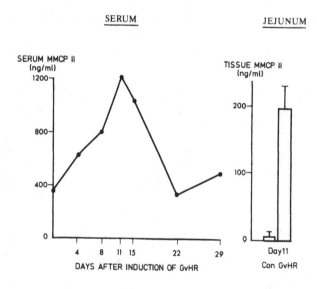

Figure 7.7 Increased mouse mucosal mast cell-specific protease II levels in the serum and small intestinal mucosa of adult (CBA × BALB/c)F$_1$ mice with proliferative GVH reaction

Immunological consequences of intestinal GVH disease

The depletion of local lymphoid cells in established GVH disease is associated with mucosal immunodeficiency, which is manifested by reduced levels of both secretory and serum IgA levels[77]. These abnormalities will add to the generalized immune deficiency seen in GVH disease, and seem likely to be important factors in the development of secondary intestinal infection. However, as with other features of mucosal pathology, the late immune defects are preceded by an early stage of immune enhancement. Thus, total secretory IgA responses may be increased early in murine GVH disease (Fig. 7.5; Watret and Ferguson, unpublished observations), while immunity to dietary antigens may be altered. Humans with acute GVH disease have raised serum antibodies against food proteins[43], while GVH disease in animals produces enhanced local and systemic immunity to dietary proteins[44]. These phenomena could reflect increased absorption of antigen through damaged mucosa or increased antigen presentation within the systemic immune system[44] or by the Ia-expressing enterocytes themselves. Irrespective of the mechanism involved, there is experimental evidence that the unusually powerful immune responses to food antigens in GVH disease may produce a local hypersensitivity reaction which adds to the mucosal damage[78].

MECHANISMS OF INTESTINAL GVH DISEASE

Cellular and genetic basis of intestinal GVH disease

All the consequences of GVH disease are absolutely dependent on recognition of host alloantigens by donor T lymphocytes. The exact nature of the T cells responsible for inducing the systemic disease remains controversial, but both CD8+ and CD4+ T cells can induce GVH disease, depending on the circumstances[79].

Initial studies of small intestinal GVH disease in mice indicated that CD8− T cells played the major role[80], but subsequent work has suggested that both CD4+ and CD8+ T cells may be required (Fig. 7.8)[60,81]. Nevertheless, CD4+ T cells seem to be much more effective, and sometimes are alone sufficient to induce a full intestinal lesion. In contrast, CD8+ T cells are rarely capable of causing gut pathology on their own. A similar pattern is found in experimental studies of colonic GVH disease, where CD4+ T cells are much more effective inducers of pathology than CD8+ T cells[48]. The two T cell subsets may play different roles in the pathogenesis of intestinal GVH disease. Thus, CD4+ T cells are sufficient and necessary to induce several small intestinal alterations, such as the increases in IEL count and MMC hyperplasia, and alone can produce significant crypt hyperplasia, villus atrophy and enhanced epithelial expression of Class II MHC[68,80]. However, CD8+ T cells are usually required for these last changes to develop fully.

In experimental animals, incompatibility at Class II MHC loci is normally sufficient and necessary for induction of all aspects of intestinal pathology[40,68,80,81], supporting the principal role of CD4+ T cells. Although Class I MHC alloantigens can induce intestinal GVH disease under some

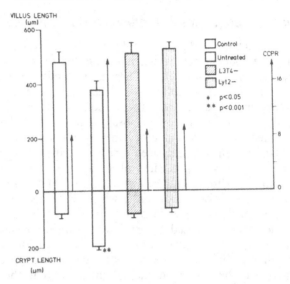

Figure 7.8 Requirement for both CD8 + and CD4 + donor T cells in the induction of intestinal GVH reaction in (CBA × BALB/c)F$_1$ mice. Villus and crypt lengths and CCPR in jejunum of mice given unseparated, CD4- or CD8-depleted donor cells

circumstances, this usually requires a large number of donor T cells[40], or a powerful Class I MHC alloantigen which is capable of activating the rare CD8 + T cells with helper cell function[81]. Even under these conditions, Class I MHC alloantigens are much less efficient than Class II antigens at

stimulating intestinal GVH disease. The ability of non-MHC alloantigens to induce intestinal GVH disease has not been studied in detail. Nevertheless, diarrhoea and crypt hyperplasia have been reported in some animal models of MHC-compatible GVH disease[63], while the relatively high incidence of intestinal GVH disease after HLA-matched BMT in humans shows that minor histocompatibility differences must be capable of inducing this form of pathology.

Together, these findings indicate that Class II MHC-restricted donor CD4 + T cells are the predominant T cell required for the induction of intestinal GVH disease. However, Class I MHC-restricted CD8 + T cells may also be important in amplifying the disease, and may also play a critical role in particular aspects of the pathology.

Nature of the local immune response in intestinal GVH disease

The fact that Class II MHC-restricted T cells are particularly important for the induction of intestinal GVH disease does not predict the exact nature of the pathogenic immune response which causes local tissue damage. In addition, there is no absolute correlation between the phenotype and function of individual T cell subsets. This section will discuss the effector mechanisms which may act locally in the intestine during GVH disease.

Organ destruction in many forms of immunopathology is often ascribed to a direct attack on tissue cells by specific cytotoxic T lymphocytes (CTL). Nevertheless, although T cells with CTL activity have been isolated from the mucosa of mice with acute GVH disease[60], several pieces of evidence argue against a role for specific CTL in intestinal GVH disease. First, as discussed above, epithelial cell destruction is not a feature of intestinal GVH disease, even when severe mucosal damage is present. Secondly, intestinal GVH disease in mice can occur in the absence of anti-host CTL in the gut or other lymphoid tissues[82]. Even when CTL can be demonstrated, their presence often does not correlate with the intestinal pathology[55,56,81], while several immunomodulatory agents can prevent intestinal GVH disease without inhibiting the generation of CTL[83,84]. Colonic GVH disease is also not affected by treating the donor lymphocytes with a lysosomotropic ester which prevents the generation of anti-host CTL *in vivo*[48].

The most persuasive evidence against a role for CTL is that the intestinal epithelium is damaged in a non-antigen-specific manner. Thus, intestinal GVH disease occurs in parental strain mice made chimeric for F_1 bone marrow cells, despite the fact that the intestinal epithelium of the host animals remains syngeneic to the parental donor T cells. In contrast, F_1 mice made chimeric for parental BM have no evidence of intestinal GVH disease after injection of parental T cells, indicating that the intestinal epithelium cannot stimulate GVH disease-inducing T cells[85]. The stimulus for this intestinal GVH disease is allogeneic Class II MHC molecules expressed on BM-derived

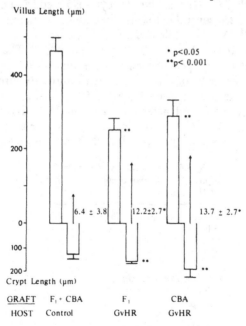

Villus Length (μm)

* p<0.05
**p< 0.001

6.4 ± 3.8   12.2±2.7*   13.7 ± 2.7*

Crypt Length (μm)

| GRAFT | F_1 + CBA | F_1 | CBA |
| HOST | Control | GvHR | GvHR |

Figure 7.9 Intestinal GVH reaction occurs as a 'bystander phenomenon'. Mucosal architecture in grafts of fetal (CBA × BALB/c)F_1 or CBA small intestine implanted in irradiated (CBA × BALB/c)F_1 mice given CBA donor cells. Villus atrophy, as well as increases in CCPR and crypt length, occur, irrespective of whether the gut grafts are syngeneic to the donor

cells ('passenger leukocytes'). Although an earlier study did not find intestinal GVH disease in $F_1 \rightarrow$parent BM chimeras[86], the 'bystander effect' of GVH disease on the gut has been confirmed by an alternative type of experiment (Fig. 7.9). In these studies, pieces of fetal small intestine of parental-type are implanted under the kidney capsule of adult F_1 hybrid mice. The grafts develop relatively normally over the space of a few weeks and are infiltrated by recirculating BM-derived cells of host origin. When a GVH disease is induced in the F_1 host animals by injection of parental lymphocytes, the donor-type grafts develop a full range of intestinal pathology, including crypt hyperplasia, increases in IEL count, crypt cell apoptosis and villus atrophy[51,54,57,58,65]. Once again, these experiments show that the gut itself does not need to present an allogeneic stimulus to the alloreactive donor cells for intestinal GVH disease to occur. It seems more likely that the pathological lesions are due to non-specific soluble mediators released during a DTH response initially directed at BM-derived cells.

Role of soluble mediators

If intestinal GVH disease can occur in the absence of specific CTL, the mechanisms responsible for the pathology must be non-specific. There is now considerable evidence that cytokines released during a local DTH response are involved (Table 7.6). Mucosal lymphocytes isolated from mice with acute GVH disease produce several cytokines, including interleukin-2 (IL-2), IL-3 and interferon-γ (IFN-γ)[67], while acute GVH disease in mice and humans is associated with increased levels of TNF-α in serum[45,87]. That at least some of these cytokines have a primary role in intestinal GVH disease is shown by the fact that treatment of mice *in vivo* with antibody directed at IFN-γ prevents all the intestinal consequences of GVH disease, including villus atrophy, crypt hyperplasia and increased IEL counts[88]. Anti-TNF-α antibodies also ameliorate intestinal GVH disease, but in this case only villus atrophy and crypt cell apoptosis are prevented, and there is no effect on the early

Table 7.6 Cytokines which have been implicated in the pathogenesis of intestinal GVH disease

---

Depletion inhibits pathology
IFN-γ
TNFα
IL-1

Cytokine exacerbates pathology
IFN-α/β
TGF-β

Cytokine enteropathic
IFN-α/β
TNF-α
IFN-γ

---

crypt hyperplasia and increased IEL counts[27] (also unpublished results). Thus, production of IFN-γ and TNF-α is an essential prerequisite for intestinal GVH disease, but these mediators may act at different stages of the pathology, IFN-γ being important for initiating the early proliferative phase and TNF-α being responsible for the later, destructive lesions. This hypothesis is supported by the findings that administration of TNF-α to normal mice produces both crypt hyperplasia and villus atrophy, while IFN-γ causes crypt hyperplasia alone[89].

Other cytokines may also be important for the enteropathy of GVH disease. Depletion of IL-1α *in vivo* partially inhibits intestinal GVH disease in mice (Table 7.7), while treatment of mice with the IFN-α/β inducer, poly-inosinic:polycytydylic acid (poly-I:C) exacerbates the systemic and intestinal consequences of acute GVH disease[83]. Normal animals given poly-I:C or IFN-α/β also develop jejunal villus atrophy and crypt hyperplasia (Fig. 7.10)[83], suggesting that IFN-α/β may be an effector molecule in the enteropathy of GVH disease. These studies suggest that a cascade of different cytokines may be important in intestinal GVH disease.

Cytokines could induce intestinal damage either by direct effects on enterocytes or indirectly via effects on other components of the mucosa. There is now ample evidence that mediators such as IFN-γ, TNF-α, IL-1, IL-6 and IFN-α/β are involved in autoimmunity and other inflammatory diseases by virtue of direct effects on tissue cells[90]. Recently it has been shown that these actions may extend to the intestine. IFN-γ is cytostatic to colonic carcinoma cells *in vitro*[91], enhances their expression of secretory component and of Class I and II MHC molecules[92] and alters transport of ions across the cell membrane[93]. IFN-γ is also cytostatic to small bowel crypt cells *in vitro*, and enhances their expression of MHC molecules (Fig. 7.11). TNF-α enhances many of these effects of IFN-γ (Fig. 7.12)[91,92] and is itself cytotoxic to crypt cells *in vitro*[89]. These findings show that enterocytes probably have receptors for cytokines, and indicate that the role of cytokines in GVH disease could partly reflect direct effects on epithelial cells.

An additional way in which cytokines could damage the gut directly is by interfering with the function of mesenchymal cells such as endothelial cells and fibroblasts. Both these cell types are known to be targets for cytokines such as TNF-α[28] and mesenchymal function is essential for maintenance of

Table 7.7 Effects of anti-interleukin-1 on intestinal GVH reaction

Group	Villus length (μm)	Crypt length (μm)	CCPR
NRS control	630.9 ± 34.8	81.9 ± 3.9	5.4 ± 1.3
NRS GVH reaction	636.8 ± 33.9	$110.6 \pm 4.7**$	$13.6 \pm 0.6*$
Anti-IL1α control	695.3 ± 33.3	85.6 ± 5.7	6.0 ± 1.3
Anti-IL1α GVH reaction	718.2 ± 14.5	$98.9 \pm 5*$	6.4 ± 1.5

$*p < 0.02$; $**p < 0.001$ vs controls.
Treatment of $(CBA \times BALB/c)F_1$ mice with rabbit anti-IL1α antibody reduces the crypt hypertrophy and abolishes the increase in crypt cell production rate which occur in GVH-reactive mice treated with normal rabbit serum (NRS) as a control

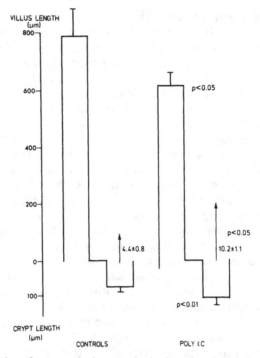

Figure 7.10 Induction of enteropathy in normal mice by enhancing production of IFN-α/β. Mice given the IFN-inducer polyinosinic:polycytydylic acid (poly-I:C) develop significant villus atrophy and crypt hyperplasia compared with controls

normal mucosal architecture[94]. Pericryptal fibroblasts seem particularly likely to be important intermediate targets of cytokine effects, and their involvement could include production of further inflammatory mediators[90].

Non-specific effector cells in intestinal GVH disease

One of the most important effects of cytokines in the immune response is to recruit and activate non-specific inflammatory cells, and this provides an additional way in which cytokines could produce gut damage in GVH disease. The potential importance of this pathway is suggested by the large number of macrophages, eosinophils and other inflammatory cells normally present in the intestinal mucosa. Recent work indicates that depletion of macrophages or interference with their production of nitric oxide inhibits intestinal GVH disease in mice (our unpublished observations). As discussed above, hyperplasia of mucosal mast cells is a feature of many experimental models of GVH disease. This probably reflects recruitment by IL-3 and not only involves increased numbers of MMC, but is also accompanied by activation of these cells, as evidenced by the increased amounts of MMC-specific protease in the serum and intestinal mucosa of rodents with GVH disease (Fig. 7.8)[70,71,73]. In addition, the release of protease parallels the development of

INTESTINAL GRAFT-VERSUS-HOST DISEASE

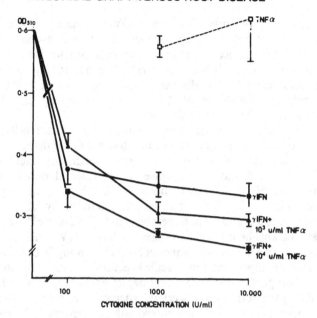

A

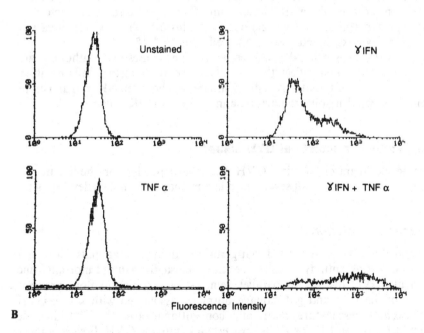

B

Figure 7.11 Direct effects of IFN-γ and TNF-α on crypt cells *in vitro*. IFN-γ is cytostatic to the RIE cell line (**A**) and induces expression of Class II MHC antigens (**B**). TNF-α alone has no effect on growth, but synergizes with the cytostatic effect of IFN-γ. It also augments the effects of IFN-γ on Class II MHC expression

crypt hyperplasia and other features of GVH disease[73]. However, it seems that MMC do not act as pathogenic effector cells in intestinal GVH disease, as mast cell-deficient mice suffer more severe enteropathy during GVH disease than mice with normal MMC numbers[73]. Furthermore, irradiated animals develop more intense GVH disease, despite their lack of MMC[70,71]. Thus, the hyperplasia of MMC in intestinal GVH disease may actually reflect an attempt to repair the mucosal damage.

One group of cytokine-dependent non-specific effector cells which does seem to be of pathogenic importance in intestinal GVH disease are NK cells. These lymphocytes are activated by several mediators, including TNF-α, IFN-γ and IFN-α/β, and GVH disease in experimental animals is associated with enhanced NK cell activity both by peripheral lymphocytes and by intestinal IEL[81,95,96]. The enhanced NK activity by IEL parallels the increased IEL count and crypt hyperplasia in GVH disease[81], and is preceded by a systemic anti-host DTH response[97]. Clinical GVH disease may also be associated with an increased number of NK cells among IEL[67]. That activated NK cells are an important non-specific effector mechanism in intestinal GVH reaction is supported by the fact that depletion of NK cells with anti-asialo G_{M1} (AsG_{M1}) antibody prevents crypt hyperplasia in murine GVH disease[98]. This antibody also prevents the enteropathy caused by IFN-α/β in normal animals, suggesting that the effects of these cytokines depends on their ability to activate NK cells[88]. It should be noted that NK cells may be of most importance during the early phase of intestinal GVH disease characterized by crypt hyperplasia. Indeed, the onset of villus atrophy in GVH disease is associated with complete loss of NK cell activity[54-56].

The ways in which NK cells could influence intestinal pathology are unknown, but could reflect their ability to produce further inflammatory cytokines[99,100]. Alternatively, a direct interaction between NK cells and crypt stem cells could involve the cytolytic machinery of NK cells.

Host factors in intestinal GVH disease

The development of intestinal GVH disease is dependent on the function of donor T lymphocytes, but several host factors may influence its development.

Intestinal microflora

Several studies have suggested that germ-free animals or animals with a gut flora consisting entirely of anaerobes have markedly reduced mortality due to acute GVH disease. In parallel, removal of aerobic gut flora prevents much of the liver and gut damage normally associated with severe GVH disease, and these features return after conventionalization[101,102]. Deliberate administration of LPS or *E. coli* exacerbates systemic GVH disease in mice, while passive immunization with antibody to *E. coli* has a mild, beneficial effect[103,104]. Together, these findings suggest that Gram-negative aerobes in the gut flora are critical for the pathogenesis of GVH disease. Nevertheless, it should be noted that, in animals, the beneficial effect of the germ-free state is generally small, and applies only to the early stages of acute GVH disease. Eventually, these animals show mortality rates and pathology which are similar to, if not higher than, those in conventional hosts[101,102,105]. Furthermore, recent studies have not confirmed initial reports that elimination of gut flora has a beneficial effect on BMT patients[7].

Local infection also does not play a primary role in the development of intestinal pathology in GVH disease, as intestinal GVH disease develops in sterile grafts of small intestine implanted under the kidney capsule of mice with GVH disease (Fig. 7.9)[57,58]. Nevertheless, intestinal bacteria could have two indirect effects. First, it seems probable that direct infection of gut damaged by the GVH disease will exacerbate the enteropathy. This is supported by the local abscesses which form round invading organisms late in GVH disease[102]. Secondly, it has been shown that crypt degeneration occurs only in sterile explants of gut if these are placed in hosts with a conventional microflora[51], suggesting that bacterial products may influence the level of systemic anti-host immune responsiveness. Enterobacteria produce several agents with adjuvant activity, and it has long been known that animals with GVH reaction have increased levels of circulating endotoxin[42]. Thus, initial damage to the gut caused by GVH disease may allow increased absorption of bacterial products which then exacerbate the tissue lesions by virtue of their ability to enhance ongoing immune responses. A related, but not exclusive, possibility is that the increased levels of bacterial endotoxin cause release of TNF-α or other enteropathic cytokines[45,105,106].

Virus infections are extremely common in patients with clinical GVH disease and Coxsackie virus A1 has been shown to cause intestinal damage in these patients[107]. Mucosal infections with herpes simplex virus and CMV are not uncommonly superimposed on intestinal GVH disease in humans[34] and CMV clearly enhances the lung disease of GVH disease[22]. Thus, both bacteria and viruses may exacerbate the mucosal pathology of GVH disease. Finally, intestinal parasites may also colonize the damaged mucosa[7,34] and it has been shown in mice that GVH disease and giardiasis may produce synergistic damage in the gut (Gillon, J. and Ferguson, A., unpublished).

Other host factors in intestinal GVH disease

Other endogenous host factors may also influence the evolution of intestinal GVH disease. Experimental studies have shown that intestinal pathology is much more severe when the hosts used are irradiated, athymic or very immature[48,54,55,108]. One explanation for these findings may be that certain host lymphoid cells, such as T lymphocytes or NK cells can resist the proliferation of alloreactive donor T cells and hence protect the gut[109]. Alternatively, the intestine of compromised hosts may be unusually susceptible to the effects of GVH disease. Irradiation has particularly profound effects on the function and renewal of the intestinal epithelium, while rapid alterations in mucosal architecture occur during the early neonatal period. These phenomena may therefore synergize with the enteropathic effects of GVH disease on the mucosa. Irrespective of the mechanisms involved, the exacerbated intestinal GVH disease in compromised hosts has important implications for the conditioning regimes used in human BMT.

SUMMARY AND CONCLUSIONS

This review has outlined the pathological effects of GVH disease on the intestine and has attempted to define some of the immunological mechanisms involved. Figure 7.12 summarizes what we consider to be the most likely pathogenesis of enteropathy in GVH disease. The scheme assumes that self-renewing crypt stem cells are the principal target of harmful immune response which depends on the production of inflammatory cytokines. The first stage of the disease involves infiltration of the mucosa by activated T lymphocytes and cytokine-mediated stimulation of crypt cell proliferation. During this proliferative phase no damage to mature enterocytes can be observed, and villus atrophy is absent. However, there may be enhanced expression of Class II MHC antigens and unusually immature enterocytes may be present on the villus surface, with concomitant alterations in digestion, absorption and fluid balance. This pattern of enteropathy seems to require IFN-γ-producing cells and may involve IFN-activated NK cells. In mild cases the intestinal GVH disease may resolve at this stage, but in severe GVH disease the cryupt hyperplasia progresses to villus atrophy. This still does not involve damage to enterocytes, but may either reflect an unstable, hyperdynamic state caused by intense crypt cell mitotic activity or is secondary to abnormalities in endothelial or fibroblast function. Finally, apoptosis occurs in crypt stem cells, terminating epithelial cell renewal and resulting ultimately in mucosal necrosis. These destructive events are associated with depletion of mucosal lymphoid cells and systemic manifestations of severe GVH disease such as anaemia. Destructive enteropathy may reflect the effects of additional cytokines, or synergistic interactions between a number of mediators. All these changes occur as a 'bystander phenomenon', in which the intestinal tissues do not stimulate the alloreactive response, but are the targets of non-specific effector mechanisms provoked by stimulation of donor T cells by bone-marrow-derived leukocytes.

The findings discussed here have several implications for clinical disease. First, they raise the possibility that immunotherapy targeted at cytokines might prove useful in treating the intestinal manifestations of GVH disease after BMT. Antibodies reactive with T cells, adhesion molecules and IL-2 (or its receptor) have all raised interest as possible therapeutic agents for immunopathological conditions, but all these strategies would carry the risk of non-specific immunosuppression. We would propose that depletion of pathogenic cytokines such as TNF-α may be a more specific approach to this problem.

Elucidating the immunopathogenesis of intestinal GVH disease may also help understand and treat other forms of tissue damage in GVH disease, including that found in the liver and skin. GVH disease in these organs has many similarities to intestinal GVH disease, with marked epithelial abnormalities and evidence for a pathogenic role for cytokines[26,28]. As intestinal GVH

PHASE 1 – PROLIFERATIVE

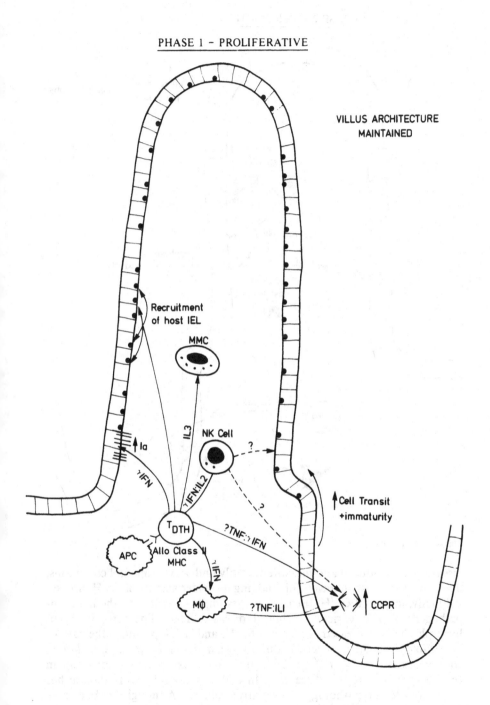

Figure 7.12 Mechanisms of enteropathy in GVH reaction. See text for details

PHASE 2 – DESTRUCTIVE

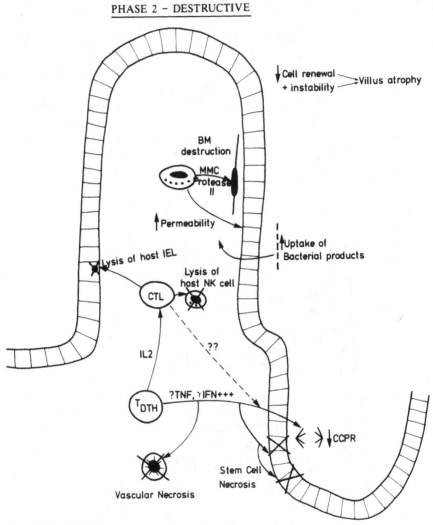

Figure 7.12 (*Contd*)

disease can be induced and measured readily under experimental conditions, it may provide a useful means for studying the wider aspects of GVH disease.

Finally, intestinal GVH disease provides important clues to the immuno-pathogenesis of a variety of clinical diseases. The villus atrophy, crypt hyperplasia and increased numbers of MMC and IEL reproduces the pattern of pathology found in several naturally occurring enteropathies, including coeliac disease, cows' milk protein intolerance, parasite infections and in certain areas of Crohn's disease[110]. In addition, colonic GVH disease has similarities to the pathology of ulcerative colitis[52]. Although GVH disease is obviously an artificial situation, it demonstrates that the intestine can be damaged during an immune response initially directed at an unrelated antigen, as clearly happens in the majority of the clinical diseases. The evidence from GVH disease that cytokines can cause enteropathy has been extended recently by the demonstration of increased local TNF-α production in inflammatory bowel disease[111]. Intestinal GVH disease should provide a useful means of investigating the pathogenesis of clinical enteropathy under experimental conditions.

References

1. Billingham, R. E., Brent, L. and Medawar, P. B. (1955). Acquired tolerance of skin homografts. *Ann. NY Acad. Sci.*, **59**, 409–98
2. Billingham, R. E. (1967). The biology of graft-versus-host reactions. *Harvey Lectures*, **62**, 21–79
3. Spitzer, T. R. (1990). Transfusion induced graft-vs-host disease. In Burakoff, S. J., Deeg, H. J., Ferrara, J. and Atkinson, K. (eds), *Graft-vs-Host Disease: Immunology, Pathophysiology and Treatment*. New York: Marcel Dekker, pp. 539–50
4. Pomposelli, F., Maki, T., Kiyoizumi, T., Gaver, L., Balogh, K. and Monaco, A. P. (1985). Induction of graft-versus-host disease by small intestinal allotransplantation in rats. *Transplantation*, **40**, 343–7
5. Schraut, W. H., Lee, K. K. W., Dawson, J. and Hurst, R. D. (1986). Graft-versus-host disease induced by small bowel allografts. *Transplantation*, **41**, 286–90
6. Deeg, H. J. and Cottler-Fax, M. (1990). Clinical spectrum and pathophysiology of acute graft-vs-host disease. In Burakoff, S. J., Deeg, H. J., Ferrara, J. and Atkinson, K. (eds), *Graft-vs-Host Disease: Immunology, Pathophysiology and Treatment*. New York: Marcel Dekker, pp. 311–35
7. Cox, G. J. and McDonald, G. B. (1990). Graft-versus-host disease of the intestine. *Springer Semin. Immunpathol.*, **12**, 283–99
8. Slavin, R. E. and Santos, G. W. (1973). The graft-versus-host reaction in man after bone marrow transplantation: pathology, pathogenesis, clinical features and implications. *Clin. Immunol. Immunopathol.*, **1**, 472–98
9. Slavin, R. E. and Woodruff, J. M. (1974). The pathology of bone-marrow transplantation. In Sommers, S. C. (ed.), *Pathology Annual*. New York: Appleton-Century-Crofts, pp. 291–344
10. Storb, R. and Thomas, E. D. (1983). Allogeneic bone marrow transplantation. *Immunol. Rev.*, **71**, 77
11. Herve, P., Cahn, J.-Y. and Beatty, P. G. (1990). Graft-vs-host disease after bone marrow transplantation from donors other than HLA-identical siblings. In Burakoff, S. J., Deeg, H. J., Ferrara, J. and Atkinson, K. (eds), *Graft-vs-Host Disease. Immunology, Pathology and Treatment*. New York: Marcel Dekker, pp. 425–54
12. Mowat, A. McI., MacKenzie, S., Baca, M. E., Felstein, M. V. and Parrott, D. M. V. (1987). Functional characteristics of intraepithelial lymphocytes from mouse small intestine. II. *In vivo* and *in vitro* responses of intraepithelial lymphocytes to mitogenic and allogeneic stimuli. *Immunology*, **58**, 627–34
13. Davies, M. D. J. and Parrott, D. M. V. (1981). Cytotoxic T cells in small intestinal epithelial, lamina propria and lung lymphocytes. *Immunology*, **44**, 367–71
14. Kernan, N. A. (1990). Graft failure following transplantation of T-cell-depleted marrow. In Burakoff, S. J., Deeg, H. J., Ferrara, J. and Atkinson, K. (eds), *Graft-versus-Host Disease: Immunology, Pathology and Treatment*. New York: Marcel Dekker, pp. 557–68
15. Dosch, H.-M. and Gelfand, E. W. (1981). Failure of T and B cell cooperation during graft-versus-host disease. *Transplant*, **31**, 48–50
16. Korsmeyer, S. J., Elfenbein, G. J., Godlman, C. K., Marshall, S. L., Santos, G. W. and Waldmann, T. A. (1982). B cell, helper T cells and suppressor T cell abnormalities contribute to disordered immunoglobulin synthesis in patients following bone marrow transplantation. *Transplant*, **33**, 184–90
17. Ferrara, J. L. M., Daley, J. P., Burakoff, S. J. and Miller, R. A. (1987). Functional T cell deficits after bone marrow transplantation across minor histocompatibility barriers: effects of graft-vs-host disease on precursor frequency of reactive cells. *J. Immunol.*, **138**, 3598–603
18. Moser, M., Sharrow, S. O. and Shearer, G. M. (1988). Role of L3T4$^+$ and Lyt2$^+$ donor

cells in graft-versus-host immune deficiency induced across a class I, class II, or whole H-2 difference. *J. Immunol.*, **140**, 2600–08

19. Levy, R. B., Jones, M. and Gray, C. (1990). Isolated peripheral T cells from GvHR recipients exhibit defective IL-2R expression IL-2 production and proliferation in response to activation stimuli. *J. Immunol.*, **145**, 3998–4005

20. Lapp, W. S., Ghayur, T., Mendes, M., Seddik, M. and Seemayer, T. A. (1985). The functional and histological basis for graft-versus-host induced immunosuppression. *Immunol. Rev.*, **88**, 107–33

21. Piguet, P. F., Grau, G. E., Collart, M. A., Vassalli, P. and Kapanci, Y. (1989). Pneumopathies of the graft-versus-host reaction: alveolitis associated with an increased level of TNF mRNA and chronic interstitial pneumonitis. *Lab. Invest.*, **61**, 37–45

22. Grundy, J. E., Shanley, J. D. and Shearer, G. M. (1985). Augmentation of graft-versus-host reaction by cytomegalovirus infections resulting in interstitial pneumonitis. *Transplantation*, **39**, 548–53

23. Beschorner, W. E., Saral, R., Hutchins, G. M., Tutschka, P. J. and Santos, G. W. (1978). Lymphocytic bronchitis associated with graft-vs-host disease in recipients of bone marrow transplants. *N. Engl. J. Med.*, **299**, 1030–36

24. Parfrey, N. A., Ste-Croix, H. and Prudhomme, G. J. (1989). Evidence that nonlymphoid tissue injury in acute graft-versus-host disease is limited to epithelial cells aberrantly expressing MHC antigens. *Transplantation*, **48**, 655–60

25. Vok-Platzer, B. and Singl, G. (1990). Cutaneous graft-vs-host disease. In Burakoff, S. J., Deeg, H. J., Ferrara, J. and Atkinson, K. (eds), *Graft-versus-Host Disease: Immunology, Pathology and Treatment*. New York: Marcel Dekker, pp. 245–54

26. Piguet, P. F., Janin-Mercier, A., Vassalli, P. and Saurat, J. H. (1987). Epidermal lesions of the GvHR: evaluation of the role of different MHC and non MHC loci and of the Lyt-2[+] and L3T4[+] T lymphocytes. *J. Immunol.*, **139**, 406–10

27. Piguet, P.-F., Grau, G. E., Allet, B. and Vassalli, P. (1987). Tumor necrosis factor/cachectin is an effector of skin and gut lesions of the acute phase of graft-vs-host disease. *J. Exp. Med.*, **166**, 1280–9

28. Piguet, P.-F. (1990). Tumor necrosis factor and graft-vs-host disease. In Burakoff, S. J., Deeg, H. J., Ferrara, J. and Atkinson, K. (eds), *Graft-vs-Host Disease: Immunology, Pathology and Treatment*. New York: Marcel Dekker, pp. 255–76

29. Snover, D. C., Weisdorf, S. A., Ramsay, N. K. C., McGlave, P. and Kersey, J. H. (1984). Hepatic graft versus host disease: a study of the predictive value of liver biopsy in diagnosis. *Hepatology*, **4**, 123–30

30. Shulman, H. M., Sharma, P., Amos, D., Fenster, L. F. and McDonald, G. B. (1988). A coded histologic study of hepatic graft-versus-host disease after human bone marrow transplantation. *Hepatology*, **8**, 463–70

31. McDonald, G. B., Shulman, H. M., Sullivan, K. M. and Spencer, G. D. (1986). Intestinal and hepatic complication of human bone marrow transplantation. *Gastroenterology*, **90**, 460

32. Snover, D. C. (1990). The pathology of acute graft-vs-host disease. In Burakoff, S. J., Deeg, H. J., Ferrara, J. and Atkinson, K. (eds), *Graft-versus-host Disease: Immunology, Pathology and Treatment*. New York: Marcel Dekker, pp. 337–53

33. McDonald, G. V. and Sale, G. E. (1984). The gastrointestinal tract after allogeneic bone marrow transplantation in humans. In Sale, G. E. and Shulman, H. M. (eds), *The Pathology of Bone Marrow Transplantation*. New York: Masson, pp. 77–103

34. Spencer, G. D., Shulman, H. M., Myerson, D., Thomas, E. D. and McDonald, G. B. (1986). Diffuse intestinal ulceration after marrow transplantation. *Human Pathol.*, **17**, 621–33

35. Simonsen, M. (1962). Graft versus host reactions. Their natural history and applicability as tools of research. *Progr. Allergy*, **6**, 349–467

36. Cornelius, E. A. (1970). Protein-losing enteropathy in the graft-versus-host reaction. *Transplant*, **9**, 247–52

37. Hedberg, C. A., Reiser, S. and Reilly, R. W. (1968). Intestinal phase of the runting syndrome in mice. II. Observations on nutrient absorption and certain disaccharidase abnormalities. *Transplantation*, **6**, 104–10

38. Lund, E. K., Bruce, M. G., Smith, M. W. and Ferguson, A. (1986). Selective effects of graft-versus-host reaction on disaccharidase expression by mouse jejunal enterocytes. *Clin. Sci.*, **71**, 189–98

39. Weisdorf, S. A., Salati, L. M., Longsdorf, J. A., Ramsay, N. K. C. and Sharp, H. L. (1988). Graft-versus-host disease of the intestine: a protein losing enteropathy characterized by fecal α_1-anti-trypsin. *Gastroenterology*, **85**, 1076–81

40. Piguet, P.-F. (1985). GvHR elicited by products of class I or class II loci of the MHC: analysis of the response of mouse T lymphocytes to products of class I and class II loci of the MHC in correlation with GvHR-induced mortality, medullary aplasia and enteropathy. *J. Immunol.*, **135**, 1637–43

41. Turner, M. W., Boulton, P., Shields, J. G., Strobel, S., Gibson, S., Miller, H. R. P. and Levinsky, R. J. (1988). Intestinal hypersensitivity reactions in the rat. I. Uptake of intact protein, permeability to sugars and their correlation with mucosal mast cell activation. *Immunology*, **63**, 119–24

42. Walker, R. I. (1978). The contribution of intestinal endotoxin to mortality in hosts with compromised resistance. A review. *Exp. Haematol.*, **6**, 172–84

43. Cunningham-Rundles, C., Brandeis, W. E., Safai, B., O'Reilly, R., Day, N. K. and Good, R. A. (1979). Selective IgA deficiency and circulating immune complexes containing bovine proteins in a child with chronic graft-versus-host disease. *Am. J. Med.*, **67**, 883–90

44. Strobel, S., Mowat, A. McI. and Ferguson, A. (1985). Prevention of oral tolerance induction to ovalbumin and enhanced antigen presentation during a graft-versus-host reaction in mice. *Immunology*, **56**, 57–64

45. Via, C. S., Sharrow, S. O. and Shearer, G. M. (1987). Role of cytotoxic T lymphocytes in the prevention of lupus-like disease occurring in a murine model of graft-versus-host disease. *J. Immunol.*, **139**, 1840–9

46. Sviland, L., Pearson, A. D. J., Eastham, E. J., Hamilton, P. J., Proctor, S. J., Malcolm, A. J. and the Newcastle upon Tyne Bone Marrow Transplant Group (1988). Histological features of skin and rectal biopsy specimens after autologous and allogeneic bone marrow transplantation. *J. Clin. Pathol.*, **41**, 148–54

47. Reilly, R. W. and Kirsner, J. B. (1965). Runt intestinal disease. *Lab. Invest.*, **14**, 102–7

48. Thiele, D. L., Eigenbrodt, M. L., Bryde, S. E., Eigenbrodt, E. H. and Lipsky, P. E. (1989). Intestinal graft-versus-host disease is initiated by donor T cell distinct from classic cytotoxic T lymphocytes. *J. Clin. Invest.*, **84**, 1947–56

49. Gorer, P. A. and Boyse, E. A. (1959). Pathological changes in F_1 hybrid mice following transplantation of spleen cells from donors of the parental strains. *Immunology*, **2**, 182–93

50. Wall, A. J., Rosenberg, J. L. and Reilly, R. W. (1971). Small intestinal injury in the immunologically runted mouse. Morphologic and autoradiographic studies. *J. Lab. Clin. Med.*, **78**, 833–4A

51. van Bekkum, D. W. and Knaan, S. (1977). Role of bacterial microflora in development of intestinal lesions from GvHR. *J. Natl. Cancer Inst.*, **58**, 787–90

52. Eigenbrodt, M. L., Eigenbrodt, E. H. and Thiele, D. L. (1991). Histologic similarity of murine colonic graft-versus-host disease (GvHD) to human colonic GvHD and inflammatory bowel disease. *Am. J. Pathol.* (In press)

53. MacDonald, T. T. and Ferguson, A. (1977). Hypersensitivity reactions in the small intestine. III. The effects of allograft rejection and of GvHD on epithelial cell kinetics. *Cell Tiss. Kinet.*, **10**, 301–12

54. Mowat, A. McI. and Ferguson, A. (1982). Intraepithelial lymphocyte count and crypt hyperplasia measure the mucosal component of the graft-versus-host reaction in mouse small intestine. *Gastroenterology*, **83**, 417–23

55. Mowat, A. McI., Felstein, M. V., Borland, A. and Parrott, D. M. V. (1988). Experimental studies of immunologically mediated enteropathy. Delayed type hypersensitivity is responsible for the proliferative and destructive enteropathy in irradiated mice with graft-versus-host reaction. *Gut*, **29**, 949–56

56. Felstein, M. V. and Mowat, A. McI. (1988). Experimental studies of immunologically mediated enteropthy. IV. Correlation between immune effector mechanisms and type of enteropathy during a graft-versus-host reaction in neonatal mice of different ages. *Clin. Exp. Immunol.*, **72**, 108

57. Mowat, A. McI. and Felstein, M. V. (1990). Experimental studies of immunologically mediated enteropathy. V. Destructive enteropathy during an acute graft-versus-host reaction in adult BDF_1 mice. *Clin. Exp. Immunol.*, **79**, 279–84

58. Mowat, A. McI. and Ferguson, A. (1981). Hypersensitivity reactions in the small intestine.

6. Pathogenesis of the graft-versus-host reaction in the small intestinal mucosa of the mouse. *Transplantation*, **32**, 238–43

59. Elson, C. O., Reilly, R. W. and Rosenberg, I. H. (1977). Small intestinal injury in the GvHR: an innocent bystander phenomenon. *Gastroenterology*, **72**, 886–9

60. Barclay, A. N. and Mason, D. W. (1982). Induction of Ia antigen in rat epidermal cells and gut epithelium by immunological stimuli. *J. Exp. Med.*, **156**, 1665–76

61. Sviland, L., Pearson, A. D., Eastham, E. J., Green, M. A., Hamilton, P. J., Proctor, S. J. and Malcolm, A. J. (1988). Class II antigen expression by keratinocytes and enterocytes – an early feature of graft-versus-host disease. *Transplantation*, **46**, 402

62. Nakhleh, R. E., Snover, D. C., Weisdorf, S. and Platt, J. L. (1989). Immunopathology of graft-versus-host disease in the upper gastrointestinal tract. *Transplantation*, **48**, 61–5

63. Rappaport, H., Khalil, A., Halle-Pannenko, O., Pritchard, L., Dantchev, D. and Mathe, G. (1979). Histopathologic sequence of events in adult mice undergoing lethal graft-versus-host reaction developed across H-1 and/or non-H-2 histocompatibility barriers. *Am. J. Pathol.*, **96**, 121–42

64. Nowell, P. C. and Cole, L. J. (1959). Lymphoid pathology in homologous disease of mice. *Transplant. Bull.*, **6**, 435

65. Simonsen, M. (1962). Graft-versus-host reactions. Their natural history and applicability as tools of research. *Progr. Allergy*, **6**, 349–467

66. Gold, J. A., Kosek, J., Wanek, N. and Bauer, S. (1976). Duodenal immunoglobulin deficiency in graft-versus-host disease (GvHD) mice. *J. Immunol.*, **117**, 471–476

67. Guy-Grand, D., Griscelli, C. and Vassalli, P. (1978). The mouse gut T-lymphocyte, a novel type of T-cell: nature, origin and traffic in mice in normal and graft-versus-host conditions. *J. Exp. Med.*, **148**, 1661–77

68. Guy-Grand, D. and Vassalli, P. (1986). Gut injury in mouse graft-versus-host reaction. Study of its occurrence and mechanisms. *J. Clin. Invest.*, **77**, 1584–95

69. Dilly, S. A. and Sloane, J. P. (1987). Changes in rectal leukocytes after allogeneic bone marrow transplantation. *Clin. Exp. Immunol.*, **62**, 545

70. Guy-Grand, D., Cerf-Bensussan, N., Malissen, B., Malassis-Seris, M., Briottet, C. and Vassalli, P.l (1991). Two gut intraepithelial CD8$^+$ lymphocyte populations with different T cell recptors: a role for the gut epithelium in T cell differentiation. *J. Exp. Med.*, **173**, 471–81

71. Sprent, J. (1976). Fate of H-2 activated T-lymphocytes in Syngeneic Hosts. I. Fate in lymphoid tissues and intestines traced with ^{3}H-thymidine, ^{125}I-deoxy-uridine and ^{51}chromium. *Cell Immunol.*, **21**, 278–302

72. Ferguson, A., Cummins, A. G., Munro, G. H., Gibson, S. and Miller, H. R. P. (1988). Intestinal mucosal mast cells in rats with graft-versus-host reaction. *Adv. Exp. Med. Biol.*, **216A**, 625–34

73. Cummins, A. G., Munro, G. H., Miller, H. R. P. and Ferguson, A. (1989). Effect of cyclosporin A treatment on the enteropathy of graft-versus-host reaction in the rat: a quantitative study of intestinal morphology, epithelial cell kinetics and mucosal immune activity. *Immunol. Cell Biol.*, **67**, 153–60

74. Crapper, R. M. and Schrader, J. W. (1986). Evidence for the *in vivo* production and release into the serum of a T cell lymphokine, persisting-cell stimulating factor (PSF), during graft-versus-host reactions. *Immunology*, **57**, 553–8

75. Newlands, G. J., Mowat, A. McI., Felstein, M. V. and Miller, H. R. P. (1990). Role of mucosal mast cells in intestinal graft-versus-host reaction in mice. *Int. Arch. Allergy Appl. Immunol.*, **98**, 308–13

76. Klein, R. M., Clancy, J. and Sheridan, K. (1984). Acute lethal graft-versus-host disease stimulates cellular proliferation in Peyer's patches and follicle associated ileal epithelium of adult rats. *Virch. Arch. (B)*, **47**, 303–11

77. Abedi, M. R., Hammarstrom, L., Ringden, O. and Smith, C. I. E. (1990). Development of IgA deficiency after bone marrow transplantation. The influence of acute and chronic graft-versus-host disease. *Transplantation*, **50**, 415–21

78. Strobel, S. (1984). PhD thesis, University of Edinburgh

79. Korngold, R. and Sprent, J. (1987). T cell subsets and graft-versus-host disease. *Transplantation*, **44**, 335–9

80. Mowat, A. McI., Borland, A. and Parrott, D. M. V. (1986). Hypersensitivity reactions in the small intestine. 7. The intestinal phase of murine graft-versus-host reactions is induced

by Lyt2⁻ T cells activated by I-A alloantigens. *Transplantation*, **4**, 192–8

81. Mowat, A. McI. and Sprent, J. (1989). Induction of intestinal graft-versus-host reactions across mutant major histocompatibility antigens by T lymphocyte subsets in mice. *Transplant*, **47**, 857–63

82. Borland, A., Mowat, A. McI. and Parrott, D. M. V. (1983). Augmentation of intestinal and peripheral natural killer cell activity during the graft-versus-host reaction in mice. *Transplantation*, **36**, 513–19

83. Felstein, M. V. and Mowat, A. McI. (1990). Experimental studies of immunologically mediated enteropathy. VI. Inhibition of acute intestinal graft-versus-host reaction in mice by 2'-deoxyguanosine. *Scand. J. Immunol.*, **32**, 461–9

84. Garside, P., Felstein, M. V., Green, E. A. and Mowat, A. McI. (1991). The role of interferon α/β in the induction of intestinal pathology in mice. *Immunology* (In press)

85. Mowat, A. McI. (1986). Ia⁺ bone marrow derived cells are the stimulus for the intestinal phase of murine graft-versus-host reaction. *Transplantation*, **42**, 141–4

86. Cornelius, E. A., Martinez, C., Yunis, E. J. and Good, R. A. (1968). Haematological and pathological changes induced in tolerant mice by the injection of syngeneic lymphoid cells. *Transplant*, **6**, 33–44

87. Symington, F. W., Pepe, M. S., Chen, A. B. and Deliganis, A. (1990). Serum tumor necrosis factor alpha associated with acute graft-versus-host disease in humans. *Transplantation*, **50**, 518–21

88. Mowat, A. McI. (1989). Antibodies to γ-interferon prevent immunologically mediated intestinal damage in murine graft-versus-host reaction. *Immunology*, **68**, 18–23

89. Garside, P. A. and Mowat, A. McI. (1991). Pathological effects of tumour necrosis factor α on the intestinal epithelium (Submitted)

90. Schoenfeld, Y. and Isenberg, D. A. (1989). The mosaic of autoimmunity. *Immunol. Today*, **10**, 123–8

91. Browning, J. and Ribolini, A. (1989). Studies on the differing effects of tumor necrosis factor and lymphotoxin on the growth of several human tumor lines. *J. Immunol.*, **143**, 1859–67

92. Kvale, D., Lovhaug, D., Sollid, L. M. and Brandtzaeg, P. (1988). Tumor necrosis factor-α up-regulates expression of secretory component, the epithelial receptor for polymeric Ig. *J. Immunol.*, **140**, 3086–9

93. Madara, J. L. and Stafford, J. (1989). Interferon-γ directly affects barrier function of cultured intestinal epithelial monolayers. *J. Clin. Invest.*, **83**, 724–7

94. Haffen, K., Kedinger, M. and Simon-Assmann, P. (1989). Cell contact dependent regulation of enterocytic differentiation. In Lebenthal, E. (ed.), *Human Gastrointestinal Development*. New York: Raven Press, pp. 19–39

95. Roy, C., Ghayur, T., Kongshavn, P. A. L. and Lapp, W. S. (1982). Natural killer activity by spleen lymph node and thymus cells during the graft-versus-host reaction. *Transplantation*, **34**, 144–6

96. Kubota, E., Ishikawa, H. and Saito, K. (1983). Modulation of F₁ cytotoxic potentials by GvHR. Host and donor-derived cytotoxic lymphocytes arise in the unirradiated F₁ host spleens under the condition of GvHR-associated immunosuppression. *J. Immunol.*, **131**, 1142–8

97. Mowat, A. McI., Borland, A. and Parrott, D. M. V. (1985). Augmentation of natural killer cell activity by anti-host delayed-type hypersensitivity during the graft-versus-host reaction in mice. *Scand. J. Immunol.*, **22**, 389–99

98. Mowat, A. McI. and Felstein, M. V. (1987). Experimental studies of immunologically mediated enteropathy. II. Role of natural killer cells in the intestinal phase of murine graft-versus-host reaction. *Immunology*, **68**, 179–83

99. Handa, K., Suzuki, R., Matsui, H., Shimizu, Y. and Kumagi, K. (1983). Natural killer (NK) cells as a responder to interleukin 2 (IL2). II. IL2-induced interferon production. *J. Immunol.*, **130**, 988–92

100. Kasahara, T., Djeu, J. Y., Dougherty, S. F. and Oppenheim, J. J. (1983). Capacity of human large granular lymphocytes to produce multiple lymphokines: interleukin 2, interferon and colony stimulating factor. *J. Immunol.*, **131**, 2379–85

101. Jones, J. M., Wilson, R. and Bealmear, P. M. (1971). Mortality and gross pathology of secondary disease in germfree mouse radiation chimeras. *Radiat. Res.*, **45**, 577–88

102. van Bekkum, D. W., Roodenburg, J., Heidt, P. J. and van der Waalt, D. (1974). Mitigation of secondary disease of allogeneic mouse radiation chimeras by modification of the intestinal

microflora. *J. Natl. Cancer Inst.*, **52**, 401

103. Moore, R. H., Lampert, I. A., Chia, Y., Aber, V. R. and Cohen, J. (1987). Influence of endotoxin on graft-versus-host disease after bone marrow transplantation across major histocompatibility barriers in mice. *Transplantation*, **43**, 731–6

104. Moore, R. H., Mapert, I. A., Chia, Y., Aber, V. R. and Cohen, J. (1987). Effect of immunisation with Escherichia coli J5 on graft-versus-host disease induced by minor histocompatibility antigens in mice. *Transplantation*, **44**, 249–53

105. Kawakami, M. and Cerami, A. (1981). Studies of endotoxin-induced decrease in lipoprotein lipase activity. *J. Exp. Med.*, **154**, 631

106. Le, J. and Vilcek, J. (1987). Tumor necrosis factor and interleukin 1: cytokines with multiple overlapping biological activities. *Lab. Invest.*, **56**, 234–48

107. Buckner, C. D., Clift, R. A., Sanders, J. E., Meyers, J. D., Counts, G. W., Farewell, V. T. and Thomas, E. D. (1978). Protective environment for marrow transplant recipients. A prospective study. *Ann. Intern. Med.*, **89**, 893–901

108. Mowat, A. McI., Felstein, M. V. and Baca, M. E. (1987). Experimental studies of immunologically mediated enteropathy. III. Severe and progressive enteropathy during a graft-versus-host reaction in athymic mice. *Immunology*, **61**, 185–8

109. Bellgrau, D. and Wilson, D. B. (1978). Immunological studies of T-cell receptors. I. Specifically induced resistance to graft-versus-host disease in rats mediated by host T-cell immunity to alloreactive parental T cells. *J. Exp. Med.*, **148**, 103–14

110. Mowat, A. McI. (1984). The immunopathogenesis of food sensitive enteropathies. In Newby, T. J. and Stokes, C. R. (eds), *Local Immune Responses of the Gut*. Boca Raton, FL: CRC Press, pp. 199–225

111. MacDonald, T. T., Hutchings, P., Choy, M.-Y., Murch, S. and Cooke, A. (1990). Tumour necrosis factor-alpha and interferon-gamma production measured at the single cell level in normal and inflamed human intestine. *Clin. Exp. Immunol.*, **81**, 301–5

8
In vitro enteropathy

C. P. BRAEGGER and T. T. MACDONALD

INTRODUCTION

Intestinal damage due to food hypersensitivity is a major cause of gastrointestinal morbidity in humans, especially in children. In the classical, delayed-onset intestinal hypersensitivities to dietary antigens (e.g. cereals and milk), the histopathological features associated with disease are small intestinal villous atrophy, crypt epithelial cell hyperplasia and crypt hypertrophy. There may also be abnormalities of surface epithelial cell structure and function. The clinical consequences of this enteropathy are malabsorption due to decreased absorptive surface, deficiency of digestive enzymes and steatorrhoea. The relative inaccessibility of clinical material from the intestine, and the difficulty in performing time-course studies in patients, has meant that our understanding of the development of the intestinal lesion in food-sensitive enteropathy is fragmentary. In addition, the immunological mechanisms which could cause tissue damage in the gut are not known, due to difficulties in obtaining lymphocytes from human gut and generating specific immune responses.

There is good evidence to suggest that T cell-mediated immune reactions can cause gut damage. Diseases such as coeliac disease, cows' milk protein intolerance and chronic inflammatory bowel disease (Crohn's disease) are associated with increased numbers of lamina propria and intraepithelial T lymphocytes[1,25]. In addition, these T lymphocytes show phenotypic markers of activation and secrete lymphokines. An important question in mucosal immunology is whether these T lymphocytes are of primary importance in mediating intestinal damage, or if they represent a secondary phenomenon. The development of an *in vitro* model of human fetal intestinal organ culture described here[2] has proved to be a useful tool to investigate the relationships between mucosal T lymphocyte activation and intestinal structure and function.

In vitro culture of jejunal biopsies from coeliac patients has also been of use in following the consequences of the mucosal cell-mediated immune response to gluten[3]. This has the advantage that the responses are antigen-specific, but has the problem that the viability of jejunal biopsies in culture is poor and cultures can be maintained for only 24–48 h before the specimens become necrotic.

IN VITRO ENTEROPATHY IN HUMAN FETAL ORGAN CULTURE

This model depends on two critical factors: first, that human fetal intestine can be grown in explant culture for long periods and second, that early in fetal life the intestine is structurally similar to adult intestine and contains abundant lymphocytes.

Development of the gut immune system

Gut epithelium

Columnar epithelium and villi develop at 9–10 weeks gestation in the human fetal gastrointestinal tract[4]. Crypt formation begins in the proximal small bowel at 10–11 weeks gestation and develops distally. Paneth cells are present in crypts at this time and the surface epithelium contains mature goblet cells.

Intraepithelial lymphocytes

Intraepithelial lymphocytes (IEL) cannot be identified morphologically in human small bowel until 11 weeks gestation, when there are three lymphocytes for every 1000 epithelial cells[5]. Their numbers increase thereafter. These results have been confirmed and extended in more recent immunohistochemical studies[6]. At 11 weeks gestation CD3+ IEL can be identified. Some of these are CD4+ and some are CD8+; however, the numbers are too low to reliably determine the relative proportions of each subset. CD3+ IEL increase in number with time (Table 8.1) and by 17–19 weeks there are two to five CD3+ IEL per 100 epithelial cells. The number of CD8+ lymphocytes

Table 8.1 T lymphocyte subclasses in human fetal ileal epithelium

Age of tissue	Number of immunostained cells as a percentage of the number of epithelial cell nuclei		
	CD3	CD4	CD8
11 weeks	1.5	1.4	0.3
12 weeks	1.1	0	0.3
14 weeks	1.8	0.6	0.9
16 weeks	2.9	0.4	1.3
17 weeks	3.2	0.9	2.1
19 weeks	2.3	0.2	1.1
8 years	15.1	3.2	13.7

Data adapted from ref. 6

exceeds the number of CD4+ IEL, as is the case in postnatal bowel. About 50% of fetal IEL are CD4− and CD8−[7]. Cells of this phenotype make up only 6% of IEL in postnatal gut[8].

In postnatal intestine there is a large population of CD3− CD7+ IEL, which are not T lymphocytes[8]. These cells are conspicuously absent from fetal intestinal IEL.

Lamina propria lymphocytes

At the earliest time studied (11 weeks gestation), there are virtually no T or B lymphocytes in fetal lamina propria. Many of the cells in the lamina propria have macrophage-like morphology, while others are spindle-shaped[9]. These cells are strongly CD45+, HLA-DR+, HLA-DP+, CD4+, and RFD1+. They are therefore probably macrophages and dendritic cells. The extent of this non-lymphoid infiltrate increased with the age of the fetus. At 11 weeks gestation there are clusters of HLA-DR+ CD4+ cells in the lamina propria which may be a Peyer's patch *anlage*[10].

At 14 weeks gestation small clusters of T and B lymphocytes are present in regions of the lamina propria which are also strongly HLA-DR+[10]. This is probably the earliest influx of lymphoid cells into the Peyer's patch *anlage* described above. B lymphocytes are not present outside these clusters in the lamina propria in many fetuses up to 22 weeks gestation. Plasma cells are not seen in healthy fetal lamina propria. From 14 weeks gestation, however, there are numerous CD3+ cells in the lamina propria (Fig. 8.1). Most of these are CD4+[6].

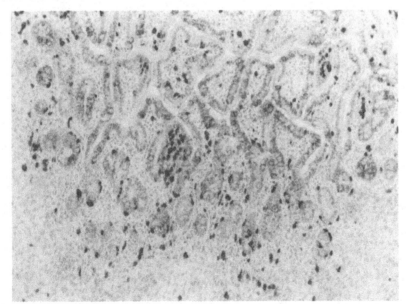

Figure 8.1 CD3+ cells in the lamina propria and epithelium of 18-week-old fetal gut. Immunoperoxidase, ×65

Peyer's patches

Peyer's patches (PP) are macroscopically identifiable in fetal human intestine at 24 weeks gestation[11]. Even in the fetus they predominate in the ileum as compared to the jejunum or duodenum. The first identifiable clusters of T and B lymphocytes, forming around groups of accessory cells, can be seen at 14 weeks gestation[10]. These increase in number and size at 16 weeks gestation. The T lymphocytes are mostly CD4+ and the B lymphocytes are surface IgM+, IgD+[12]. There is no cellular zonation. By 19 weeks well-defined PP have formed. A striking feature of these is that virtually every cell in the PP (including T lymphocytes, B lymphocytes and accessory cells) is major histocompatibility antigen (MHC) Class II positive. The PP contain well-defined, central B lymphocyte zones containing follicular dendritic cells. The follicle B lymphocytes are surface IgM+, IgD+ and express CD5. Surrounding the follicles are well-defined T lymphocyte zones, most of the cells being CD4+ (Fig. 8.2). A follicle-associated epithelium also develops by this time, characterized by a more cuboidal epithelium and a relative sparsity of goblet cells. Putative M-cells have been identified in follicle-associated epithelium[4].

There is no evidence of PP germinal centre formation in healthy human fetal small intestine. After birth these develop rapidly due to antigenic stimulation from luminal bacteria[13].

Fetal colon

Fetal colon is different from postnatal colon in that it has villi. The surface

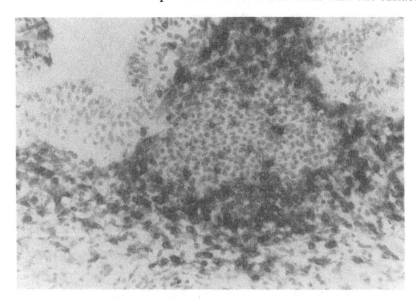

Figure 8.2 CD3+ cells in a Peyer's patch of a 19-week-old fetus. Note the occasional T lymphocyte in the primary follicle. Immunoperoxidase, ×260

epithelial cells also contain the disaccharidases usually only found in the small bowel in postnatal life. The development of IEL and lamina propria T lymphocytes follows that of the small bowel; however, there are conspicuously fewer follicles in colon than in ileum.

Summary

It is clear that by 20 weeks gestation the human intestinal immune system is well-developed, although in a state of inactivity since it is not exposed to antigenic stimulus from the lumen.

Organ culture of human fetal small and large intestine

Small explants (1–2 mm across) of human fetal gut can be maintained in organ culture for several weeks with retention of morphology, epithelial cell renewal and enterocyte function. An *in vitro* system has therefore been developed[2] to study T lymphocyte–epithelial interactions in small and large intestine. Explants of human fetal intestine (small and large bowel) containing T lymphocytes (15–20 weeks gestation) can be cultured in the presence of pokeweek mitogen or monoclonal anti-CD3 antibodies to directly activate mucosal T lymphocytes *in situ*.

Evidence for local T lymphocytes activation

T lymphocyte activation can be measured by immunohistochemical staining for T lymphocyte activation markers such as interleukin-2 receptor (CD25). CD25 is the α-chain of the interleukin-2 receptor and therefore a useful activation marker of lymphoid cells. Interleukin-2 receptors are expressed very early after lymphocyte activation. Lymphokines can also be measured directly in the culture supernatants.

After 6–72 h of culture of 18–22-week-old fetal gut, the explants were snap-frozen and sections were cut and stained immunohistochemically with anti-CD25 antibody[2]. CD25 + cells were not seen in the unstimulated control cultures. In explants stimulated with anti-CD3 or pokeweed mitogen, CD25 + cells were detectable in the lamina propria as early as 6 h (Fig. 8.3)[14]. Their number increased until 24 h of culture and remained the same thereafter (Table 8.2). CD25 + cells were rare in the epithelium. Some of the CD25 + cells were morphologically small and round, with only a small cytoplasm; others were large and had the appearance of macrophages. The small cells were CD3 +, CD4 +. Supernatants of stimulated gut cultures (taken on day 2–3 of culture) contained interleukin-2 and interferon-γ, whereas unstimulated cultures had no detectable lymphokine production. The same experiments were carried out with fetal gut aged 12–14 weeks, which contains no or only very few T lymphocytes. In this case the addition of pokeweed mitogen or anti-CD3 induced no CD25 + cells in the lamina propria and no lymphokines were detectable in the supernatants.

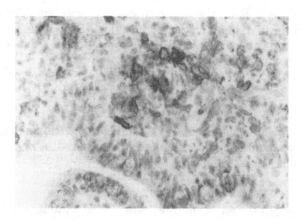

Figure 8.3 CD25+ cells in the lamina propria of a 19-week-old fetal gut explant stimulated with anti-CD3. These cells were not detected in explants cultured in normal medium. Immunoperoxidase, ×400

Consequences of T lymphocyte activation

Mucosal morphology. Examination of the gross appearance of the explants from 18–20-week-old fetuses treated with pokeweed mitogen or anti-CD3 showed major differences from controls[2]. In controls the villi were shorter than usual due to water absorption, but they were clearly visible. In T lymphocyte-stimulated cultures the surface of the mucosa was obscured by a layer of cellular debris, but short villi could be seen underneath the debris (Fig. 8.4a, b). Immunohistochemical analysis of the tissues showed that in control cultures the villi were tall, and that epithelial cell division (detected with the monoclonal antibody Ki67) was in the crypts. In contrast in T lymphocyte-stimulated cultures villi were short and the crypts were hypertrophic. The most dramatic feature, however, was the increase in epithelial cell proliferation induced by T lymphocyte stimulation. This was apparent by a 10-fold increase in epithelial Ki67+ cells and a similar increase in the rate of epithelial crypt cell production as measured by stathmokinetic techniques (Fig. 8.5a, b).

Table 8.2 Number of CD25+ cells (immunostaining with monoclonal anti-CD25 antibody) in the lamina propria of fetal small intestinal organ cultures of various ages after culture with pokeweed mitogen (15 μg/ml) for 3 days; there were no CD25+ cells in the lamina propria of any of the control organ cultures

Age of tissue (weeks)	CD25+ cells/×40 field
14	0
16	2.3 ± 1.3
17	2.3 ± 0.9
18	12.5 ± 1.5
20	15.9 ± 4.4
22	21.3 ± 2.6

Data adapted from ref. 2

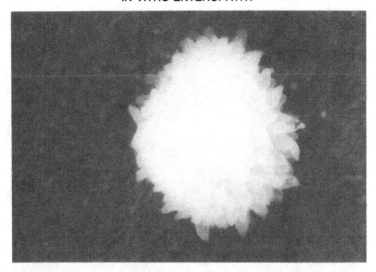

a

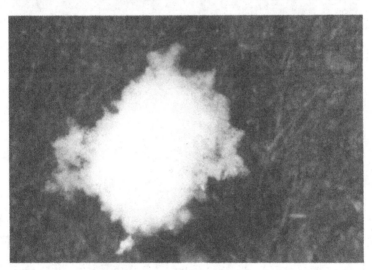

b

Figure 8.4 Morphological appearance of explants of human small intestine of 18-week gestation, cultured for 72 h in normal medium (**a**), and in medium containing 15 µg/ml pokeweed mitogen (**b**). In the pokeweed mitogen-treated culture the surface is covered with epithelial debris. ×24

Mucosal lymphocytes. As might be expected, the addition of T lymphocyte mitogens led to an increase in the density of T lymphocytes in the lamina propria[7], (Fig. 8.6a,b). In control cultures, over the initial 72 h of culture, IEL levels decreased dramatically. In contrast, in anti-CD3-treated cultures IEL levels remained high and even increased in some experiments. These IEL had the unusual phenotype of CD3+, 4−, 8−, and most of them used the $\alpha\beta$ T cell receptor. Many of these IEL appeared highly motile and could even occasionally be seen crossing from the epithelium onto the villous surface.

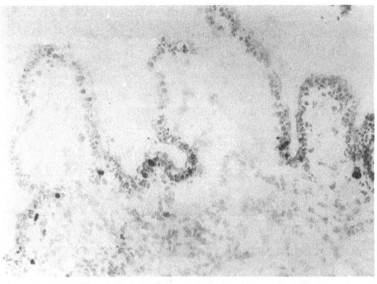

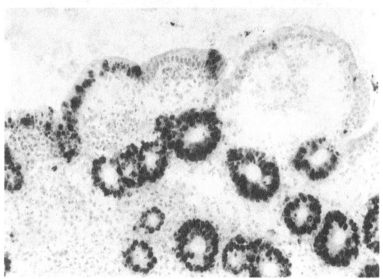

Figure 8.5 Ki67-staining of sections of explants of human fetal small bowel of 18-week gestation, cultured for 72 h in medium alone (a), or in medium containing 15 µg/ml pokeweed mitogen (b). Notice the morphological changes (villous atrophy), and the intense epithelial cell proliferation in the crypts in the pokeweed mitogen-treated cultures. Immunoperoxidase. ×70

Other epithelial change. The local T lymphocyte inflammatory response also led to a dramatic increase in HLA-DR expression on lamina propria cells and crypt epithelial cells, which are usually HLA-DR negative[16] (Fig. 8.7). This was probably due to the local production of interferon-γ. Although the

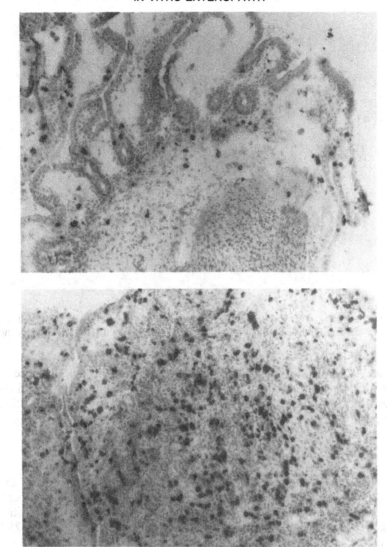

a

b

Figure 8.6 CD3 + cells in explants of human fetal small intestine of 18-week gestation, cultured for 3 days in medium alone (**a**), or with anti-CD3 (**b**). Notice the increased number of T lymphocytes in the anti-CD3-stimulated cultures. Immunoperoxidase. ×60

epithelial cells were hyperplastic they were morphologically normal, and no damage was seen to either crypt or surface epithelial cells in T lymphocyte-stimulated cultures.

Effects of cyclosporin A. To ensure that the effects were due to activated T lymphocytes, cyclosporin A was added at the onset of culture to inhibit T

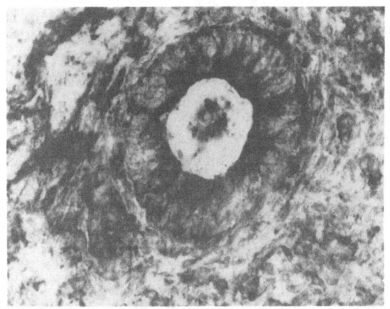

Figure 8.7 HLA-DR + crypt epithelial cells in 18-week-old fetal gut explants, stimulated with pokeweed mitogen. Epithelial cells of unstimulated explants were all HLA-DR negative (not shown). Immunoperoxidase. ×260

lymphocyte activation[2]. This was effective in that in the presence of cyclosporin A, the number of CD25 + cells in the lamina propria and the amount of interleukin-2 in the supernatants was diminished. In addition, cyclosporin A inhibited the mucosal damage and the increase in Ki67 + cells in the crypts (Table 8.3).

Fetal colon. Similar experiments were carried out using explants of fetal colon, the only major difference between fetal colon and small bowel being that goblet cells are much more abundant in the former tissue. The addition of pokeweed mitogen to explants of 17–20-week-old fetal colon led to CD25 + cells in the lamina propria. There was also an increase in epithelial cell proliferation in the glands, which was not so obvious as in the small bowel because of the higher rate of proliferation seen in control cultures of fetal

Table 8.3 Effect of cyclosporin A on the development of crypt epithelial hyperplasia and the appearance of CD25 + cells in pokeweed mitogen-treated human fetal small intestinal organ cultures of 20-week gestation

	Ki67 + cells/crypt	CD25 + cells/field
Control	0.4 ± 0.2	0
Pokeweed mitogen (15 µg/ml)	35.2 ± 2.7	15.8 ± 4.4
Cyclosporin A (15 µg/ml)	1.6 ± 0.6	0
Pokeweed mitogen + cyclosporin A	1.0 ± 0.5	2.2 ± 0.5

Data adapted from Table 2 of ref. 2

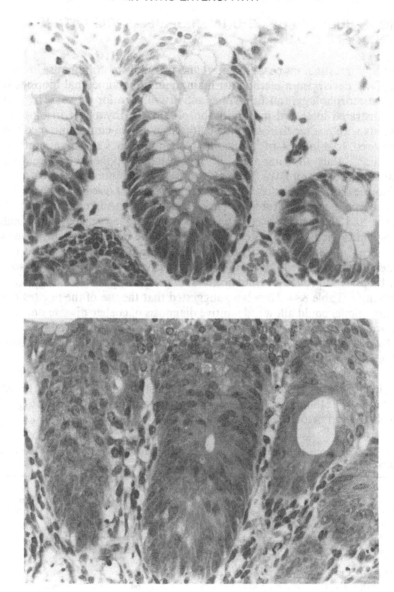

a

b

Figure 8.8 Sections of explants of human fetal colon of 20-week gestation, cultured for 72 h in medium alone (**a**), and in medium containing 15 µg/ml pokeweed mitogen (**b**). Notice the goblet cell depletion in pokeweed mitogen-treated cultures. H&E, ×240

colon. The most striking feature, however, of T lymphocyte-stimulated fetal colon was the rapid decrease in epithelial goblet cells which were replaced with columnar cells[16] (Fig. 8.8a, b).

ORGAN CULTURE OF JEJUNAL BIOPSIES FROM PATIENTS WITH COELIAC DISEASE

To study intestinal mucosal function and metabolism in humans, Browning and Trier developed a method for maintaining human jejunal biopsies with normal morphology and functional activity *in vitro* for up to 72 h[17]. They demonstrated increased incorporation of tritiated thymidine in biopsies of patients with coeliac disease when cultured in gluten-containing medium as compared to biopsies of the same patients when kept in a gluten-free medium[18], thus showing that the high rate of epithelial cell renewal – characteristic of untreated coeliac disease – was maintained *in vitro*.

Biopsies from patients with untreated coeliac disease showed some improvement when cultured *in vitro*. There was an increase in enterocyte height and the height of the brush border, and an increase in alkaline phosphatase activity. If gluten was added to the cultures, no improvement was seen[19]. The same investigators demonstrated that cortisol added to the gluten-containing medium could completely reverse the gluten effects, so that the biopsies improved biochemically and morphologically as in gluten-free medium[20] (Table 8.4). They later suggested that the use of the *in vitro* organ culture model could allow a definitive diagnosis of coeliac disease on a single biopsy[21]; however, this has not proved to be a practical procedure.

To assess the role of different gluten fractions in producing enteropathy in patients with coeliac disease, the organ culture model was used to test *in vitro* cytotoxicity of several gluten fractions, some of them known to be toxic *in vivo*[22]. None of the gluten fractions tested were cytotoxic *in vitro*. Nevertheless, other investigators were able to produce peptides from α-gliadin which showed cytotoxicity to coeliac biopsies[23].

Table 8.4 Biochemical and morphological changes of jejunal biopsies *in vitro* in presence and absence of gluten and cortisol

	Alkaline phosphatase activity ($\mu mol\ PNP/g$ protein per min)	Sucrase ($\mu mol\ glucose/$ g per min)	Enterocyte height (μm)
Normal controls			
0 h	400	58	28
24–28 h/ – gliadin	580	62	26
24–48 h/ + gliadin	590	64	26
24–48 h/ + gliadin/			
+ cortisol	480	n.d.	n.d.
Untreated coeliac disease			
0 h	100	15	20
24–48 h/ – gliadin	400	19	24
24–48 h/ + gliadin	200	10	19
24–48 h/ + gliadin/			
+ cortisol	470	n.d.	n.d.

n.d. = Not done
Data adapted from refs 17 and 18

Another interesting observation was the demonstration of migration-inhibition factor (MIF) activity in the culture medium of biopsies from patients with coeliac disease when cultured with gliadin, but absence of MIF activity when cultured in the absence of gliadin[3]. These observations supported the theory that coeliac disease is caused by a cell-mediated immune response of gut lymphocytes to gliadin, and that this process causes crypt hyperplasia and villous atrophy.

CONCLUSIONS

Activated T lymphocytes can be detected by immunohistochemistry using monoclonal anti-CD25 antibody, which is an *in vivo* marker of lymphoid cells that have recently been exposed to their specific antigen presented in the context of MHC molecules. In the mucosa in some enteropathies, CD25-positive cells can be found. In Crohn's disease, CD25-positive cells are abundant in the lamina propria of the inflamed mucosa, but are absent in the uninflamed parts of the gut[1]. Double-staining showed that most of these cells are T lymphocytes[24]. In coeliac disease, CD25-positive cells are also found in the lamina propria[25]. Some infants with intractable diarrhoea also have increased numbers of activated T lymphocytes in their intestinal mucosa[26].

The *in vitro* organ culture model of human fetal intestine has proved to be a useful instrument to investigate the role of mucosal T cells in the pathogenesis of small bowel enteropathy. *In situ* activation of T lymphocytes causes a severe crypt hyperplasia and villous atrophy, features very similar to coeliac disease and early stages of small bowel Crohn's disease. In fetal colon, activation of T lymphocytes produces additionally a severe goblet lymphocyte depletion, which can typically be found in ulcerative colitis. These observations emphasize the important role of lymphocyte-mediated immunity and T lymphocytes in chronic inflammatory bowel diseases and in food-sensitive enteropathies such as coeliac disease, and indicate that these cells are of primary importance and not just a secondary phenomenon.

Organ cultures of jejunal biopsies of patients with coeliac disease and normal controls also proved to be a useful tool for investigating the immunological basis of food sensitive enteropathies, although the system is limited due to short periods of tissue survival *in vitro*.

REFERENCES

1. Selby, W. S., Janossy, G., Bofill, M. and Jewell, D. P. (1984). Intestinal lymphocyte subpopulations in inflammatory bowel disease. *Gut*, **25**, 32–40
2. MacDonald, T. T. and Spencer, J. (1988). Evidence that activated mucosal T cells play a role in the pathogenesis of enteropathy in human small intestine. *J. Exp. Med.*, **167**, 1341–9
3. Ferguson, A., MacDonald, T. T., McClure, J. P. and Holden, R. J. (1975). Cell-mediated immunity to gliadin within the small-intestinal mucosa in coeliac disease. *Lancet*, **1**, 895–902
4. Moxey, P. C. and Trier, J. S. (1979). Specialised cell types in the human fetal intestine. *Anat. Rec.*, **191**, 269–85

5. Orlic, D. and Lev, R. (1977). An electron microscopic study of intraepithelial lymphocytes in human fetal small intestine. *Lab. Invest.*, **37**, 554–61

6. Spencer, J., Dillon, S. B., Isaacson, P. G. and MacDonald, T. T. (1986). T cell subclasses in human fetal ileum. *Clin. Exp. Immunol.*, **65**, 553–8

7. Monk, T. J., Spencer, J., Cerf-Bensussan, N. and MacDonald, T. T. (1988). Activation of mucosal T-cells in situ with anti-CD3 antibody: phenotype of the activated T cells and their distribution within the mucosal micro-environment. *Clin. Exp. Immunol.*, **74**, 216–22

8. Spencer, J., Isaacson, P. G. and MacDonald, T. T. (1989). Heterogeneity in intraepithelial lymphocyte subpopulations in fetal and post-natal human small intestine. *J. Paediatr. Gastrointest. Nutr.*, **9**, 173–7

9. Spencer, J., MacDonald, T. T. and Isaacson, P. G. (1987). Heterogeneity of non-lymphoid cells expressing HLA-D region antigens in human fetal gut. *Clin. Exp. Immunol.*, **67**, 415–24

10. Spencer, J., MacDonald, T. T., Finn, T. T. and Isaacson, P. G. (1986). Development of Peyer's patches in human fetal terminal ileum. *Clin. Exp. Immunol.*, **64**, 536–43

11. Cornes, J. S. (1965). Number, size, and distribution of Peyer's patches in the human small intestine. Part 1. The development of Peyer's patches. *Gut*, **6**, 225–9. Part 2. The effect of age on Peyer's patches. *Gut*, **6**, 230–3

12. Perkkio, M. and Savilahti, E. (1980). Time of appearance of immunoglobulin-containing cells in the mucosa of the neonatal intestine. *Pediatr. Res.*, **14**, 953–5

13. Bridges, R. L., Condie, R. M., Zak, S. J. and Good, R. A. (1957). The morphologic basis of antibody formation development during the neonatal period. *J. Lab. Clin. Med.*, **53**, 331–57

14. Ferreira, R. daC., Forsyth, L. A., Richman, P., Wells, C., Spencer, J. and MacDonald, T. T. (1990). Changes in mucosal morphology and the rate of epithelial cell renewal induced by a T cell mediated immune response in human small intestine *in vitro*. *Gastroenterology*, **98**, 1255–63

15. MacDonald, T. T., Weinel, A. and Spencer, J. M. (1988). HLA-DR expression in human fetal intestinal epithelium. *Gut*, **29**, 1342–8

16. Evans, C. M., Phillips, A., Walker-Smith, J. A. and MacDonald, T. T. (1991). Activation of lamina propria T cells causes crypt cell proliferation and goblet cell depletion in human fetal colon. *Gut* (in press)

17. Browning, T. H. and Trier, J. S. (1969). Organ culture of mucosal biopsies of human small intestine. *J. Clin. Invest.*, **48**, 1423–32

18. Trier, T. S. and Browning, T. H. (1970). Epithelial cell renewal in cultured duodenal biopsies in coeliac sprue. *N. Engl. J. Med.*, **233**, 1245–50

19. Falchuk, Z. M., Gebhard, R. L., Sessoms, C. and Strober, W. (1974). An *in vitro* model of gluten-sensitive enteropathy. *J. Clin. Invest.*, **53**, 487–500

20. Katz, A. J., Falchuk, Z. M., Strober, W. and Shwachman, H. (1976). Inhibition by cortisol of the effect of gluten protein in vitro. *N. Engl. J. Med.*, **295**, 131–135

21. Katz, A. J. and Falchuk, Z. M. (1978). Definitive diagnosis of gluten-sensitive enteropathy. *Gastroenterology*, **75**, 695–700

22. Hauri, H. P., Kedinger, M., Haffen, K. *et al.* (1978). Re-evaluation of the technique of organ culture for studying gluten toxicity in coeliac disease. *Gut*, **19**, 1090–8

23. DeRitis, G., Auricchio, S., Jones, H. W. *et al.* (1988). *In vitro* (organ culture) studies of the toxicity of specific A-gliadin peptides in celiac disease. *Gastroenterology*, **94**, 41–9

24. Choy, M.-Y., Richman, P. I., Walker-Smith, J. A. and MacDonald, T. T. (1991). Differential expression of CD25 on mucosal T cells and macrophages distinguishes the lesions in ulcerative colitis and Crohn's disease. *Gut*, **31**, 1365–70

25. MacDonald, T. T. (1990). The role of activated T lymphocytes in gastrointestinal disease. *Clin. Exp. Allergy*, **20**, 247–52

26. Cuenod, B., Brousse, N., Goulet, O. *et al.* (1990). Classification of intractable diarrhoea in infancy using clinical and immunohistological criteria. *Gastroenterology*, **99**, 1037–43

9
Molecular basis of cell migration into normal and inflamed gut

M. SALMI and S. JALKANEN

The mucosal immune system functions as the first line of defence against microbes. It includes the gut-associated lymphatic sites and some anatomically remote tissues such as the lactating mammary gland. The gut-associated lymphoid tissue consists of organized lymphoid tissues with well-defined B and T cell areas (Peyer's patches and appendix) and the lamina propria. The mucosal immune system has some special features distinct from its non-mucosal counterparts. For example, IgA is produced in the form of dimers and larger polymers, and intraepithelial T cells of the mucosal epithelium represent a unique T cell subpopulation[1,2]. The special nature of the intestinal immune system is largely based on selective migration of effector and memory cells to mucosal sites. A critical step controlling this migration is binding of lymphocytes to vascular endothelium at sites of lymphocyte exit from the blood. Several adhesion molecules, both on the lymphocyte and endothelial cell surfaces, are required for this interaction. In inflammatory conditions, expression of these molecules may change. Furthermore, some other adhesion molecules are induced only at sites of inflammation to facilitate the traffic of lymphocytes and other leukocytes into the tissue. Recently, new molecules involved in this process have been reported, and functional and other properties of the known ones have been elucidated in more detail. This review will focus on the recent progress in research on leukocyte traffic to mucosal lymphatic tissues both in physiological and inflammatory conditions. Especially, the molecular interactions between leukocytes and vascular endothelium will be discussed.

RECIRCULATION PATHWAYS

The starting point for the research on lymphocyte recirculation was the fundamental discovery of Gowans and Knight[3]. They found that large thoracic duct lymphocytes of rat home to intestinal lymphoid tissues when injected back into the animals, whereas small lymphocytes can enter any lymphoid tissue of the body. Since this discovery, several elegant *in vivo* studies using different animal models have further increased our knowledge on non-random migration of lymphocytes. These studies have created the basis for the current concept of lymphocyte recirculation[4-7]: most mature lymphocytes recirculate continuously between the blood and lymphoid organs. They leave the blood by binding to specialized venules, called high endothelial venules (HEV) in organized lymphatic tissues[8]. From there, they drain into efferent lymphatics that return the cells via the thoracic duct back to the blood circulation. Virgin lymphocytes can freely migrate through different organs in the body in the search of antigen, but after antigen activation they selectively migrate to sites where they first encountered their cognate antigen.

At mucosal sites, after differentiation in the organized lymphoid organs (Peyer's patches/appendix) the lymphocytes drain into the intestinal lymphatics, pass via the mesenteric nodes and enter the thoracic duct and the systemic circulation. Finally, they leave the blood at mucosal sites. According to the concept of the common mucosal immune system[9,10], this type of migration system distributes cells sensitized at one mucosal surface to other mucosal sites. Its importance is clearly demonstrated by the finding that the lactating mammary gland secretes antibodies specific to antigens encountered in the mother's gastrointestinal tract, thus providing protection for the suckling. Moreover, after oral immunizations, specific antibodies can be found in secretions of anatomically distant exocrine glands[9].

After entering the intestinal area, most B cells localize in the lamina propria where they further proliferate and differentiate. In contrast, many T cells migrate further into the intestinal epithelium. This phenomenon is at least partially antigen-dependent, because luminal antigens determine the magnitude of the intraepithelial migration[11]. On the other hand, intraepithelial lymphocytes are found before the birth, indicating that the migration can also occur independently of the antigen[12]. Moreover, epithelial homing of γ/δ T cells has been shown to be independent of T cell receptor specificity[13]. Intraepithelial lymphocytes are usually found along the basement membrane, and can probably cross it to either direction[14]. Therefore, it seems possible that the intraepithelial T lymphocytes re-enter the lamina propria for some immunoregulatory function. The mucosal recirculation route is illustrated in Fig. 9.1.

Even though lymphocyte recirculation occurs almost entirely via HEV and venules functioning like HEV, there is a continuous low-grade migration of lymphocytes and monocytes from the blood to afferent lymph at vascular beds in non-lymphoid tissues[15]. Interestingly, cells of the memory phenotype have been found to accumulate in the afferent lymph[16]. This indicates that at least the memory cells are able to use this alternative pathway from the

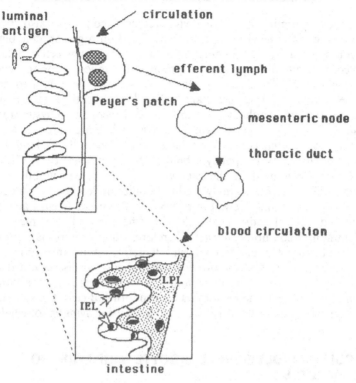

Figure 9.1 Recirculation pathways of precursors of intraepithelial lymphocytes (IEL) and lamina propria lymphocytes (LPL). Naive lymphocytes first encounter antigen and differentiate in the Peyer's patch. These activated lymphocytes then return back to the blood via the lymphatic system. Finally, they reenter the mucosa and home into the lamina propria or into the epithelium

blood to non-lymphoid tissues at vascular beds. In contrast, cells of the naive phenotype accumulate in the efferent lymph, suggesting that their recirculation pathway mainly is from the blood to lymph nodes via HEV[16].

ASSAYS FOR LEUKOCYTE–ENDOTHELIAL CELL INTERACTION

Interaction between the lymphocyte and the vascular endothelial cell is an essential step controlling lymphocyte recirculation and their extravasation to sites of inflammation. Molecular interactions between lymphocytes and HEV can be studied using an *in vitro* assay, originally developed by Stamper and Woodruff[17]. In this assay, lymphocytes are incubated on frozen sections of lymphoid organs. During this incubation, lymphocytes selectively bind to HEV in the tissue. The binding of lymphocytes to HEV in this assay system has been shown to correlate extremely well to the homing capacity of different lymphocyte populations *in vivo*[18]. Development of this HEV-binding assay has been invaluable for human studies because of the experimental limitations inherent in human *in vivo* studies. Using this assay the original observation of non-random homing of lymphocytes has been confirmed also in man. Lymphocyte homing has been shown to be based on organ-specific binding of recirculating cells to HEV in different organs[18,19]. Certain cell populations bind selectively either to peripheral lymph node, mucosal, or to synovial HEV *in vitro*[20,21]. Furthermore, this binding can be inhibited in an organ-specific manner by different antibodies[20,21]. Recently, evidence for the existence of specific lymphocyte–endothelial cell recognition systems in the skin and in the lung-associated lymphatic tissues has been presented[22,23].

Different endothelial cell cultures have been used instead of the frozen section assay to study lymphocyte binding to endothelial cells. HEV cell cultures have been used in the rat system[24,25], whereas umbilical cord endothelial cells have been widely used for studies on leukocyte–endothelial cell interaction in man (reviewed in ref. 26). Furthermore, *in vitro* activation of the umbilical cord endothelial cells with different mediators may mimic the inflammatory conditions *in vivo*. Therefore, valuable information on the regulation of leukocyte–endothelial cell interactions in inflammation can be obtained. These assay systems provide a useful tool to dissect out distinct steps in leukocyte extravasation. In addition to analysis of recognition and stable binding between the leukocytes and endothelial cells, the subsequent transmigration of leukocytes can also be evaluated using living endothelial cells.

MOLECULES INVOLVED IN LEUKOCYTE MIGRATION TO MUCOSAL SITES

As early as the late 1960s it was postulated that lymphocyte homing is dependent on certain sugar-containing receptors on the lymphocyte surface[27]. However, it was not until 1983 that Gallatin and his co-workers[28] reported the MEL-14 antibody that blocked lymphocyte binding to mouse peripheral lymph node HEV *in vitro*, and inhibited lymphocyte homing to peripheral lymph nodes *in vivo*. This was the first direct evidence for the existence of specific molecules mediating lymphocyte binding to HEV. After this initial discovery, several other surface molecules on lymphocytes and endothelial cells have been reported to be important in lymphocyte–HEV interaction in different species[21,29-31]. Similarly, a number of molecules have been shown to be involved in neutrophil binding to normal and/or activated endothelium[32,33]. The leukocyte surface molecules found to play a part in this type of interaction have been called homing receptors, and their organ-specific ligands on endothelial cells have been designated addressins. This nomenclature has turned out to be somewhat misleading for some of the molecules, because these molecules also have other functions (discussed below). Moreover, the nomenclature of these molecules has been very confusing because of their independent identification in several laboratories, and the lack of knowledge on their multifunctional nature at the time when the molecules were named. They should rather be called homing-associated molecules.

Some important molecules involved in leukocyte traffic into mucosal sites have so far been found only in animal species. It is, however, very likely that equivalent molecules will also be discovered in humans; therefore, descriptions of these molecules have been included herein. Some of the molecules presented below are important in mediating leukocyte traffic to sites of inflammation. At mucosal sites their role in mediating leukocyte traffic in inflammatory conditions has not formally been proven. However, due to their general functional nature it is most likely that they also play an important part in mucosa; they have therefore been included in this presentation. In the literature there are reports of still other molecules involved in the process of leukocyte–endothelial cell adhesion. Because the structural characterizations of these molecules are still incomplete, their identity in relation to the known adhesion molecules is unclear; therefore they are not included in this review. The human homing-associated antigens on leukocytes and endothelial cells are listed in Table 9.1 and Table 9.2, respectively.

Homing-associated molecules on leukocytes

Very late activation antigen-4 (VLA-4; CD49d/CD29)

VLA-4 is a member of the integrin family consisting of one α and one β subunit[34]. It shares the β subunit (β-1) with five other VLA proteins. Three different forms of the VLA-4 α subunit have been reported. Molecular weights of these forms are 180, 150 (the main form) and 70/80 kD. VLA-4 is almost exclusively expressed on cells of haematopoietic origin such as peripheral blood lymphocytes, monocytes and thymocytes. Fibroblasts and epithelial cells are usually negative. The involvement of this group of molecules in lymphocyte binding to mucosal HEV was first reported in mouse. Holzmann and Weissman reported[31] that a molecule called lymphocyte Peyer's patch adhesion molecule-1 (LPAM-1) functions as a mouse lymphocyte homing receptor for mucosal HEV. Later, Holzmann and co-workers have shown that LPAM-2 in mouse, and VLA-4 in human, mediate lymphocyte adherence to mucosal endothelium[35]. LPAM-1 shares the α-4 subunit with mouse VLA-4 (LPAM-2), but has a unique beta chain, β-p. Interestingly, not all human α-4 chains are associated with β-1 chains, suggesting that the human equivalent for the mouse β-p may exist.

The known ligands of VLA-4 are the vascular cell adhesion molecule-1 (VCAM-1) on endothelial cells and an extracellular matrix molecule, fibronectin[34,36,37]. Based on inhibition studies using monoclonal antibodies against different epitopes of VLA-4, interactions with these two ligands seem to be mediated via different domains of the VLA-4 molecule[34,37]. It is possible that these interactions are differentially regulated *in vivo* depending on the function required. For example, expression of the domain binding to VCAM-1 may be responsible for the enhanced traffic of lymphocytes to sites of inflammation. When the lymphocyte is inside the lymphoid tissue, interaction with fibronectin via another domain is relevant. It is currently not known whether VCAM-1 is the only ligand for VLA-4 on the endothelial cell surface. Neither is the ligand molecule for the α-4 associated with β-p known. It may well be that α-4/β-p uses different ligands than the α-4/β-1 form. In addition to the homing-associated functions, VLA-4 has also been reported to mediate both heterotypic and homotypic aggregation of lymphocytes[38,39]. To what extent different structural forms of VLA-4 are responsible for these versatile functions needs to be resolved.

CD44 (Hermes, ECMR III, Pgp-1, Hutch-1, In(Lu)-related antigen)

Evidence for the association of CD44 to lymphocyte binding to HEV came from the studies in which the expression of CD44 correlated remarkably well with the HEV-binding capacity of normal lymphocytes and lymphoblastoid cell lines. Moreover, one of the monoclonal antibodies used in the expression studies, Hermes-3, inhibited lymphocyte binding to mucosal HEV and a polyclonal anti-CD44 antibody blocked lymphocyte binding to peripheral lymph node, mucosal and synovial HEV[21]. These inhibition studies suggest that some determinant(s) of the lymphocyte CD44 molecule is involved in organ-specific HEV interactions. Direct evidence for the involvement of the lymphocyte CD44 in HEV binding came from the studies in which purified human lymphocyte CD44 was demonstrated to bind to mouse mucosal addressin, MAd[40]. This interaction could also be inhibited by the Hermes-3 monoclonal antibody. In contrast, CD44 isolated from the epithelial cells failed to bind to MAd, indicating that the presence of the HEV-binding epitope(s) of CD44 is dependent on the cell type. Since these binding studies were performed using MAd of mouse origin, the results suggest that structurally a very similar endothelial ligand molecule also exists in humans.

CD44 is widely expressed on several haematopoietic and non-haematopoietic cell lines[41,42]. It has been described to be involved in several functions including T cell activation, lateral movement of cells, erythrocyte rosetting, and binding to extracellular matrix molecules such as hyaluronate, collagen and fibronectin[43-46] (Jalkanen and Jalkanen, *J. Cell. Biol.*, in press); therefore it is clearly one of the multifunctional homing-associated molecules. CD44 is structurally a very heterogeneous molecule due both to post-translational modifications and different sizes of core proteins. The lymphocyte form of the molecule has the major form of 90 kD and a chondroitin sulphate-containing form yielding the molecular weight of 180–200 kD[47]. Recent studies suggest that the 90 kD form (the Hermes-3 defined region) is involved in lymphocyte–HEV interaction, whereas the chondroitin sulphate side-chains mediate lymphocyte binding to fibronectin when the lymphocyte is inside the lymphatic tissue. Hyaluronate binding that may also occur at the endothelial cell level probably strengthens the adhesion. Some of the divergent functions have been connected to certain structural domains of the molecule. They are illustrated in Fig. 9.2. Despite much knowledge on the properties of CD44, intensive research is still needed to resolve how all the different functional characteristics of CD44 are regulated at the structural level.

Lymphocyte function-associated antigen-1 (LFA-1; CD11a/CD18)

The LFA-1 molecule is an important adhesion molecule in diverse immune functions[33]. It shares a common β-chain (β-2) with other leukocyte integrins (MAC-1 and p150/90). Like MAC-1 and p150/90, LFA-1 is expressed on

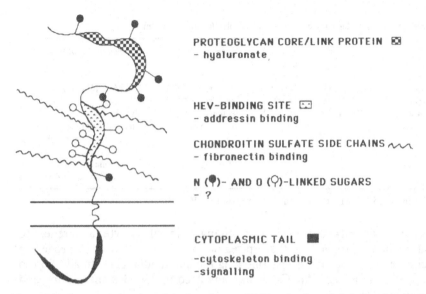

PROTEOGLYCAN CORE/LINK PROTEIN ▨
- hyaluronate,

HEV-BINDING SITE ⊡
- addressin binding

CHONDROITIN SULFATE SIDE CHAINS ∿
- fibronectin binding

N (●)- AND O (♀)-LINKED SUGARS
- ?

CYTOPLASMIC TAIL ■

-cytoskeleton binding
-signalling

Figure 9.2 Structural domains of the lymphocyte CD44 molecule and their functional roles. The structure is based on the data reported by Goldstein *et al.*[48] and Stamenkovic *et al.*[49]

monocytes and polymorphonuclear leukocytes, but it is the only leukocyte integrin that is significantly expressed on lymphocytes[33]. In lymphocyte–HEV interaction, LFA-1 may play an adhesion-strengthening role in a non-organ-specific fashion[50,51]. The known ligands for LFA-1 are the intercellular adhesion molecules (ICAM-1 and ICAM-2)[33]. Whether they also serve as ligands for LFA-1 on non-inflamed HEV is not known. The importance of leukocyte integrins in leukocyte extravasation is clearly illustrated in patients whose cells do not express this group of molecules due to defects in the synthesis of the β-chain. These patients suffer from life-threatening infections and die at an early age, because especially their neutrophils are not capable of entering the inflammation sites.

MAC-1 (CD11b/CD18, CR3)

MAC-1 is expressed mainly on granulocytes and monocytes[26]. Like LFA-1, it is an important adhesion molecule, but has a much larger ligand repertoire including at least iC3b, factor X, leishmania gp63, zymosan and fibrinogen[33,52]. ICAM-1 may serve as its endothelial cell ligand[26]. MAC-1 is an important molecule mediating neutrophil and monocyte adherence to activated endothelium at sites of inflammation, and it may also participate in the subsequent transmigration. The main function of MAC-1 may be to cement the neutrophil adhesion after the first recognition via other molecules, and it is possibly not involved in the initial recognition at all[53]. Neutrophil activation leads to an increased expression of MAC-1. In experimental conditions, expression of MAC-1 can be induced up to 10-fold by phorbol esters and chemoattractants[26]. However, the increased expression of MAC-1

Table 9.1 Human leukocyte adhesion molecules for endothelium

Molecule	CD	Molecular weight (kD)	Family	Ligands on endothelium
LFA-1	CD11a/18	180/95	Integrin ($\alpha^L/\beta2$)	ICAM-1, ICAM-2
Mac-1	CD11b/18	160/95	Integrin ($\alpha^M/\beta2$)	ICAM-1
VLA-4	CD49d/29	150/130	Integrin ($\alpha4/\beta1$)	VCAM-1
LECAM-1[a]		90	LECCAM	Charged (sulphate, phosphate NeuNac) oligosaccharides with fucose?
Hermes	CD44	90	Proteoglycan	Hyaluronate, human equivalent of MAd?

[a] Not involved in lymphocyte binding to mucosal HEV

may not directly correlate with changes in phagocyte adherence to endothelium[26], suggesting that up-regulation of MAC-1 may be needed to facilitate the subsequent steps following the initial adherence. In addition to phagocyte adherence, MAC-1 is also involved in complement binding and phagocytosis[52].

ENDOTHELIAL CELL LIGANDS FOR LEUKOCYTE RECEPTORS

Mucosal vascular addressin (MAd)

MAd was the first organ-specific endothelial cell ligand described. The role of MAd as a mucosal endothelial cell ligand for the lymphocyte homing receptor(s) has been demonstrated both *in vitro* and *in vivo*[54]. MECA-367, a monoclonal antibody against the MAd, inhibits mouse lymphocyte binding to Peyer's patch HEV in the frozen section assay, and blocks the homing of small lymphocytes to Peyer's patches almost completely *in vivo*. In contrast, MECA-367 does not have any effect on lymphocyte binding to peripheral lymph node HEV, or on homing to peripheral lymph nodes[54]. The human equivalent for the MAd has not yet been found.

Expression of MAd is developmentally regulated. In normal adult mice the MAd is selectively expressed on HEV in Peyer's patches and on flat-walled venules in the lamina propria[54]. Moreover, venules in the lactating mammary gland stain positively with the anti-MAd antibodies[54]. Interestingly, at birth also the venules in peripheral lymph nodes express the MAd. The expression gradually decreases, and the adult pattern is reached at the age of 4–6 weeks[55]. Wide expression of the MAd in infancy may be significant for the development of immunity, because it allows distribution of the antigen-activated cells from the mucosal sites to the lymphoid organs throughout the body.

Intercellular adhesion molecules (ICAM-1 and ICAM-2)

These molecules belong to the immunoglobulin superfamily and are important ligands for LFA-1[33,56]. ICAM-1 is normally expressed on some lymphocytes, monocytes and vascular endothelium (Fig. 9.3), but its expression can be up-regulated by inflammatory mediators on a wide variety of cells[33]. ICAM-2 is a truncated form of ICAM-1 with only two variable domains instead of the five domains present in ICAM-1[57]. ICAM-2 is basally expressed on endothelial cells and its expression cannot be up-regulated by cytokines[33]. Both these ICAMs mediate lymphocyte binding to human umbilical vein endothelial cells. Although it is very likely that they also function as ligands for LFA-1 on mucosal endothelium, their role in lymphocyte homing to mucosal sites has not yet been demonstrated. Interestingly, ICAM-1 also functions as a virus receptor mediating the entrance of the rhinovirus into the cells[33].

Vascular cell adhesion molecule-1 (VCAM-1; INCAM-110)

VCAM-1, the endothelial cell ligand for VLA-4, is expressed on cytokine-stimulated endothelial cells *in vitro*. Lipopolysaccharide and cytokines such as interleukin-1 and tumour necrosis factor-α up-regulate its expression[58]. *In vivo*, VCAM-1 is highly expressed on dendritic cells in a variety of lymphoid tissues, on arterial endothelium and on small vessels[59]. Interestingly, only some postcapillary venules are positive with anti-VCAM-1 antibodies, suggesting the possibility that on endothelial cells other ligands for VLA-4 may exist.

Endothelial leukocyte adhesion molecule-1 (ELAM-1; LECAM-2)

ELAM-1 belongs to the LEC-CAM family together with the peripheral lymph node homing receptor (LAM-1, MEL-14, Leu-8, TQ1, LECAM-1) and GMP-140 (LECAM-3)[60], a protein of endothelial cells and platelets. An interesting structural feature of these molecules is that they all contain a lectin-like domain. This lectin-binding domain is most likely crucial for adhesion. Recent reports from independent laboratories have shown that the receptor for ELAM-1 may contain the sialyl-Lewis X carbohydrate determinant[60]. ELAM-1 is present only on activated endothelium both *in vitro* and *in vivo*[61]. Its expression can be up-regulated by inflammatory mediators such as interleukin-1 and tumour necrosis factor-α. Most reports have described ELAM-1 as an adhesion ligand for monocytes and neutrophils[32]. However, *in vitro* experiments suggest that it may also mediate binding of T cells to the endothelium[62].

HECA-452

HECA-452 antigen was originally identified as a marker for HEV in organized lymphoid tissues[63]. For example, it is highly expressed on venules in large bowel specimens. It is also induced on vascular endothelium in non-lymphoid organs infiltrated by large numbers of lymphocytes[63]. Although HECA-452

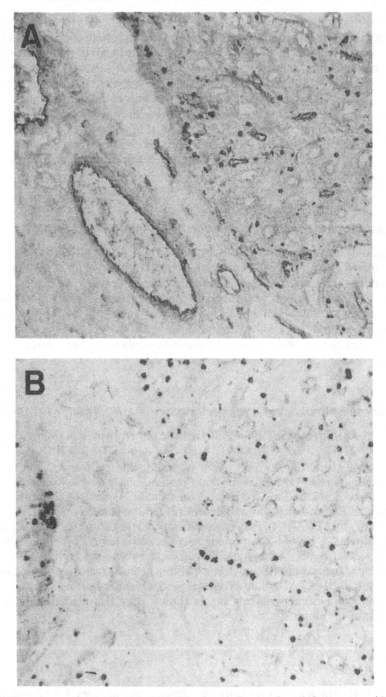

Figure 9.3 Phenotype of the vessels in the lamina propria of a normal gut. **A**: Immunoperoxidase staining with anti-Factor VIII antibody showing all the vessels in the area; **B**: all the vessels are negative with an anti-ELAM-1 antibody; **C**: Some of the vessels show positive staining with a monoclonal antibody against ICAM-1 (arrows). ×100

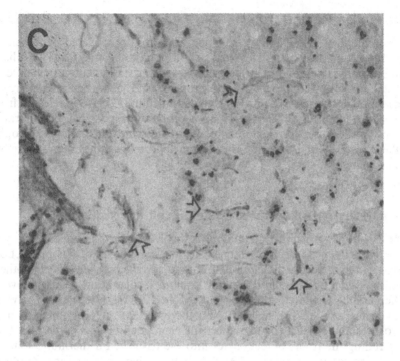

Figure 9.3 (*Contd*)

may serve as a useful tool for identification of the venules mediating lymphocyte homing, its direct role as an endothelial cell ligand for the lymphocyte homing receptors has not been proven. Moreover, it is also expressed on the cells belonging to the myeloid and monocyte/macrophage lineages. Recently, HECA-452 has been described to be specifically expressed on the lymphocytes migrating into the skin[64]. The structural properties of this molecule are not well known.

MHC Class II and LFA-3

MHC Class II and LFA-3 molecules have been described to mediate lymphocyte adherence to endothelium[65-67]. However, MHC Class II is not constitutively expressed on endothelial cells, and therefore cannot play a role in HEV-mediated homing of lymphocytes. On the other hand, endothelial cells can be induced to express MHC Class II by interferon-γ. Activated endothelial cells then can present antigen in an MHC-restricted manner both to resting and to antigen-specific T cells[67]. Endothelial LFA-3 may also be involved in this antigen presentation by binding to its ligand, CD2, on the T lymphocyte. Interaction based on antigen presentation between T cells and endothelial cells may be critical in mediating the migration of antigen-specific helper T cells into the tissue at sites of inflammation.

Granule membrane protein (GMP-140; CD62, LECAM-3, PADGEM)

Involvement of GMP-140 in neutrophil binding to activated endothelium has been suggested by studies in which antibodies against GMP-140 have inhibited this interaction between leukocytes and endothelium (reviewed in ref. 26). Various activators such as thrombin and leukotrienes cause rapid (<30 min) adherence of neutrophils to endothelium. GMP-140 released from the storage granules in minutes is very probably responsible for this rapid adhesion, because up-regulation of other molecules mediating neutrophil adherence (ELAM-1 and ICAM-1) requires protein synthesis, and therefore takes longer.

Complexity of leukocyte–endothelial cell interaction

The constantly growing list of molecules involved in the binding of leukocytes to endothelial cells clearly demonstrates the complexity of this interaction. Some of the molecules function in an organ-specific manner, whereas others mediate binding in a more general fashion. Cooperation between several differentially regulated molecules is required for stable binding between leukocytes and endothelial cells. Furthermore, at sites of inflammation, cytokines and other mediators affect the expression of these molecules, thus controlling the traffic of leukocytes into the tissue[68]. Furthermore, some of the molecules are up-regulated extremely fast, whereas appearance of others may take several hours or even days. This may critically determine the cell composition seen at sites of inflammation at various time points. Locally, the vascular endothelium is the target for that type of regulation; it may therefore be the key factor in controlling the non-random cell migration. Thus, the endothelial cells in different locations may express different numbers

Table 9.2 Human endothelial adhesion molecules for leukocytes

Molecule	CD	Molecular weight (kD)	Family	Mucosa	Basal	Upreg.	Ligand(s)	Cells
ICAM-1	CD54	100	Ig	+	+	+	LFA-1, MAC-1	L,G,M
ICAM-2		55	Ig	?	+	−	LFA-1	L,G,M
VCAM-1		100	Ig	+	+	+	VLA-4	L,M
ELAM-1		115	LECCAM	+	−	+	sialyl-Le^x	G,M,L?
GMP-140	CD62	140	LECCAM	?	−[a]	+	LNF III (CD15)	G,M

Ig, immunoglobulin superfamily; LECCAM, leukocyte endothelial cell adhesion molecules, or selectin family; mucosa, expressed on endothelium at mucosal sites; basal, expression on normal, unstimulated endothelium; upreg., expression upregulated by inflammatory mediators; sialyl-Le^x, sialyl-Lewis X (NeuNacα2-3Galβ1-4(Fucα1-3)GlcNac); LNF III, lacto-N-fucopentaose III (Galβ1-4(Fucα1-3)GlcNacβ1-3Galβ1–4Glc); ligand(s), leukocyte ligands of the endothelial adhesion molecule; cells, ligand cell types; L, lymphocytes; G, granulocytes; M, monocytes
[a] Present in storage granules in endothelial cells

of organ-specific and common endothelial cell adhesion molecules comple-
mentary to a set of homing-associated cell surface molecules specific for each
leukocyte subset.

PHENOTYPE AND FUNCTION OF VENULES AT MUCOSAL SITES

Lymphocytes enter the mucosal sites using two morphologically different
types of venules. Entrance into the Peyer's patches and the appendix occur
via HEV, whereas the lymphocytes enter the lamina propria via flat-walled
venules that function in an HEV-like manner[69]. It is not currently known
whether the flat-walled venules are functionally identical with HEV in
organized mucosal lymphoid tissues or whether they have – besides common
properties – some unique ones that selectively direct the traffic of certain
lymphocyte populations into the lamina propria instead of the Peyer's
patches. The recent phenotypic analyses speak for similarities between the
venules, because the flat-walled venules in the lamina propria bear the same
mucosal addressin as the Peyer's patch HEV, and so far no homing-associated
antigens discriminating these morphologically different types of venules have
been found. Functionally, this issue is difficult to study, especially in humans,
because the frozen section assay widely used to study molecular interactions
between lymphocytes and HEV encounters specific problems when binding
to lamina propria vessels is studied. For example, lymphocyte binding to
flat-walled venules is difficult to assess due to the excessive background
adhesion to other structures in the lamina propria. Also confident identification
of the thin-walled vessels might sometimes be troublesome in frozen sections
of the lamina propria in the assay conditions. Therefore, we chose Peyer's
patch and appendix HEV to study the binding of lamina propria lymphocyte
populations[70]. The results of these studies provided further evidence for
similarities between the HEV and the flat-walled venules in functional means
also. The normal lamina propria immunoblasts (IgA-positive blasts and T
cell blasts) bound extremely well to HEV in Peyer's patches and appendix,
but did not bind at all to HEV in peripheral lymph nodes. One interpretation
of these results is that the immunoblasts have recently entered the lamina
propria *in vivo* using the same molecules as they now in this *in vitro* assay
use for binding to appendix/Peyer's patch HEV. It is also possible that these
cells bear two sets of receptors. One is for binding to HEV in Peyer's patches
and the other one is for binding to flat-walled endothelium in the lamina
propria. On the basis of *in vivo* murine studies the MAd is responsible for
the traffic of gut-homing blasts both to the Peyer's patches and the lamina
propria, but additional mechanisms, not yet identified, may exist[53]. Whether
the mechanisms are similar for binding to endothelium in the Peyer's patches
and in the lamina propria remains to be determined. It is also possible that
other factors such as chemotaxis and interactions with microenvironmental
elements contribute to the final distribution of lymphocyte subsets observed
in vivo.

LEUKOCYTE MIGRATION IN INTESTINAL DISEASES

In inflammatory conditions, such as in ulcerative colitis and Crohn's disease, the number of lymphocytes in inflamed areas may increase up to four-fold[71]. Also the normal predominance of IgA-secreting cells disappears and the cells secrete mainly IgG. In Crohn's disease especially elevated secretion of IgG2 is observed, whereas in ulcerative colitis IgG1 and IgG3 production is significantly increased[71]. Moreover, the typical mucosal IgA production pattern, consisting mainly of polymeric IgA and subclass 2, shifts to the systemic type monomeric IgA1 production[71]. Besides lymphocytes, inflammatory infiltrates contain monocytes and macrophages. Large numbers of polymorphonuclear leukocytes also extravasate into the inflamed mucosa and submucosa. The increased traffic of leukocytes partly depends on

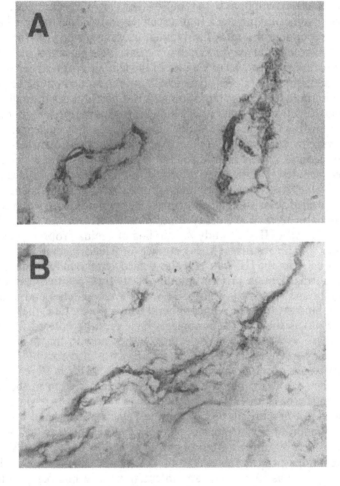

Figure 9.4 Phenotype of the vessels in the lamina propria affected by Crohn's disease. The vessels are brightly positive with antibodies against ELAM-1 (**A**) and ICAM-1 (**B**). ×400

secretion of inflammatory mediators in the area, which up-regulate certain adhesion molecules on vascular endothelial cells. Such endothelial cell molecules include at least ICAM-1 and ELAM-1, as shown in Fig. 9.4. It is very likely that other molecules, some of which have not yet been identified, may also be involved in the process of leukocyte extravasation. Appearance of new molecules not normally expressed on endothelial cells may allow the entrance of cells that would not be able to home to non-inflamed mucosal tissues. This idea is supported by phenotypic analyses of cells found in the inflamed areas and also our own binding studies (Salmi *et al.*, manuscript in preparation). We have found that the HEV-binding properties of lamina propria cells of patients suffering from inflammatory bowel diseases are different from those of normal lamina propria cells. Small lymphocytes have partially lost their preferential binding to mucosal tissues, and some large immunoblasts also bind – unlike normal lamina propria immunoblasts – to peripheral lymph node HEV. The situation may be analogous to that described by Rose *et al.*[6] They found that lymphoblasts originating from peripheral lymph nodes do not migrate into the non-inflamed gut. However, in inflammation caused by *Trichinella spiralis* the same cells were able to home into the intestine. Homing of the cells not normally present in the lamina propria to mucosal sites may be largely responsible for the immunopathological phenomena seen in inflammatory bowel diseases. Accumulation of cells in the tissue is clearly dependent on the input of leukocytes, but it may be also regulated by decreased output of leukocytes. These distinct steps are most probably regulated independently. Mechanisms controlling the output of cells are largely unknown.

Inflammatory and infectious bowel diseases are sometimes complicated by extraintestinal manifestations such as arthritis, skin lesions and eye symptoms. In our studies we found that both normal and inflamed gut contains immunoblasts that are able to bind to HEV in inflamed synovium. These types of binding properties may have clinical importance, because it is theoretically possible that the same pathogen or antigen first enters the gut, and thereafter gets trapped in, or is transported into, the synovial tissue. In this case the antigen-activated blasts from the mucosal tissues that also have the synovial homing receptor(s) would be able to home either to the mucosal sites or to the synovial tissue. Antigen-activated blasts would then, inside the synovium, be extremely effective in starting the immune response against their cognate antigen. If the antigen persists[72], or crossreactive host antigens are present, the situation can become chronic, with all the consequences. The immunopathogenetic mechanisms may be analogous in other extraintestinal manifestations. A schematic model of the recirculation routes in infectious bowel diseases with extraintestinal manifestations is presented in Fig. 9.5.

Lymphocyte infiltrates are also found in the intestine of patients suffering from coeliac disease or dermatitis herpetiformis. In duodenal biopsies obtained from these patients all the infiltrating leukocytes bear the CD44 antigen[73]. ICAM-1 is expressed on infiltrating plasma cells and endothelial cells. The level of expression seems to depend on the extent of inflammation[73]. In contrast, anti-HECA-452 antibody, a marker for the vessels mediating lymphocyte traffic, does not stain any vessels in the duodenal area despite

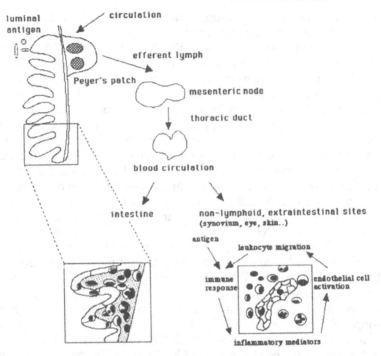

Figure 9.5 A schematic model describing the development of extraintestinal manifestations after infectious bowel diseases. Freely recirculating lymphocytes encounter a mucosal pathogen, after which they differentiate in the microenvironment of Peyer's patches and become antigen-specific. From the Peyer's patches these cells drain into the intestinal lymphatics, pass through the mesenteric lymph nodes and enter the thoracic duct and the blood circulation. The same pathogen or its antigenic fractions have entered the extraintestinal tissues as a free antigen, in the form of immune complexes, or inside the cells. Because the antigen-activated lymphocytes also have homing receptors for binding to HEV in these organs (shown in the case of the synovium), they can leave the blood, besides in the mucosal lymphoid tissues, also in the extraintestinal sites as, for example, in the synovium. The inflammation is initiated by a specific pathogen, but can be continued by immune response against crossreactive host antigens

heavy lymphocytic infiltrations, even though it nicely stains the vessels in large bowel samples of non-inflamed gut and in biopsies obtained from the gut affected by inflammatory bowel diseases[73]. These findings suggest that CD44 and ICAM-1 may be involved in lymphocyte traffic to the duodenal area. Moreover, HECA-452 is not a prerequisite for lymphocyte extravasation into the duodenum, and venules mediating lymphocyte traffic are not antigenically identical in all mucosal sites.

DIAGNOSTIC AND THERAPEUTIC IMPLICATIONS BASED ON LEUKOCYTE TRAFFIC

Lymphocyte recirculation can be utilized to study immune responses at certain areas of the body. The method is based on the migration of mucosal lymphocytes. The activated cells are captured from the blood on their way back to the mucosal sites, and their antibody production is investigated *in vitro*. This approach has been successfully used to study the mucosal immune responses to oral vaccinations[74]. It may also be applicable for studies on the persistence of microbial antigens during mucosal infections.

Another fascinating field based on leukocyte extravasation is the development of anti-adhesion therapy to inhibit harmful leukocyte migration. Since the initial binding of leukocytes to endothelial cells is the prerequisite for their extravasation, inhibition of leukocyte adherence will prevent the tissue damage. If we take inflammatory bowel diseases and other chronic inflammations into consideration it is possible to target either the migrating lymphocytes with specific antibodies or ligand analogues, or the endothelial cell surface ligands with the small inhibitory molecules mimicking the receptor. Theoretically, the easiest approach would probably be to develop drugs that make the endothelial cell ligands non-functional. Before such a therapy can be applied to patient care a considerable amount of research is needed to resolve the complex regulation mechanisms of leukocyte–endothelial cell interactions.

CONCLUSION

Several molecules have been described to mediate leukocyte binding to endothelial cells. They include molecules that control the entrance of recirculating lymphocytes from the blood into the mucosal tissues. Others are inflammation-induced molecules that mediate traffic of granulocytes, monocytes and also lymphocytes into the tissue in inflammatory conditions. The first set of molecules is important in determining the unique characteristics of normal mucosal immune responses, and the second set is responsible for the immunopathological features seen, for example, in infectious and inflammatory bowel diseases. Studies of these molecules have increased our understanding on the mechanisms behind the phenomena described in animal models more than 25 years ago. They have also provided future views for invention of therapeutic agents that would allow manipulation of the homing-associated molecules, and thus the nature of local inflammatory responses.

Acknowledgements

We wish to thank all our colleagues who have participated in our original work summarized here, and especially Dr Haskard for providing anti-ELAM-1 and anti-ICAM-1 antibodies used for staining of the gut specimens in Figs 9.3 and 9.4. Our work has been supported by grants from the Finnish Academy, the Finnish Cancer Foundation, the Sigrid Juselius Foundation, and the Yrjö Jahnsson Foundation.

References

1. Brandtzaeg, P., Halstensen, T. S., Kett, K., Krajci, P., Kvale, D., Rognum, T. O., Scott, H. and Sollid, L. M. (1989). Immunobiology and immunopathology of human gut mucosa: humoral immunity and intraepithelial lymphocytes. *Gastroenterology*, **97**, 1562–84
2. Mowat, A. McI. (1990). Human intraepithelial lymphocytes. *Springer Sem. Immunopathol.*, **12**, 165–90
3. Gowans, J. L. and Knight, E. J. (1964). The route of recirculation of lymphocytes in the rat. *Proc. R. Soc. Lond.*, **159**, 257–82
4. Griscelli, C., Vassalli, P. and McCluskey, R. T. (1969). The distribution of large dividing lymph node cells in syngeneic recipient rats after intravenous injection. *J. Exp. Med.*, **130**, 1427–42
5. Parrott, D. M. V. and Ferguson, A. (1974). Selective migration of lymphocytes within the mouse small intestine. *Immunology*, **26**, 571–88
6. Rose, M. L., Parrott, D. M. V. and Bruce, R. G. (1976). Migration of lymphoblasts to the small intestine. II. Divergent migration of mesenteric and peripheral immunoblasts to sites of inflammation in the mouse. *Cell. Immunol.*, **27**, 36–46
7. Chin, W. and Hay, J. B. (1980). A comparison of lymphocyte migration through intestinal lymph nodes, subcutaneous lymph nodes, and chronic inflammatory sites of sheep. *Gastroenterology*, **79**, 1231–42
8. Anderson, A. O. and Anderson, N. D. (1976). Lymphocyte emigration from high endothelial venules in rat lymph nodes. *Immunology*, **31**, 731–48
9. Mestecky, J. (1987). The common mucosal immune system and current strategies for induction of immune responses in external secretions. *J. Clin. Immunol.*, **7**, 265–75
10. Bienenstock, J., McDermott, M., Befus, D. and O'Neill, M. (1978). A common mucosal immunological system involving the bronchus, breast and bowel. *Adv. Exp. Med. Biol.*, **107**, 53–9
11. Ferguson, A. and Parrott, D. M. V. (1972). The effect of antigen deprivation on thymus-dependent and thymus-independent lymphocytes in the small intestine of the mouse. *Clin. Exp. Immunol.*, **12**, 477–88
12. Spencer, J., Dillon, S. B. and MacDonald, T. T. (1986). T cell subclasses in fetal human ileum. *Clin. Exp. Immunol.*, **65**, 553–8
13. Bonneville, M., Itohara, S., Krecko, E. G., Mombaerts, P., Ishida, I., Katsuki, M., Berns, A., Farr, A. G., Janeway, C. A. and Tonegawa, S. (1990). Transgenic mice demonstrate that epithelial homing of gamma/delta T cells is determined by cell lineages independent of T cell receptor specificity. *J. Exp. Med.*, **171**, 1015–26
14. Marsh, M. N. (1975). Studies of intestinal lymphoid tissue. II. Aspects of proliferation and migration of epithelial lymphocytes in the small intestine of mice. *Gut*, **16**, 674–82
15. Mackay, C. R., Kimpton, W. G., Brandon, M. R. and Cahill, R. N. P. (1988). Lymphocyte subsets show marked differences in their distribution between blood and the afferent and efferent lymph of peripheral lymph nodes. *J. Exp. Med.*, **167**, 1755–65
16. Mackay, C. R., Marston, W. and Dudler, L. (1990). Naive and memory T cells show distinct pathways of lymphocyte recirculation. *J. Exp. Med.*, **171**, 801–17
17. Stamper, H. B. and Woodruff, J. J. (1976). Lymphocyte homing into lymph nodes: In vitro demonstration of the selective affinity of recirculating lymphocytes for high-endothelial venules. *J. Exp. Med.*, **144**, 828–33
18. Butcher, E. C. (1986). The regulation of lymphocyte traffic. *Curr. Top. Microbiol. Immunol.*, **128**, 85–122
19. Butcher, E. C., Scollay, R. G. and Weissman, I. L. (1980). Organ specificity of lymphocyte migration: mediation by highly selective lymphocyte interaction with organ-specific determinants on high endothelial venules. *Eur. J. Immunol.*, **10**, 556–61
20. Jalkanen, S., Steere, A. C., Fox, R. I. and Butcher, E. C. (1986). A distinct endothelial cell recognition system that controls lymphocyte traffic into inflamed synovium. *Science*, **233**, 556–8
21. Jalkanen, S., Bargatze, R. F., de los Toyos, J. and Butcher, E. C. (1987). Lymphocyte recognition of high endothelium: Antibodies to distinct epitopes of an 85-95 kD glycoprotein antigen differentially inhibit lymphocyte binding to lymph node, mucosal, or synovial endothelial cells. *J. Cell. Biol.*, **105**, 983–90
22. Sackstein, R., Falanga, V., Streilein, J. W. and Chin, Y.-H. (1988). Lymphocyte adhesion to psoriatic dermal endothelium is mediated by a tissue-specific receptor/ligand interaction. *J. Invest. Dermatol.*, **91**, 423–8

23. Geoffroy, J. S., Yednock, T. A., Curtis, J. L. and Rosen, S. D. (1988). Evidence for a distinct lymphocyte homing specificity involved in lymphocyte migration to lung-associated lymph nodes. *FASEB J.*, **2**, A667

24. Ager, A. and Mistry, S. (1988). Interaction between lymphocytes and cultured high endothelial cells: an in vitro model of lymphocyte migration across high endothelial venule endothelium. *Eur. J. Immunol.*, **18**, 1265–74

25. Ise, Y., Yamaguchi, K., Sato, K., Yamamura, Y., Kitamura, F., Tamatani, T. and Miyasaka, M. (1988). Molecular mechanisms underlying lymphocyte recirculation. I. Functional, phenotypical and morphological characterization of high endothelial cells cultured in vitro. *Eur. J. Immunol.*, **18**, 1235–44

26. Carlos, T. M. and Harlan, J. M. (1990). Membrane proteins involved in phagocyte adherence to endothelium. *Immunol. Rev.*, **114**, 5–28

27. Woodruff, J. J. and Gesner, M. (1969). The effect of neuraminidase on the fate of transfused lymphocytes. *J. Exp. Med.*, **129**, 551–62

28. Gallatin, W. M., Butcher, E. C. and Weissman, I. L. (1983). A cell surface molecule involved in organ-specific homing of lymphocytes. *Nature*, **304**, 30–4

29. Chin, Y. H., Rasmussen, R. A., Woodruff, J. J. and Easton, T. G. (1986). A monoclonal anti-HEBFpp antibody with specificity for lymphocyte surface molecules mediating adhesion to Peyer's patch high endothelium of the rat. *J. Immunol.*, **136**, 2556–61

30. Kraal, G., Twisk, A., Tan, B. and Scheper, R. (1986). A surface molecule on guinea pig lymphocytes involved in adhesion and homing. *Eur. J. Immunol.*, **16**, 1515–19

31. Holzmann, B. and Weissman, I. L. (1989). Integrin molecules involved in lymphocyte homing to Peyer's patches. *Immunol. Rev.*, **108**, 45–61

32. Osborn, L. (1990). Leukocyte adhesion to endothelium in inflammation. *Cell*, **62**, 3–6

33. Springer, T. A. (1990). Adhesion receptors of the immune system. *Nature*, **346**, 425–34

34. Hemler, M. E., Elices, M. J., Parker, C. and Takada, Y. (1990). Structure of the integrin VLA-4 and its cell–cell and cell–matrix adhesion functions. *Immunol. Rev.*, **114**, 46–65

35. Holzmann, B., McIntyre, B. W. and Weissman, I. L. (1989). Identification of a murine Peyer's patch-specific lymphocyte homing receptor as an integrin molecule with an alfa chain homologous to human VLA-4 alfa. *Cell*, **56**, 37–46

36. Wayner, E. A., Carcia-Pardo, A., Humpries, M. J., McDonald, J. A. and Carter, W. G. (1989). Identification and characterization of the T lymphocyte adhesion receptor for an alternative cell attachment domain (CS-1) in plasma fibronectin. *J. Cell Biol.*, **109**, 1321–30

37. Elices, M., Osborn, L., Takada, Y., Crouse, C., Luhowskyj, S., Hemler, M. E. and Lobb, R. R. (1990). VCAM-1 on activated endothelium interacts with the leukocyte integrin VLA-4 at a site distinct from the VLA-4/fibronectin binding site. *Cell*, **60**, 577–84

38. Clayberger, C., Krensky, A., McIntyre, B. W., Koller, T. S., Parham, P., Brodsky, F., Linn, D. J. and Evans, E. L. (1987). Identification and characterization of two novel lymphocyte function-associated antigens, L24 and L25. *J. Immunol.*, **138**, 1510–14

39. Campanero, M. R., Pulido, R., Ursa, M. A., Rodriquez-Moya, M., de Landazuri, M. O. and Sanchez-Madrid, F. (1990). An alternative leukocyte homotypic adhesion mechanism, LFA-1/ICAM-1-independent, triggered through the human VLA-4 integrin. *J. Cell Biol.*, **110**, 324–32

40. Berg, E. L., Goldstein, L. A., Jutila, M. A., Nakache, M., Picker, L. J., Streeter, P. R., Wu, N., Zhou, D. and Butcher, E. C. (1989). Homing receptors and vascular addressins: cell adhesion molecules that direct lymphocyte traffic. *Immunol. Rev.*, **108**, 5–18

41. Picker, L. J., Nakache, M. and Butcher, E. C. (1989). Monoclonal antibodies to human lymphocyte homing receptors define a novel class of adhesion molecules on diverse cell types. *J. Cell Biol.*, **109**, 927–38

42. Kansas, G. S., Wood, G. and Dailey, M. O. (1989). A family of cell-surface glycoproteins defined by a putative anti-endothelial cell receptor antibody in man. *J. Immunol.*, **142**, 3050–7

43. Haynes, B. F., Telen, M. J., Hale, L. P. and Denning, S. M. (1989). CD44 – a molecule involved in leukocyte adherence and T-cell activation. *Immunol. Today*, **10**, 423–8

44. Carter, W. G. and Wayner, E. A. (1988). Characterization of the class III collagen receptor, a phosphorylated, transmembrane glycoprotein expressed in nucleated human cells. *J. Biol. Chem.*, **263**, 4193–4201

45. Aruffo, A., Stamenkovic, I., Melnick, M., Underhill, C. B. and Seed, B. (1990). CD44 is the principal cell surface receptor for hyaluronate. *Cell*, **61**, 1303–13

46. Jacobson, K., O'Dell, D. and August, T. J. (1984). Lateral diffusion of an 80,000-dalton glycoprotein in the plasma membrane of murine fibroblasts: relationships to cell structure and function. J. Cell. Biol., 99, 1624–33

47. Jalkanen, S., Jalkanen, M., Bargatze, R. F., Tammi, M. and Butcher, E. C. (1988). Biochemical properties of glycoproteins involved in lymphocyte recognition of high endothelial venules in man. J. Immunol., 141, 1615–23

48. Goldstein, L. A., Zhou, D. F. H., Picker, L. J., Minty, C. N., Bargatze, R. F., Ding, J. F. and Butcher, E. C. (1989). A human lymphocyte homing receptor, the Hermes antigen is related to cartilage proteoglycan core and link proteins. Cell, 56, 1063–72

49. Stamenkovic, I., Amiot, M., Pesando, J. M. and Seed, B. (1989). A lymphocyte molecule implicated in lymph node homing is a member of the cartilage link protein family. Cell, 56, 1057–62

50. Hamann, A., Jablonski-Westrich, D., Duijvestijn, A. M., Butcher, E. C., Baisch, H., Harder, R. and Thiele, H. G. (1988). Evidence for an accessory role of LFA-1 in lymphocyte-high endothelium interaction during homing. J. Immunol., 140, 693–9

51. Pals, S. T., den Otter, A., Miedema, F., Kabel, P., Keizer, G. D., Scheper, R. J. and Meijer, C. J. L. M. (1988). Evidence that leukocyte function-associated antigen-1 is involved in recirculation and homing of human lymphocytes via high endothelial venules. J. Immunol., 140, 1851–3

52. Albelda, S. M. and Buck, C. A. (1990). Integrins and other cell adhesion molecules. FASEB J., 4, 2868–80

53. Butcher, E. C. (1990). Cellular and molecular mechanisms that direct leukocyte traffic. Am. J. Pathol., 136, 3–11

54. Streeter, P. R., Berg, E. L., Rouse, B. T. N. and Butcher, E. C. (1988). A tissue-specific endothelial cell molecule involved in lymphocyte homing. Nature, 331, 41–6

55. Streeter, P. R. and Butcher, E. C. (1988). Developmental alterations in the spatial distribution of tissue specific endothelial cell differentiation antigens involved in lymphocyte homing. J. Cell. Biol., 107, 553A

56. Dustin, M. L. and Springer, T. A. (1988). Lymphocyte function-associated antigen-1 (LFA-1) interaction with intercellular adhesion molecule (ICAM-1) is one of at least three mechanisms for lymphocyte adhesion to cultured endothelial cells. J. Cell. Biol., 107, 321–9

57. Staunton, D. E., Dustin, M. L. and Springer, T. A. (1989). Functional cloning of ICAM-2 cell adhesion ligand for LFA-1 homologous to ICAM-1. Nature, 339, 61–4

58. Wellicome, S. M., Thornhill, M. H., Pitzalis, C., Thomas, D. S., Lanchbury, J. S. S., Panayi, G. S. and Haskard, D. O. (1990). A monoclonal antibody that detects a novel antigen on endothelial cells that is induced by tumor necrosis factor, IL-1, or lipopolysaccharide. J. Immunol., 144, 2558–65

59. Rice, G. E. and Bevilacqua, M. P. (1989). An inducible endothelial cell surface glycoprotein mediates melanoma adhesion. Science, 246, 1303–5

60. Brandley, B. K., Swiedler, S. J. and Robbins, P. W. (1990). Carbohydrate ligands of the LEC cell adhesion molecules. Cell, 63, 861–3

61. Cotran, R., Gimborne, Jr, M. A., Bevilacqua, M. P., Mendrik, D. L. and Pober, J. S. (1986). Induction and detection of a human endothelial activation antigen in vivo. J. Exp. Med., 164, 661–5

62. Graber, N., Venkat Copal, T., Wilson, D., Beall, L. D., Polte, T. and Newman, W. (1990). T cells bind to cytokine-activated endothelium via novel inducible sialoglycoprotein and endothelial leukocyte adhesion molecule-1. J. Immunol., 145, 819–30

63. Duijvestijn, A. M., Horst, E., Pals, S. T., Rouse, B. N., Steere, A. C., Picker, L. J., Meijer, C. J. L. M. and Butcher, E. C. (1988). High endothelial differentiation in human lymphoid and inflammatory tissues defined by monoclonal antibody HECA-452. Am. J. Pathol., 130, 147–55

64. Picker, L. J., Terstappen, L., Rott, L. S., Streeter, P. R., Stein, H. and Butcher, E. C. (1990). Differential expression of homing-associated adhesion molecules by T cell subsets in man. J. Immunol., 145, 3247–55

65. Manolios, N., Geczy, C. and Schrieber, L. (1988). Anti-Ia monoclonal antibody (10-2.16) inhibits lymphocyte-high endothelial venule (HEV) interaction. Cell. Immunol., 117, 152–61

66. Masuyama, J., Minato, N. and Kano, S. (1986). Mechanisms of lymphocyte adhesion to human vascular endothelial cells in culture. T lymphocyte adhesion to endothelial cells

through endothelial HLA-DR antigens induced by gamma interferon. *J. Clin. Invest.*, 7, 1596–1601

67. Hughes, C. C. W., Savage, C. O. S. and Pober, J. S. (1990). The endothelial cell as a regulator of T-cell function. *Immunol. Rev.*, 117, 85–102

68. Issekutz, T. B. (1990). Effects of six different cytokines on lymphocyte adherence to microvascular endothelium and in vivo lymphocyte migration in the rat. *J. Immunol.*, 144, 2140–6

69. Jeurissen, S. H., Duijvestijn, A. M., Sontag, Y. and Kraal, G. (1987). Lymphocyte migration into lamina propria of the gut is mediated by specialized HEV-like blood vessels. *Immunology*, 62, 273–7

70. Jalkanen, S., Nash, G. S., de los Toyos, J., MacDermott, R. P. and Butcher, E. C. (1989). Human lamina propria lymphocytes bear homing receptors and bind selectively to mucosal high endothelium. *Eur. J. Immunol.*, 19, 63–8

71. MacDermott, R. P. and Stenson, W. F. (1986). The immunology of idiopathic inflammatory bowel disease. *Hosp. Pract.*, 15 Nov., pp. 97–116

72. Granfors, K., Jalkanen, S., von Essen, R., Lahesmaa-Rantala, R., Isomäki, O., Pekkola-Heino, K., Merilahti-Palo, R., Saario, R., Isomäki, H. and Toivanen, A. (1989). Yersinia antigens in synovial-fluid cells from patients with reactive arthritis. *N. Engl. J. Med.*, 320, 216–21

73. Jalkanen, S., Saari, S., Kalimo, H., Lammintausta, K., Vainio, E., Leino, R., Duijvestijn, A. and Kalimo, K. (1990). Lymphocyte migration into the skin: the role of lymphocyte homing receptor (CD44) and endothelial cell antigen (HECA-452). *J. Invest. Dermatol.*, 94, 786–92

74. Kantele, A. (1990). Antibody-secreting cells in the evaluation of the immunogenicity of an oral vaccine. *Vaccine*, 8, 321–6

10
Intestinal permeation of molecules in health and disease

I. S. MENZIES and M. W. TURNER

INTRODUCTION

The mammalian gut must provide an effective barrier to the penetration of food proteins and their intermediate breakdown fragments as well as to pathogens and their toxic products. For example, relatively small peptides of molecular weight 2000–8000 derived from wheat gluten are still potentially toxic when absorbed by the patient with coeliac disease[1]. Nevertheless, even the healthy intestinal tract has been shown in many species to permit the passage of small amounts of undegraded macromolecular dietary antigen. The uptake of such material is influenced by the permeability of the gut and by both local and systemic immune responses. The complexities of the immune defence mechanisms which have been developed at gut mucosal surfaces are reviewed elsewhere in this volume, and are not further discussed here. This chapter will address the question of the intestinal uptake of macromolecules, and in particular the use of various probes to evaluate molecular permeation in health and disease.

Evidence quoted for intestinal uptake of antigens depends either upon the appearance of circulating antibodies, or upon detection of the antigen itself in body fluids (e.g. plasma) following ingestion. Unfortunately the appearance of circulating antibody, though indicating immunologically significant entry, does not distinguish arrival by the intestinal from the dermal or respiratory route. However, this criticism is more relevant to environmental antigens such as house dust mite and pollen allergens. Though measurements of the antigen itself provide more direct evidence of entry this is difficult in practice because intestinal permeation of such large molecules is very limited (much less than 0.5% of the amount ingested), space distribution after absorption is large (at least 14 litres in the average human adult), and sequestration by the tissues considerable. Renal excretion of such macromolecules is negligible

173

so that measurement of recovery in urine is not an option. This means that analytical techniques of very great sensitivity are required to quantify, or even detect, the entry of protein antigens which may, in addition, become degraded to an uncertain extent by intestinal proteolytic enzymes following oral administration.

In this chapter consideration is first given to the choice of probes for the assessment of intestinal permeability and our understanding of the basic mechanisms underlying permeability. After discussing the measurement of protein uptake in both humans and experimental animals the last section is devoted to causes of abnormal intestinal permeability in both health and disease.

THE USE OF NON-METABOLIZABLE PROBES FOR ASSESSING INTESTINAL PERMEABILITY

Early studies of human small intestinal permeability by Fordtran et al. exploiting the principles of reflection coefficient[2] and restrictive diffusion[3], taken in conjunction with later studies[4,5], clearly demonstrate that while permeation of biologically inert lipid-insoluble polar molecules below 0.4 nm radius ($\leqslant$ MW 180) is substantial, the permeation of those with a molecular radius above 0.5 nm ($\leqslant$ MW 342) is very restricted. The findings suggest the presence of at least two distinct pathways of 'aqueous permeation' in the small intestinal mucosa, one a high-incidence 'small-pore' pathway accommodating molecules such as water, urea, erythritol, rhamnose and mannitol (MW 18, 60, 118, 164 and 182) and the other a low-incidence 'large-pore' pathway accommodating larger molecules such as oligosaccharides (lactulose, melibiose, cellobiose, raffinose, stachyose; MW 342, 342, 342, 508, 674), dextran MW 3000) and [^{51}Cr]EDTA (MW about 340) in addition, of course, to the smaller molecules.

Figure 10.1 illustrates some of the pathways which are available for passive (unmediated) permeation of molecules across the intestinal epithelium. In addition to the pinocytotic route indicated, several other biochemically and physically mediated mucosal pathways are also recognized. For example, there is a directional sodium-dependent pathway requiring energy which appears to be involved in the absorption of D-glucose and D-galactose. In contrast, the uptake of D-fructose and D-xylose is apparently a passive non-directional and non-sodium-dependent process. Some of the characteristics of various test molecules which have been used to assess intestinal absorption are summarized in Table 10.1.

Probe-markers that are fully excreted by the kidney after absorption become concentrated in the urine to levels about 100-fold higher than those in the plasma, a fact that can be exploited to estimate the often very small quantities that permeate the intestine. Renal excretion of orally administered non-metabolizable test molecules with unrestricted glomerular permeation (i.e. MW < 20 000) therefore provides an effective non-invasive method for assessing human intestinal permeation. Though this may also apply for somewhat larger molecules, restriction to diffusion across the glomerular

INTESTINAL PERMEATION OF MOLECULES

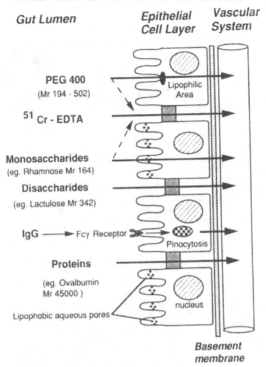

Figure 10.1 Diagram showing the pathways available for passive (unmediated) permeation of molecules across the intestinal epithelium. The major pathways illustrated are: (i) a 'small-pore' pathway (molecular radius ≤ 0.4 nm, polar) used by monosaccharides; (ii) a 'large-pore' pathway (molecular radius ≥ 0.5 nm, polar) used by disaccharides, [⁹¹Cr]-EDTA and probably proteins; (iii) a lipid pathway (molecules soluble in membrane lipid) used by PEG 400. In addition a route available for mediated uptake of selected protein antigens by pinocytosis is also illustrated. Note, however, that the IgG-Fcγ receptor observed in rodents and piglets has no human equivalent. (Figure modified from an original by Dr. S. Strobel)

barrier increases above MW 20 000 and becomes complete at about MW 70 000. Permeation (i.e. the quantity absorbed) depends, as illustrated in Fig. 10.2, not upon mucosal permeability alone, but also on the state of 'exposure factors' such as time (transit rate), mucosal surface area, and concentration gradient, which are difficult to control or measure *in vivo*.

The principle of 'differential absorption', also illustrated in Fig. 10.2, can be applied to overcome the effect of these premucosal variables by administering small and large molecular probes in combination (MW 182 and 164) combined with either lactulose, melibiose or cellobiose (MW 342). When administered in such pairs diffusion of the probes is affected equally by the premucosal factors, and the absorption ratio is determined solely by the state of the intestinal large/small-pore permeability profile. Provided that the selected probes resist metabolic degradation and have a similar space distribution and renal clearance following absorption, ratios of urinary excretion should correspond to intestinal absorption ratios (for review of methods see Menzies[9]).

Table 10.1 Behaviour of test molecules employed for assessing intestinal absorption

Test probe	Molecular weight (Daltons)	Jejunal absorption		Colonic absorption[b]	Recovery in urine	
		Mechanism	Relative rate[a]		Percentage of i.v. dose excreted in 24 h	Percentage of oral dose excreted in 5 h (mean value)
D-glucose	180	Active mediated	100	nil	<1.0%	nil
D-galactose	180	Active mediated	85	nil	about 1.0%	1.0%
3-O-methyl-D-glucose	194	Active mediated	55	nil	>85%	50%
D-xylose	150	Passive mediated	24	nil	about 50%	30%
D-arabinose	150	Passive mediated	14	nil	about 60%	20%
L-rhamnose	164	Non-mediated	7.5	nil	about 75%	12%
D-mannitol	182	Non-mediated	7.5	nil	>90%	30%
Lactulose	342	Non-mediated	<0.1	nil	>95%	0.3%
Melibiose	342	Non-mediated	<0.1	nil	>95%	0.3%
Raffinose	508	Non-mediated	<0.07	nil	>95%	0.2%
Stachyose	674	Non-mediated	<0.03	nil	>95%	0.1%
FITC-dextran	3000	Non-mediated	<0.01	nil	>95%	0.05%
Sucrose	342 }	Hydrolysed by	Sucrase }	nil	>95%	0.05%
Lactose/cellobiose	342 }		Lactase }	nil	>95%	0.06%
Palatinose	342 }		Isomaltase }	nil	>95%	0.05%
[^{51}Cr]EDTA	340 (approx.)	Non-mediated	<0.1	about 0.7%	>95%	0–5 h 0.44% (small intestine) 5–24 h 0.70% (mainly colonic)
PEG-400						
Polymer 1	194	Non-mediated	25	?	<30%	15%
Polymer 4	326	Non-mediated	25	?	<45%	22%
Polymer 8	502	Non-mediated	6	?	about 69%	5%

[a] Average values are given for the relative rates of absorption from the jejunum (D-glucose = 100). Monosaccharide absorption was estimated by jejunal perfusion at concentrations of about 5 mmol/l, and 24 h recovery in urine following intravenous administration in healthy human volunteers[6-8]
[b] Absorption of sugars from the colon is usually negligible because of bacterial degradation

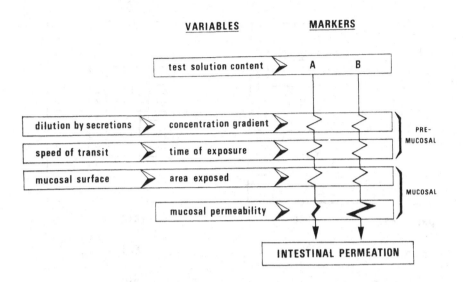

Figure 10.2 The relationship between 'permeability' (a condition of the mucosal barrier) and 'permeation' (quantity absorbed). Permeation depends not only upon the state of mucosal permeability, but also upon concentration gradient, time of exposure, and area of the absorptive surface involved. 'Differential absorption' can be assessed by combined oral administration of 'small-pore' and 'large-pore' probes (test markers 'A' and 'B') which respond identically to dilution, transit, renal clearance and other non-mucosal factors. The A/B excretion ratio (of the percentages recovered in the urine) provides a specific index of the state of intestinal permeability, unaffected by the other variables

The large-pore pathway is generally thought to be paracellular, but it is not yet clear whether the small-pore pathway, which responds to experimental stress and pathology in an entirely different way, is transcellular, paracellular or both[8].

The use of non-metabolizable probe markers provides a useful means for assessing both quantitative and qualitative aspects of intestinal permeability. However, it is doubtful whether any of the probes introduced so far can provide a reliable estimate of antigenic protein uptake. As already mentioned, such antigens may also have some ability to pass across cell membranes by virtue of lipid partition or pinocytosis (see Fig. 10.1) in addition to the pathways that the available test probes are thought to monitor.

It is necessary to emphasize here that the total *quantity* of antigen taken up by the intestine is likely to be the most important measurement from the immunological standpoint. Although abnormal permeability due, for instance, to villous atrophy is most clearly indicated by a *raised* monosaccharide/disaccharide permeation ratio, it is usually accompanied by a *reduced* absorptive area. Because of the latter, total uptake of large molecules may not be increased, even though the relative permeability of the mucosa to such molecules when expressed per unit area is markedly increased (see Fig. 10.3 and also section on coeliac disease – Figure 10.8).

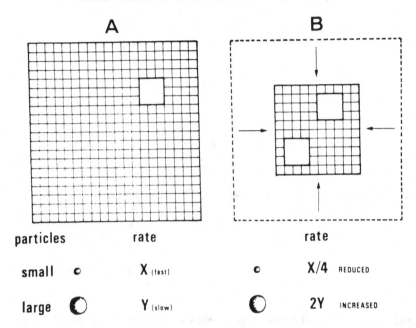

Figure 10.3 Permeation by inert molecules of differing size through a restrictive membrane with pores of differing size: **A** is a diagrammatic representation of the intestinal absorptive surface with a high incidence of water pores which admit molecules 0.4 nm radius and below, and a low incidence of larger water channels capable of accommodating larger molecules; **B** shows the effect of villous atrophy: the absorptive area is reduced with corresponding impairment of small molecular permeation, while an increased incidence of larger water channels associated with the 'mucosal damage' allows a disproportionate increase in the permeation of larger molecules

UPTAKE OF DIETARY PROTEIN ANTIGENS IN EXPERIMENTAL ANIMALS

There is a large literature describing the uptake of macromolecular antigens from the gut in various laboratory animals (see review by Husby[10]). Unfortunately, much of the earlier work is of questionable value because radiolabelled antigen was used and it was subsequently demonstrated that much of the radioactivity transferred across the gut was no longer protein-bound[11]. It now seems likely that iodinases present in the gut lumen are able to cleave ^{125}I from the labelled protein, and that the free isotope retains the ability to bind to endogenous serum proteins of the animal.

Over the past decade immunochemical techniques such as the enzyme-linked immunosorbent assay (ELISA) have been preferred for the measurement of intact dietary proteins in the blood stream. Although in general the levels of transferred protein are very low (e.g. measured in ng/ml), there remains a residual worry that some of the material detected consists of protein fragments retaining antigenicity and the ability to bind to endogenous proteins[12].

There are many other potentially confusing variables such as the species of animal used and its age at the time of study. The permeability of the gut to intact proteins is much higher before gut closure occurs, and the latter differs from species to species. Whereas in humans it appears to be complete by 34–36 weeks of gestation, or at most by the end of the neonatal period[13], it is a postnatal event in many species, particularly those with a pronounced transfer of maternal IgG from milk to offspring, e.g. the pig. The complex composition of both colostrum and milk may also significantly influence uptake at this stage.

After gut closure the immune state of an animal probably determines the fate and effect of absorbed antigen. Secretory IgA and serum IgG, IgM and IgE antibodies with specificity for the protein may be present and may form immune complexes. Sophisticated separation techniques may be required to determine whether or not a particular protein antigen is circulating as a free entity or is aggregated into immune complexes.

Despite the interpretational problems much useful work has been done with experimental animals, and many fundamental issues which have been addressed would be difficult or impossible to study in humans. For example, we have shown that in mice gavaged with ovalbumin, the protein could be detected in serum obtained as early as 2 min after the feed, and reached maximum levels at 60 min (see Fig. 10.4). Gel filtration analysis of serum obtained after 5 min revealed only intact ovalbumin when the fractions were assayed using a specific ELISA procedure (see Fig. 10.5).

Two publications have suggested that animals rendered hypersensitive to one food protein will, when challenged locally in the gut, absorb increased amounts of an unrelated 'bystander' antigen. Kilshaw and Slade[15] showed that in calves made sensitive to soya flour there was an increased uptake of the protein β-lactoglobulin when the animals were simultaneously fed soya and milk. In the following year Bloch and Walker[16] demonstrated enhanced uptake of BSA from the gut when rats presensitized to ovalbumin received

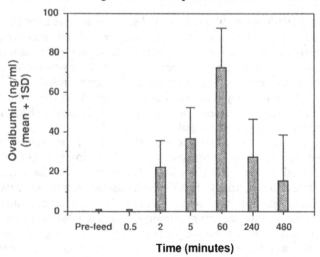

Figure 10.4 Serum concentrations of ovalbumin measured by a ELISA procedure at various times after feeding 25 mg ovalbumin to BALB/c mice. Data represent means + SD ($n = 20$ for each time point). Reproduced from Peng *et al.*[14] with permission

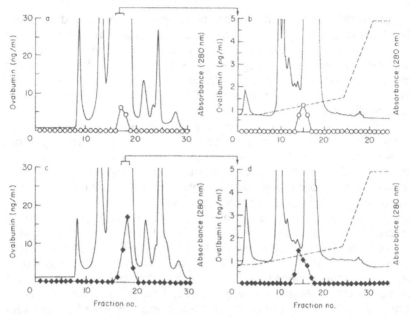

Figure 10.5 (a) Superose 6 gel filtration fractionation of pooled BALB/c serum obtained 5 min after feeding 25 mg ovalbumin. Levels of immunoreactive ovalbumin (O) were determined by sandwich ELISA. (b) Mono Q anion exchange chromatography of fraction 17 from the Superose 6 gel filtration fractionation (a). Levels of immunoreactive ovalbumin (O) were determined by sandwich ELISA. (c) Superose 6 gel filtration fractionation of pooled BALB/c serum obtained 1 h after feeding 25 mg of ovalbumin. Levels of immunoreactive ovalbumin (♦) were determined by sandwich ELISA. (d) Mono Q anion exchange chromatography of fraction 18 from the Superose 6 gel filtration fractionation (c). Levels of immunoreactive ovalbumin (♦) were determined by sandwich ELISA. Reproduced from Peng et al.[14] with permission

an intralumenal challenge with that antigen. More recently we have confirmed these observations and, in addition, demonstrated an increased lactulose/rhamnose urine excretion ratio when these sugars were administered simultaneously with the challenge antigen. However, there was no correlation between these measurements. It was possible to confirm independently that an intestinal hypersensitivity reaction was associated with the permeability changes by measuring the release of rat mast cell protease (RMCPII), a specific marker for mucosal mast cell secretion (see Fig. 10.6).

There was a significant positive correlation between the serum levels of RMCPII and the lactulose/rhamnose excretion ratios ($p < 0.05$) but no correlation existed between RMCPII and BSA levels in the challenged rats. In other studies the urinary lactulose/rhamnose ratios of rats with cetrimide-induced gut damage were found to be significantly increased, although BSA uptake into the serum remained unaltered. We concluded from these two studies that there is no simple correlation between gut permeation of low molecular weight sugars and the uptake of macromolecular proteins.

Using the neonatal guinea pig Weaver and Coombs[18] compared the uptake of the cows' milk protein β-lactoglobulin and the sugar lactulose in an attempt to address the question 'does sugar permeability reflect macromolecular

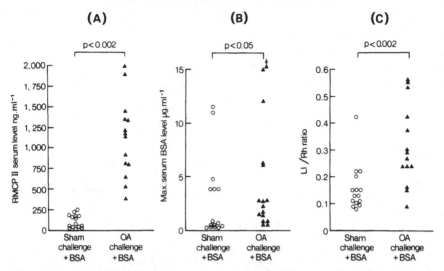

Figure 10.6 Comparison of protein uptake, sugar permeability and release of an intestinal mast cell mediator in rats undergoing antigen challenge in the small intestine. Rats were presensitized to ovalbumin and 14 days later were given an oral feed of BSA (the 'bystander' protein); 1 h later a mixture of ovalbumin, lactulose and rhamnose was instilled into the lumen of the small intestine. Panel A, rat mast cell protease II levels in serum 1 h after the ovalbumin challenge; panel B, maximum serum BSA levels observed; panel C, lactulose/rhamnose excretion ratios measured over a 6 h period. Reproduced from Turner et al.[17] with permission

absorption?' They found the gut hyperpermeable to both β-lactoglobulin and lactulose during the immediate postnatal period. After intestinal closure at 6 days protein uptake ceased, but the gut remained permeable to lactulose, suggesting that β-lactoglobulin and lactulose traverse the gastrointestinal mucosa by distinct pathways.

UPTAKE OF DIETARY PROTEIN ANTIGENS IN HUMANS

Over the past decade there have been several reported studies of dietary antigen uptake in healthy adults. The preferred antigens have been ovalbumin and the cows' milk protein β-lactoglobulin, and whereas the results with the egg protein are in broad agreement, those obtained using β-lactoglobulin are more controversial.

Husby and colleagues[19,20] have undertaken extensive investigations comparing the patterns of antigen uptake between different individuals and also in the same individual at different times. Some of the heterogeneity is illustrated in Fig. 10.7. After a test meal peak levels of ovalbumin were reached at times ranging from 120 to 240 min. The molecular size distribution of the absorbed antigen was investigated in a subsequent report, and in all of the subjects studied the immunoreactive protein was found to have either the expected, or a higher, molecular weight. The latter 'higher molecular weight' moieties were provisionally identified as immune complexes with host anti-ovalbumin antibodies. There was no evidence that low molecular weight

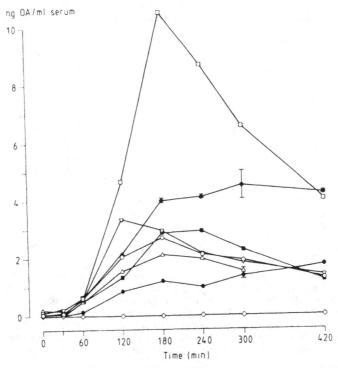

Figure 10.7   Detection of ovalbumin (OA) by an ELISA procedure in the sera of eight healthy adults after a test meal. The bars denote the range of triplicate determinations; when not indicated the range is within the symbol. Reproduced from Husby *et al.*[19] with permission

fragments of ovalbumin were present. In some individuals circulating antigen could be detected for up to 48 h after the test meal.

As mentioned previously, gut closure in humans is generally regarded as an *in utero* event, although Beach *et al.*[13] found evidence of increased intestinal permeability to lactulose during the neonatal period, and it certainly may not have occurred in preterm infants by the time of delivery. Roberton *et al.*[21] noted that following a milk feed serum levels of bovine β-lactoglobulin were much higher in preterm infants than in term infants. More recently Axelsson *et al.*[22] have confirmed these observations using α-lactalbumin as a molecular weight marker.

CAUSES OF ABNORMAL INTESTINAL PERMEABILITY

In various types of small intestinal disease there is increased urinary excretion of intact lactose and sucrose which is due to a combination of decreased hydrolysis and of increased mucosal permeability to dietary disaccharide, both being features of mucosal damage[5,23-25]. But excessive urinary excretion of intact disaccharide has also been demonstrated in healthy subjects following ingestion of very hyperosmotic solutions, and following oral administration of certain drugs, or of detergents such as cetrimide given for experimental purposes.

Studies in apparently normal individuals

Increased permeability due to hyperosmolar stress

This effect was first described in isolated frog skin preparations by Hans Ussing[26] and has subsequently been demonstrated in other mucous epithelia including the normal human intestine[5,27,28]. Ingestion of very hyperosmolar solutions ($>1500\,mOsmol/l$) temporarily increases intestinal permeability in normal subjects to large molecules such as oligosaccharide and [^{51}Cr]EDTA (molecular radius $\geqslant 0.5\,nm$) without affecting the permeation of smaller molecules such as L-rhamnose and mannitol (molecular radius $\leqslant 0.4\,nm$). This change reverts to normal within 2.5 h, and probably as soon as the hyperosmolar stress has dispersed. Hyperosmolar stress is known to increase the permeation of molecules as large as dextran MW 3000. In the presence of villous atrophy (even when mild) this effect, which may be induced by ingestion of honey, treacle, syrups or confectioneries containing crystalline sugar, becomes enhanced: it may play an aetiological role in coeliac disease by predisposing to permeation of the jejunal mucosa by toxic fractions of gluten. Though many solutes (sugars, salts, urea and glycerol) induce this effect, acute ingestion of ethanol does not[5,29].

Drugs and therapeutic agents

Oral administration of certain cytotoxic and non-steroidal anti-inflammatory drugs is known to increase intestinal permeability to oligosaccharides and [^{15}Cr]EDTA[30,31]. Some antibiotics (e.g. neomycin) are also known to induce changes in small intestinal morphology[32,33] and permeability (Menzes, I. S., unpublished observtions).

Altered intestinal permeability due to disease

Villous atrophy

There have probably been more studies of gastrointestinal permeability in patients with coeliac disease than in any other disease group. Most of the clinical effects seen in coeliac disease stem from the primary pathological manifestation, villous atrophy. Though the most important cause of persistent villous atrophy in Caucasians is coeliac disease, it is also seen in tropical sprue and enteropathy[34,35], and the most frequent cause of temporary villous atrophy is probably acute gastroenteritis[36].

The effect of villous atrophy on intestinal permeation is the result of several factors of which reduction in absorptive area and increased permeability to larger molecules are the two most important. As shown diagrammatically in

Fig. 10.3, reduction in absorptive area results in reduced permeation of all constituents, whether lipid- or non-lipid-soluble, or of large or small molecular size, and is the mechanism responsible for the 'malabsorption' associated with moderate or severe villous atrophy. Here, therefore, are two associated changes capable of exerting independent and opposite effects upon the absorption of certain dietary constituents. The outcome, as illustrated in Fig. 10.8, varies according to the balance between the *increase* in permeability and *decrease* in absorptive area in a particular patient. Figure 10.8 shows, in scattergram form, the urinary excretion of two small-molecular test molecules (D-xylose and L-rhamnose) and a large-molecular probe (lactulose) after simultaneous ingestion in a group of 19 patients with untreated coeliac disease in comparison with 24 healthy adult subjects. Whereas only nine of the patients (48%) had increased 'permeation' of the large molecular probe (lactulose) above the normal mean + 2SD (0.6% of oral dose), all had clearly abnormal lactulose/L-rhamnose and lactulose/D-xylose permeability ratios.

A third factor relating to intestinal permeation concerns the effect of hyperosmolar stress. Healthy subjects develop a temporary increase in small intestinal permeability to large-molecular probes such as lactulose, raffinose, stachyose and dextran, MW 342, 504, 666 and 3000[27,28] and [51Cr]EDTA[8] following ingestion of solutions with an osmolarity made greater than 2000 mOsmol/1 by addition of various solutes (sugars, mannitol, urea, sodium and potassium chloride, urea and glycerol). It was also noted that the majority of patients with villous atrophy, whether mild or severe, had a significantly greater susceptibility to this effect, over 90% showing clearly increased

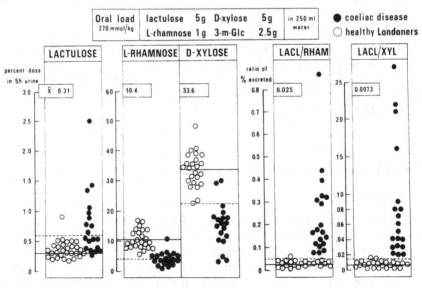

Figure 10.8 Intestinal absorption of lactulose, 1-rhamnose and D-xylose in untreated coeliac disease following ingestion of an iso-osmolar test containing these sugars. Patients with coeliac disease (n = 19) excrete more lactulose and less L-rhamnose and D-xylose than healthy subjects (n = 29). Diagnostic discrimination of the two groups is improved when results are expressed as lactulose/L-rhamnose and lactulose/D-xylose excretion ratios

lactulose permeation following ingestion of 100 ml of a test solution made moderately hyperosmolar (1500 mOsmol/1) by the addition of sugars (sucrose, etc.), urea or glycerol.

The increased permeability associated with villous atrophy affects only large polar molecules such as oligosaccharide, dextran and [^{51}Cr]EDTA which are virtually insoluble in lipid. Whether or not the permeation pathway involved relates to the entry of protein or other antigens is, at the present time, an important unresolved question. Two studies of the uptake of macromolecular dietary antigens in patients with coeliac disease reached different conclusions. A small study by Pitcher-Willmott et al.[37] failed to find any evidence of increased protein uptake in coeliac children. In contrast, Husby and colleagues[38] did find evidence of augmented antigen uptake in coeliac patients following gluten challenge; this is illustrated in Fig. 10.9.

Dermatitis herpetiformis

In an investigation of 20 patients with dermatitis herpetiformis (DH) Griffiths and co-workers[39] measured the differential absorption of D-xylose and 3-O-methyl-D-glucose and the unmediated intestinal permeation (simple diffusion) of lactulose and L-rhamnose. Both iso-osmolar and hyperosmolar test solutions were employed and the results compared with those obtained from a group of healthy adult volunteers. The findings in each patient were also correlated with small intestinal histology. The majority of patients with villous atrophy had an abnormally raised intestinal lactulose permeation and lactulose/rhamnose permeability ratios, whereas in patients with normal small intestinal morphological grading the permeability indices did not differ significantly from the healthy control group. Irrespective of the small intestinal histological findings there was a high incidence of delayed plasma D-xylose absorption peaks in the DH patients. These results suggest that abnormal intestinal permeability in DH is the result of gluten-induced damage to the mucosa rather than an inherent primary defect.

Crohn's disease

Work from several different groups suggests that this inflammatory disease is characterized by an altered gut permeability. For example Sanderson and co-workers[40] assessed the efficacy of an elemental diet in the treatment of Crohn's disease in 14 children aged 11–17 years with active small bowel disease. Iso-osmolar oral test sugar solutions were administered before and after the treatment. All 14 children had abnormally raised lactulose/rhamnose permeability ratios before treatment and these fell significantly after treatment with the elemental diet. Coincidentally there was a marked clinical improvement.

Katz and colleagues[41] have also shown that patients with Crohn's disease have an increased lactulose permeability compared with their relatives, or healthy control subjects having no family history of inflammatory bowel disease.

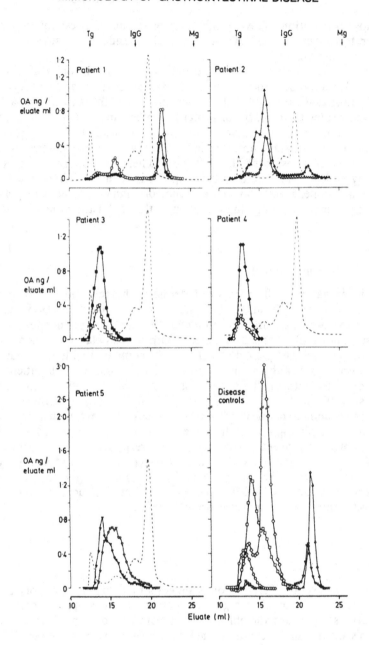

Figure 10.9 HPLC fractionation of various sera from children with coeliac disease after a test meal containing ovalbumin and β-lactoglobulin. The sera were fractionated by the HPLC technique and the protein antigens assayed by ELISA procedures. Serum levels of both proteins were increased in four out of five coeliac patients after gluten challenge (closed symbols) compared to the levels observed when the patients were on a gluten-free diet (open symbols). The elution volumes of purified thyroglobulin (Tg), IgG and myoglobulin (Mg) are indicated. Reproduced from Husby et al.[38] with permission

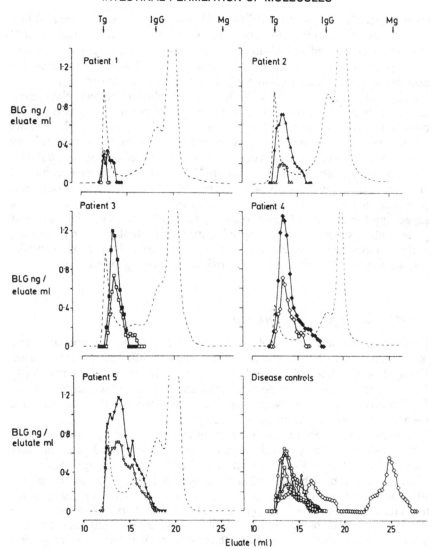

Figure 10.9 (*Contd*)

Atopic dermatitis

Following the ingestion of egg or milk the levels of the major constituent proteins (ovalbumin and β-lactoglobulin, respectively) subsequently detected in the serum of patients with atopic eczema are increased compared to the levels found in healthy individuals[42]. Since a possible explanation for such findings is an enhanced passage of food antigens across the gut wall of the atopic individuals there have been several investigations of gastrointestinal uptake using various inert molecules. Absorption of polyethylene glycol of mean molecular weight 4000 (PEG 41K) was reported to be increased in a proportion of patients with atopic eczema[43]. Subsequently Pike et al.[44] reported that the median lactulose/rhamnose ratio was greater in 26 children with atopic eczema than in a control group of 29 children which included both healthy individuals and others with various non-eczematous dermatoses. Furthermore, there was a tendency for younger children to have the highest lactulose/rhamnose ratios. Since increased sugar permeability is normally present at birth but falls to 'adult' values by the 9th day of life[13], the authors speculated that there might be a prolongation of this enhanced permeability in some individuals, with a concomitant risk of increased exposure to putative allergens in the diet. Two other groups[45,46] have also reported enhanced lactulose uptake in patients with atopic dermatitis, but any aetiological relevance of these studies must be questioned in view of the animal work suggesting the absence of any correlation between protein uptake and sugar permeability (see earlier). A prospective study is presently under way in the authors' laboratories which is attempting to measure both protein uptake and sugar permeability in infants at risk of developing atopic eczema.

Cows' milk protein intolerance

Intolerance to the proteins of cows' milk is relatively common in young infants, and up to 8% of the population may be affected to some degree. Using different-sized ethylene glycol polymers to assess gut permeability Fälth-Magnusson et al.[47] reported significant changes in the excretion of the PEG following challenge with cows' milk, and similar observations have been made by other groups using sugar probes.

A more direct approach to the problem of antigen absorption in children with cows' milk allergy was the study of Heyman et al.[48]. Jejunal biopsies were obtained from 15 children with cows' milk protein allergy at the time of diagnosis and both before and after antigen challenge, and from 18 control subjects. Fragments of the biopsy were mounted in an Ussing chamber for measurement of mucosal to serosal transport of horseradish peroxidase (HRP). At the time of diagnosis HRP fluxes were significantly higher (about 8-fold) in the children with CMA than in control children. After several months on a milk-free diet the HRP flux returned to control values. Following milk challenge a rise in HRP permeation was observed, but this did not reach significance.

One of the clinical presentations of cows' milk intolerance may be infantile colic. This association was first suggested by Jakobsson and Lindberg[49], and the same group have recently made a detailed study of macromolecular absorption in such infants[50]. Serum samples were obtained from infants 30 and 60 min after an intake of human milk and the levels of α-lactalbumin determined using a competitive radioimmunoassay. Both breast-fed and formula-fed infants with infantile colic had significantly higher serum levels of α-lactalbumin than did appropriate age-matched healthy control subjects. The findings suggest that the gut mucosa of infants with infantile colic is abnormal, but the precise nature of the abnormality remains unclear.

CONCLUSIONS

Low levels of intact protein antigens are able to cross the gastrointestinal tract of both experimental animals and healthy humans. Reproducible, sensitive immunochemical assays of the proteins suggest that uptake begins as soon as 2–5 min after ingestion and that levels may rise until a peak or plateau is reached 60–120 min later. Uptake probably occurs in part by a process of endocytosis, but there may also be some paracellular passage. There is no convincing evidence that such protein is degraded, but in some individuals much of the detected material may be in the form of circulating immune complexes.

During the past 20 years reliable techniques suitable for the clinical investigation of human intestinal permeability have been introduced. However, the abnormal permeability demonstrated by these methods in conditions such as gastroenteritis and coeliac disease is not necessarily associated with increased absorption of antigenic material, because impairment of absorption due to villous atrophy with reduction in mucosal surface is often simultaneously present. Furthermore it is not clear that the available probes are appropriate for assessing the pathways involved in the uptake of antigens, most of which are molecules of much greater dimension. Simultaneous measurement of protein uptake and intestinal permeability to 'middle' molecular-weight non-metabolizable oligosaccharides such as lactulose, both in normal guinea pigs and in rats undergoing intestinal hypersensitivity reactions, suggest that there is no simple correlation between the two measurements.

References

1. Dissanayake, A. S., Jerrome, D. W., Offord, R. E., Truelove, S. C. and Whitehead, R. (1974). Identifying toxic fractions of wheat gluten and their effect on jejunal mucosa in coeliac disease. *Gut*, **15**, 931–46
2. Fordtran, J. S., Rector, F. C., Ewton, M. F., Soter, N. and Kinney, J. (1965). Permeability characteristics of the human small intestine. *J. Clin. Invest.*, **44**, 1935–44
3. Fordtran, J. S., Rector, F. C., Locklear, T. W. and Ewton, M. F. (1967). Water and solute movement in the small intestine of patients with sprue. *J. Clin. Invest.*, **46**, 287–98
4. Loehry, C. A., Hilton, P. J., Axon, A. T. and Creamer, B. (1969). Small bowel permeability and molecular size. *Gut*, **10**, 1044–5
5. Menzies, I. S. (1974). Absorption of intact oligosaccharide in health and disease. *Biochem. Soc. Trans.*, **2**, 1042–7
6. Bull, J. and Menzies, I. S. (1979). Measurement of sugar absorption by intestinal perfusion: the use of urea to eliminate experimental variation. *Gut*, **23**, A449
7. Laker, M. F., Bull, H. J. and Menzies, I. S. (1982). Evaluation of mannitol for use as a probe-marker of gastrointestinal permeability in man. *Eur. J. Clin. Invest.*, **12**, 485–91
8. Maxton, D. G., Bjarnason, I., Reynolds, A. P., Catt, S. D., Peters, T. J. and Menzies, I. S. (1986). ^{51}Cr-EDTA, L-rhamnose and polyethyleneglycol 400 as probe markers for assessment *in vivo* of human intestinal permeability. *Clin. Sci.*, **71**, 71–80
9. Menzies, I. S. (1983). Medical importance of sugars in the alimentary tract. In Developments in Sweeteners – 2. Transmucosal passage of inert molecules in health and disease. In Skahauge, E. and Heintz, K. (eds), *Intestinal Absorption and Excretion*, Falk Symposium 36. Lancaster, MTP Press
10. Husby, S. (1988). Dietary antigens. Uptake and humoral immunity in man. *Acta Pathol. Microbiol. Immunol. Scand.*, **96** (Suppl. 1), 1–40
11. Skogh, T. (1982). Overestimate of ^{125}I-protein uptake from the adult mouse gut. *Gut*, **23**, 1077–80

12. Udall, L. N., Bloch, K. J., Fritze, L. and Walker, W. A. (1981). Binding of exogenous fragments to native proteins: possible explanation for the overestimation of uptake of extrinsically labelled macromolecules from the gut. *Immunology*, **42**, 251-7
13. Beach, R. C., Menzies, I. S., Clayden, G. S. and Scopes, J. W. (1982). Gastrointestinal permeability changes in the preterm neonate. *Arch. Dis. Child.*, **57**, 141-5
14. Peng, H-J., Turner, M. W. and Strobel, S. (1990). The generation of a 'tolerogen' after the ingestion of ovalbumin is time-dependent and unrelated to serum levels of immunoreactive antigen. *Clin. Exp. Immunol.*, **81**, 510-15
15. Kilshaw, P. J. and Slade, H. (1980). Passage of ingested protein into the blood during gastrointestinal hypersensitivity reactions: experiments in the preruminant calf. *Clin. Exp. Immunol.*, **41**, 575-82
16. Bloch, K. J. and Walker, W. A. (1981). Effect of locally induced intestinal anaphylaxis on the uptake of a bystander antigen. *J. Allergy Clin. Immunol.*, **67**, 312-16
17. Turner, M. W., Boulton, P., Shields, J. G., Strobel, S., Gibson, S., Miller, H. R. P. and Levinsky, R. J. (1988). Intestinal hypersensitivity reactions in the rat. I. Uptake of intact protein, permeability to sugars and their correlation with mucosal mast-cell activation. *Immunology*, **63**, 119-24
18. Weaver, L. T. and Coombs, R. R. A. (1988). Does 'sugar' permeability reflect macromolecular absorption? A comparison of the gastro-intestinal uptake of lactulose and beta-lactoglobulin in the neonatal guinea pig. *Int. Arch. Allergy Appl. Immunol.*, **85**, 133-5
19. Husby, S., Jensenius, J.C. and Svehag, S-E. (1985). Passage of undegraded dietary antigen into the blood of healthy adults. Quantification, estimation of size distribution, and relation of uptake to levels of specific antibodies. *Scand. J. Immunol.*, **22**, 83-92
20. Husby, S., Jensenius, J. C. and Svehag, S-E. (1985). Passage of undegraded dietary antigen into the blood of healthy adults. Further characterization of the kinetics of uptake and the size distribution of the antigen. *Scand. J. Immunol.*, **24**, 447-55
21. Roberton, D. M., Paganelli, R., Dinwiddie, R. and Levinsky, R. J. (1982). Milk antigen absorption in the preterm and term neonate. *Arch. Dis. Child.*, **57**, 369-72
22. Axelsson, I., Jakobsson, I., Lindberg, T., Polberger, S., Benediktsson, B. and Räihä, N. (1989). Macromolecular absorption in preterm and term infants. *Acta. Paediatr. Scand.*, **78**, 532-7
23. Gryboski, J. D., Thayer, W. R., Gabrielson, I. W. and Spiro, H. M. (1963). Disacchariduria in gastrointestinal disease. *Gastroenterology*, **45**, 633-7
24. Weser, E. and Sleisenger, M. H. (1965). Lactosuria and lactose deficiency in adult coeliac disease. *Gastroenterology*, **48**, 571-8
25. Menzies, I. S., Laker, M. F., Pounder, R., Ball, J., Heyer, S., Wheeler, P. G. and Creamer, B. (1979). Abnormal intestinal permeability of sugars in villous atrophy. *Lancet*, **2**, 1107-9
26. Ussing, H. (1966). Anomalous transport of electrolytes and sucrose through the isolated frog skin induced by hypertonicity of the outside bathing solution. *Ann. NY Acad. Sci.*, **137**, 543-55
27. Laker, M. F. and Menzies, I. S. (1977). Increase in human intestinal permeability following ingestion of hypertonic solutions. *J. Physiol.*, **265**, 881-94
28. Wheeler, P. G., Menzies, I. S. and Creamer, B. (1978). Effect of hyperosmolar stimuli and coeliac disease on the permeability of the human gastrointestinal tract. *Clin. Sci. Mol. Med.*, **54**, 495-501
29. Smethurst, P., Menzies, I. S., Levi, A. J. and Bjarnason, I. (1988). Is alcohol directly toxic to the small bowel? *Clin. Sci.*, **75**, 50-51P.
30. Bjarnason, I., Williams, P., Smethurst, P., Peters, T. J. and Levi, A. J. (1986). Effect of non-steroidal anti-inflammatory drugs and prostaglandins on the permeability of the human small intestine. *Gut*, **27**, 1292-7
31. Siber, G. R., Mayer, R. J. and Levin, M. J. (1980). Increased gastrointestinal absorption of large molecules in patients after 5-fluoracil therapy for metastatic colon carcinoma. *Cancer Res.*, **40**, 3430-6
32. Rogers, A. I., Vloedman, D. A., Bloom, E. C. and Kalser, M. H. (1966). Neomycin-induced steatorrhoea. *J. Am. Med. Assoc.*, **197**, 185-90
33. Dobbins, W. D., Herrero, B. A. and Mansbach, C. M. (1968). Morphological alterations associated with neomycin-induced malabsorption. *Am. J. Med. Sci.*, **255**, 63-77
34. Cook, G. C. and Menzies, I. S. (1986). Intestinal absorption and unmediated permeation of sugars in post infective tropical malabsorption and tropical sprue. *Digestion*, **33**, 109-16

35. Cook, G. C. (1980). Malabsorption in the tropics. In Cook, G. C. (ed.), *Tropical Gastroenterology*. Oxford: Oxford University Press, pp. 271–324
36. Davidson, G. P. and Barnes, G. L. (1979). Structural and functional abnormalities of the small intestine in infants and young children with rotaviral enteritis. *Acta Paediatr. Scand.*, **69**, 181–6
37. Pitcher-Wilmott, R. W., Booth, I., Harries, J. and Levinsky, R. J. (1982). Intestinal absorption of food antigens in coeliac disease. *Arch. Dis. Child.*, **57**, 462–6
38. Husby, S., Foged, N., Høst, A. and Svehag, S-E. (1987). Passage of dietary antigen into the blood of children with coeliac disease. Quantification and size of distribution of absorbed antigens. *Gut*, **28**, 1062–72
39. Griffiths, C. E. M., Menzies, I. S., Barrison, I. G., Leonard, J. N. and Fry, L. (1988). Intestinal permeability in dermatitis herpetiformis. *J. Invest. Dermatol.*, **91**, 147–9
40. Sanderson, I. R., Boulton, P., Menzies, I. and Walker-Smith, J. A. (1987). Improvement of abnormal lactulose/rhamnose permeability in active Crohn's disease of the small bowel by an elemental diet. *Gut*, **28**, 1073–6
41. Katz, K. D., Hollander, D., Vadheim, C. M., McElree, C., Delahunty, T., Dadufalza, V. D., Krugliak, P. and Rotter, J. I. (1989). Intestinal permeability in patients with Crohn's disease and their healthy relatives. *Gastroenterology*, **97**, 927–31
42. Paganelli, R., Levinsky, R. J., Brostoff, J. and Wraith, D. G. (1979). Immune complexes containing food proteins in normal and atopic subjects after oral challenge and effect of sodium cromoglycate on antigen absorption. *Lancet*, **1**, 1270–2
43. Jackson, P. G., Lessof, M. H., Baker, R. W. R., Ferrett, J. and MacDonald, D. M. (1981). Intestinal permeability in patients with eczema and food allergy. *Lancet*, **1**, 285–6
44. Pike, M. G., Heddle, R. J., Boulton, P., Turner, M. W. and Atherton, D. J. (1986). Increased intestinal permeability in atopic eczema. *J. Invest. Dermatol.*, **86**, 101–4
45. Parrilli, G., Ayola, F., Lembo, G., Cuomo, R., Budillon, G. and Santoianni, P. (1984). Abnormal intestinal permeability to lactulose in patients with atopic dermatitis. In MacDonald, D. M. (ed.), *Immunodermatology*. London: Butterworth, pp. 21–2
46. Ukabam, S. O., Mann, R. J. and Cooper, B. T. (1984). Small intestinal permeability to sugars in patients with atopic eczema. *Br. J. Dermatol.*, **110**, 649–52
47. Fälth-Magnusson, D., Kjellman, N. I. M., Odelram, H., Sundquist, T. and Magnusson, K. E. (1986). Gastrointestinal permeability in children with cows' milk allergy: effect of milk challenge and sodium cromoglycate as assessed with polyethylene glycols (PEG-400 and PEG 1000). *Clin. Allergy*, **16**, 543–55
48. Heyman, M., Grasset, E., Ducroc, R. and Desjeux, J.-F. (1988). Antigen absorption by the jejunal epithelium of children with cows' milk allergy. *Pediatr. Res.*, **24**, 197–202
49. Jakobsson, I. and Lindberg, T. (1978). Cow's milk as a cause of inhfantile colic in breast-fed infants. *Lancet*, **1**, 437–9
50. Lothe, L., Lindberg, T. and Jakobsson, I. (1990). Macromolecular absorption in infants with infantile colic. *Acta. Paediatr. Scand.*, **79**, 417–21

11
Immunology of gastrointestinal lymphoma

J. SPENCER and P. G. ISAACSON

Normal gut-associated lymphoid tissue (GALT) has distinctive features geared to its role of protecting the gastrointestinal tract from infectious agents whilst allowing nutrients to be efficiently absorbed and immunologically tolerated (Chapter 1). These characteristics are reflected by a group of equally distinctive lymphomas which arise in the gastrointestinal tract. Apart from the inherently interesting aspects of this group of malignancies, the behaviour of the tumour cells can be considered as a reflection of the behaviour of the normal cells from which they originate. The range of phenotypes observed within a lymphoid tumour probably reflects the lineage of the normal cells of origin and the changes they undergo during differentiation. Similarly, characteristic patterns of tumour dissemination are thought to reflect the migratory potential of their normal lymphoid counterparts. The characteristics of mucosal lymphomas of different histogenetic types will be considered independently.

GASTROINTESTINAL B CELL LYMPHOMAS

A clinicopathologically distinct group of low-grade extranodal B cell lymphomas has been identified whose histological features closely resemble those of the small intestinal Peyer's patches. These are termed low-grade lymphomas of mucosa-associated lymphoid tissues, or 'MALT type' lymphomas[1]. This group includes lymphomas of the gastrointestinal tract[2], lung[3,4], salivary gland[5] and thyroid[6]. Gastrointestinal lymphomas, especially gastric lymphoma, of MALT type are by far the commonest, and therefore have been the most intensively studied. Immunoproliferative small intestinal disease (IPSID) is a specific subtype of low-grade B cell MALT lymphoma, distinguished by its epidemiology and the synthesis of an abnormal immunoglobulin α heavy chain[7,8]. Low-grade B cell MALT lymphoma, including IPSID, may undergo transformation into a high-grade lymphoma. In a proportion of gastrointestinal

B cell lymphomas presenting as high-grade tumours, foci of low-grade MALT lymphoma can be identified. This strongly implies that a transition from low-to high-grade may occur as the low-grade tumour progresses[9]. It is not known whether those high-grade lymphomas in which no low-grade MALT element can be identified are derived from low-grade lymphomas, or indeed whether they are of the same lineage as MALT lymphomas. A variety of other B cell tumours arise in the gut, including multiple lymphomatous polyposis[10], which is an intestinal manifestation of centrocytic lymphoma and Burkitt's lymphoma[11,12] both of which tend to occur in the ileocaecal region. Other types of low- or high-grade B cell lymphoma corresponding to peripheral lymph node equivalents may present primarily in the gastrointestinal tract, but do so infrequently.

Lymphomas of MALT type

Low-grade B cell lymphoma of MALT

Primary B cell gastric lymphoma is the most common low-grade lymphoma of MALT type and as such will be discussed as the archetype of other lymphomas in this group. Patients with low-grade B cell gastric lymphoma often have a history of repeat endoscopic biopsies showing changes characteristic of an inflammatory response rather than lymphoma. Treatment for gastritis or peptic ulcer may be intermittently successful.

The stomach is normally devoid of lymphoid tissue. However, like most B cell lymphomas of MALT, primary B cell gastric lymphoma appears to arise from a background of acquired reactive MALT resembling small intestinal Peyer's patches[13-15] (Fig. 11.1). The acquisition of reactive lymphoid tissue including B cell follicles may be a critical factor in the pathogenesis of the tumour.

In most cases the lymphoma infiltrates around the reactive B cell follicles, spreading diffusely into the surrounding mucosa. The tumour cells are small to medium-sized, with moderately abundant cytoplasm and nuclei which have an irregular outline bearing a close resemblance to the nuclei of centrocytes (small cleaved cells in the follicle centre). The detailed cytology of these centrocyte-like (CCL) cells covers a spectrum; some are closer in appearance to small lymphocytes and others show the features of so-called monocytoid B cells with abundant rather clear cytoplasm and well-defined cell borders. A small number of transformed blasts are characteristically present. A central feature of low-grade MALT lymphomas is the presence of lymphoepithelial lesions formed by invasion of individual crypts by aggregates of CCL cells which eventually leads to disintegration of the crypt. Such lymphoepithelial lesions resemble those formed by normal marginal zone B cells in the dome epithelium of the Peyer's patches, though in normal Peyer's patches the epithelial structure remains intact[16,17] (Fig. 11.1).

Plasma cell differentiation is present to a variable degree in approximately one-third of low-grade MALT lymphomas and tends to be maximal beneath the surface (lumenal) epithelium[2].

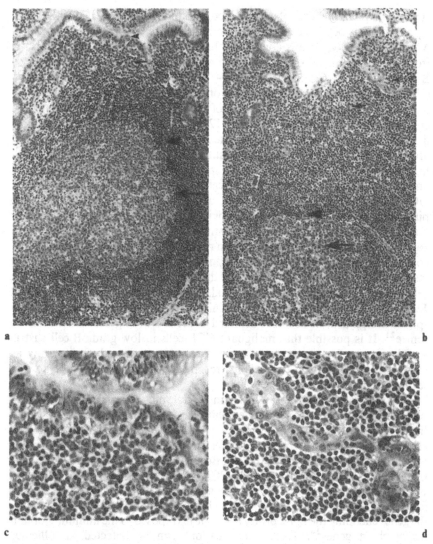

Figure 11.1 Gut-associated lymphoid tissue in (a) Peyer's patch and (b) low-grade primary B cell gastric lymphoma. Primary B cell gastric lymphoma arises from a background of acquired lymphoid tissue that resembles small intestinal Peyer's patches. Analogous zones of B cells are indicated in (a) and (b): follicle centre cells with large arrows, mantle zone B cells with large arrow heads (both populations benign in (a) and (b)), centrocyte-like cells with small arrows (benign in (a) but malignant in (b)) and the lymphoepithelial lesions with small arrow-heads. Detail of the normal lymphoepithelium and the lymphoepithelial lesion formed by malignant centrocyte-like cells in (a) and (b) are shown in (c) and (d) (H&E ×32 (a and b) ×40 (c and d))

Immunohistochemical studies and DNA analysis have allowed detailed characterization of the nature of the tumour cells in low-grade gastric lymphoma and their intriguing relationship to the reactive follicles.

The CCL cells which form the diffuse infiltrate which surrounds the follicle centres in early lymphomas, and which form the lymphoepithelial lesions, typically express markers of mature B cells including CD19, CD20 and CD22. Approximately 50% of cases express complement receptors CD21 and CD35. Most express IgM or less commonly IgA[2]. CCL cells differ phenotypically from the resting B cells in the follicular mantle zone. Whereas mantle zone B cells are IgD +, CCL cells are IgD −. In addition a monoclonal antibody (UCL-4D12) raised to tumour cells from a case of low-grade B cell MALT lymphoma recognizes 50% of cases of gastric lymphoma, whereas mantle zone B cells are consistently UCL-4D12 − [18]. Malignant CCL cells are most likely to be derived from marginal zone B cells which form a prominent zone around the mantle in normal intestinal Peyer's patches. Peyer's patch marginal zone B cells and those in the splenic white pulp are almost certainly analogous. Like the malignant CCL cells, marginal zone B cells are IgD −, UCL-4D12 + [18] (Fig. 11.2). A study using an anti-idiotypic antibody to pinpoint tumour cells immunohistologically at sites distant to the tumour bulk showed localization of small intestinal CCL cells in the splenic marginal zone[19] (Fig. 11.3). Functional studies in rats have demonstrated that marginal zone B cells are memory B cells responsible for some secondary immune responses to T-dependent antigens and that they are derived from proliferating cells in the follicle centre[20]. It has also been observed that when killed Escherishia coli organisms are administered intravenously into rats, the splenic marginal zone becomes depleted as the B cells migrate into the follicle centre[21]. It is possible that malignant CCL cells in low-grade B cell gastric lymphoma are memory B cells capable of infiltrating and proliferating as blast cells in the follicle centre, thus recapitulating the course of a normal secondary immune response.

The frequent presence of light chain monotypic CCL cells within follicle centres often imparts a follicular appearance to the tumour. This has led to the suggestion that B cell lymphomas of MALT are follicular malignancies. However, immunohistochemical studies have shown that whereas malignant follicle centres are CD10 (CALLA) +, Bcl 2 protein + and CDw32 (KB61) −, light chain restricted populations of CCL cells in follicle centres are CD10 −, Bcl 2 protein − and CDw32 + [22,23]. In addition it has been shown that most follicular lymphomas contain t(14;18) chromosomal translocations in which the genes encoding the Bcl-2 protein become juxtaposed to the immunoglobulin heavy chain genes[24]. These translocations can be detected in follicular lymphomas using both cytogenetics and Southern blotting, with probes for the joining region of the immunoglobulin heavy chains and for the Bcl-2 major and minor breakpoints. No evidence of t(14;18) translocations using either cytogenetic or Southern blot analysis has been observed in lymphomas of MALT[25]. Although the tumours themselves are not follicular malignancies, the follicle centre is undoubtedly important in the pathogenesis of the tumour.

In summary, the monotypic population of cells in low-grade gastric lymphoma shows a range in phenotype and morphology, the components of which are variably represented in different cases. The components are as follows:

1. Quiescent CCL cells which have an inter- or intrafollicular distribution. They make the characteristic lymphoepithelial lesions.

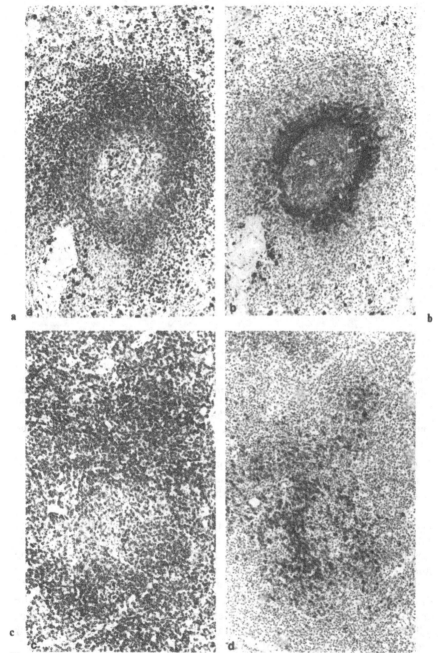

Figure 11.2 Frozen sections of spleen (**a** and **b**) and MALT lymphoma (**c** and **d**) stained with monoclonal antibodies UCL4D12 (**a** and **c**) and UCL3D3 (**b** and **d**) to marginal zone and mantle zone B cells respectively[18]. In the tumour the malignant cells, like the marginal zone B cells in the spleen, are UCL4D12+, UCL3D3− whereas the reactive cells and the mantle zone B cells are UCL4D12−, UCL3D3+. This supports the hypothesis that marginal zone B cells and mucosal centrocyte-like cells are analogous. (Immunoperoxidase ×22)

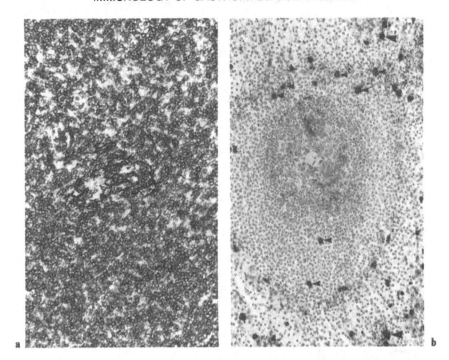

Figure 11.3 Frozen sections of (**a**) low-grade small intestinal B cell lymphoma and (**b**) normal, apparently uninvolved spleen from the same patient stained using an anti-idiotypic antibody to the malignant cells. The anti-idiotypic antibody recognizes the entire small intestinal tumour population and isolated cells in the marginal zone of the spleen (small arrow-heads) having migrated from the small intestinal tumour site[19]. Endogenous peroxidase activity in the red pulp is indicated with large arrow-heads. This implies homology between the mucosal centrocyte-like cells and marginal zone B cells, and suggests that they may share a common migratory pathway. (Immunoperoxidase ×22)

2. Large transformed cells, either concentrated in the follicle centre or interspersed amongst the CCL cells.
3. Plasma cells immediately beneath the epithelium.

The range in cellular phenotype and morphology observed and the association with the follicle centre, in particular with the follicular dendritic cells, relates closely to the range of cells and distribution which would be expected in the course of an immune response. This suggests that primary B cell gastric lymphoma is antigen-driven. We have used an anti-idiotypic antibody to study the binding of tumour-derived immunoglobulin in a case of low-grade primary B cell gastric lymphoma to determine the specificity of the tumour cells. We found that the tumour immunoglobulin recognized mucosal venular endothelium both in the patient's tissues and tissues from other individuals[26]. This supports the hypothesis that the monoclonal lymphoproliferation at sites of acquired MALT may be driven by antigen, perhaps as in the case described above by an autoantigen.

Primary B cell gastric lymphomas, like all B cell lymphomas of MALT, have a good prognosis, irrespective of grade, when compared stage for stage with lymphomas of other histogenetic types[27,28]. This is due mainly to the tendency of the tumour cells to grow slowly and remain localized so that surgery is an effective treatment. The reasons for this indolent behaviour are not known, but there are several hypotheses:

1. It is likely that malignant CCL cells are analogous to marginal zone B cells. It has been shown in rats that splenic marginal zone B cells are a non-recirculating population[29], thus the tendency of the tumour cells to remain localized may reflect the static nature of this cell type. Against this argument is the observed presence of lymphocytes within lymphatics in tissue sections which are presumably destined to leave the tumour site.
2. Adoptive transfer experiments in animals have shown that labelled activated B cells derived from GALT will 'home' to the gut when injected intravenously into recipient animals[30]. It is possible that the tendency of mucosal lymphomas to remain localized despite the presence of B cells leaving the tumour in lymphatics may reflect this phenomenon. It has been shown in experimental animals, however, using isolated loops of gut, that the homing of activated B cells involves the whole gut and not just the site of origin of the B cells. Local proliferation can occur, however, by local stimulation of the extravasated cells with antigens[31,32].
3. Studies of tumour cell migration using anti-idiotypic antibodies have shown that although tumour cells may migrate beyond the tumour site, they may differentiate into plasma cells rather than proliferating to produce tumour metastases[19]. The localized nature of B cell lymphomas of MALT may be due to their dependency on local antigenic stimulation as described above, paralleling the tendency of antigen-reactive extravasated B cells to proliferate locally at the site of antigenic challenge[31,32]

Further experiments are required before the relative contributions of these hypotheses to the overall behaviour of the tumour is understood.

High-grade B cell lymphomas of MALT

High-grade primary gastrointestinal lymphoma appears to be more common than the low-grade lesion which has been described above. This difference may be more apparent than real since, until recently, many of the low-grade tumours were not regarded as true lymphomas, being classified as examples of florid lymphoid hyperplasia or 'pseudolymphoma'[13]. Foci of high-grade lymphoma may be seen in low-grade MALT lymphoma suggesting transformation from one to the other as occurs in other low-grade lymphomas[9]. The extent of this secondary high-grade component varies; in some cases it is confined to colonized follicle centres as already described; in others there are sheets of transformed blasts within the predominantly low-grade CCL cell infiltrate while further cases are characterized by a predominance of high-grade lymphoma with only small residual foci of low-grade tumour which can be difficult to detect. Cases in which a low-grade component cannot be detected may be primary high-grade lymphomas.

The histological features of high-grade MALT lymphoma are not as distinctive as those of the low-grade tumour. Lymphoepithelial lesions are not formed by the transformed cells which infiltrate in sheets and between glands. Although follicles containing large neoplastic cells are often present, there are fewer follicles than in low-grade lymphoma. The large cells resemble centroblasts (large non-cleaved cells in the follicle centre), but tend to have more cytoplasm which may impart a plasmablastic appearance. In keeping with this, immunohistochemistry reveals abundant cytoplasmic Ig.

An important question is whether the high-grade MALT lymphomas exhibit the same favourable clinical behaviour as the low-grade tumours. Some reports suggest that this is the case, and, furthermore, that stage for stage there is no difference between the two grades of gastrointestinal lymphoma[33]. Others, however, have shown that a higher grade results in less favourable behaviour[34].

Immunoproliferative small intestinal disease

This condition is a variant of MALT lymphoma characterized by a diffuse lymphoplasmacytic (predominantly plasmacytic) infiltrate in the upper small intestine (Fig. 11.4). The disease occurs almost exclusively in the Middle East.

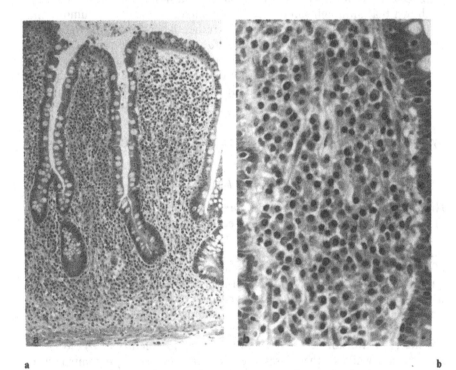

a   b

Figure 11.4 Paraffin section of small intestine from a patient with IPSID. The villi (a) become distended due to the plasma cell infiltrate shown in detail in (b). (H&E ×22 (a), ×38 (b))

An important distinguishing feature of IPSID is the synthesis of α-heavy chain, without light chain, by the plasma cells; this can be detected in the serum or duodenal juice in approximately two-thirds of cases, hence the term α-chain disease. In the remaining one-third of cases the α-chain protein is still synthesized but not secreted[35].

IPSID is a disease of young adults and usually presents with profound malabsorption. It runs a prolonged course and rarely spreads out of the abdomen until the terminal stages, when high-grade transformation may occur. There are numerous reports describing remissions or even cure of IPSID in its early stages following the use of broad-spectrum antibiotics[36]. There seems little doubt that the removal of either specific or non-specific immune stimulants from the gut lumen can have a profound effect on some cases of IPSID in the early stages. The fact that this type of MALT lymphoma is to a degree antigen-responsive may have an important bearing on MALT tumours as a whole.

The histology of IPSID exemplifies all the features of low-grade B cell lymphoma of MALT with marked plasma cell differentiation[22]. Three stages of IPSID are recognized[37]. In stage A the lymphoplasmacytic infiltrate is confined to the mucosa and mesenteric lymph nodes. In stage B nodular mucosal lymphoid infiltrates are present and the infiltrate extends below the muscularis mucosa. Stage C is characterized by the presence of lymphomatous masses and transformation to high-grade lymphoma. The plasma cell infiltrate in the mucosa causes broadening, but not shortening, of the villi. These cells are not invasive and show no evidence of mitotic division. Already present in stage A IPSID, and increasing in prominence in stage B, are aggregates of CCL B cells which cluster around epithelial crypts and form lymphoepithelial lesions. Reactive follicles vary in number, and it is colonization of these by CCL cells that results in the lymphoid nodules of stage B IPSID and the so-called follicular lymphoma variant. Intrafollicular blast transformation and plasma cell differentiation also occur. Transformation to high-grade lymphoma occurs in the same way as in gastric lymphoma except that the high-grade cells more frequently show bizarre cytological features.

Immunohistochemical and immunochemical studies have shown that the plasma cells in IPSID express only an immunoglobulin α_1-chain paraprotein and no light chain. Recent studies of the α-chain locus in a single case showed that the defects can be traced back to the α-chain genes in which most notably much of the V_H and switch $C_H 1$ regions were deleted[38]. The absence of light chain precludes the use of light chain restriction to confirm monoclonality in IPSID. Monoclonality has, however, been confirmed using Southern blotting to detect clonally rearranged immunoglobulin light chain genes[39]. One of the most intriguing aspects of stage A IPSID is its responsiveness to antibiotic therapy resulting in clinical and histological remission at least in the short term, as described above. Although there is clearly a genetic defect in the immunoglobulin genes of the tumour cells in these cases, the disease appears to be driven by bacteria or a bacterial product in its early stages. It is possible to speculate that the B cells are originally stimulated to proliferate by a factor of bacterial origin. The immunoglobulin produced is defective and therefore unable to neutralize the driving bacterial stimulus. When the stimulus is removed using antibiotics, the lymphoproliferation and production of abnormal α_1-heavy chains ceases.

Malignant lymphoma centrocytic (multiple lymphomatous polyposis)

Cases of lymphoma producing multiple lymphomatous polyps of the intestine were first described in 1961[40]. Any part of the gastrointestinal tract may be involved, but in many of the cases the largest tumours are in the ileocaecal region[10,41]. Macroscopically, the intestinal mucosa is peppered with multiple white fleshy polyps ranging in size from 0.5 to 2 cm; much larger tumours may be present especially in the ileocaecal region. The mesenteric lymph nodes are usually obviously involved.

Cytologically, the infiltrate consists of a uniform population of centrocytes. Characteristically reactive follicle centres are trapped in the lymphomatous infiltrate which appears selectively to replace their mantle zones. Intestinal glands are displaced and obliterated but lymphoepithelial lesions are not present. The tumour cells are generally surface IgM and IgD +, and express the antigen CD5 which is more commonly associated with T cells. As such these cells are phenotypically and behaviourally distinct from the CCL cells in MALT-type lymphomas described above. CD5 + B cells are rare in normal postnatal lymphoid tissues though CD5 is expressed by B cells in fetal lymphoid tissues[42,43]. Multiple lymphomatous polyposis is probably the mucosal presentation of centrocytic lymphoma which occurs in the periphery. The malignancies may be derived from CD5 + B cells, the putative precursors of recirculating mantle zone B cells present in the fetus, by maturation arrest. In postnatal tissues CD5 + B cells are involved in the production of autoantibodies. Consistent with this, immunoglobulin from cases of centrocytic lymphomas has been shown to be reactive with a spectrum of autoantigens[44].

Burkitt's lymphoma

In the Middle East primary gastrointestinal Burkitt's lymphoma is a common disease of children. It has been comprehensively studied in Algeria[11,12]. Cytogenetic defects and infection with Epstein–Barr (EB) virus are seen in most cases. The disease is more common in boys and shows a peak incidence between four and five years of age. There is predeliction for the terminal ileum, but any part of the small intestine may be involved. Histologically the mucosa is effaced by sheets of monomorphic blasts interspersed with phagocytic histiocytes (macrophages). Lymphoepithelial lesions are not present.

Burkitt's lymphoma is a tumour which may reflect the migratory behaviour of a population of mucosal B cells. Characteristic spread of the tumour to lactating breast, paralleling migration of B blasts from the gut to the mammary glands of experimental animals during lactation, has been described[45,46]. Burkitt's lymphoma is a more aggressive tumour than lymphomas of MALT. This suggests that the tumour cells are derived from another mucosal B cell population, or that the infection with EBV results in more aggressive behaviour.

GASTROINTESTINAL T CELL LYMPHOMAS OF MALT

Primary gastrointestinal T cell lymphomas are much less common than B cell tumours and do not show the same striking epidemiological features. Enteropathy-associated T cell lymphoma (EATL) is the only distinctive T cell tumour of the gut which, in some ways, is the equivalent of B cell MALT lymphoma in that it appears to arise from a gut-committed T cell. Other T cell lymphomas rarely arise in the gut.

Enteropathy-associated T cell lymphoma (EATL)

This is a small intestinal tumour previously termed malignant histiocytosis of the intestine because it was thought to be of true histiocytic (mono-cyte/macrophage) origin[47]. It was subsequently shown, using Southern blotting with a probe to the β-chain of the T cell receptor, to be a T cell tumour[48]. The tumour in EATL may occur as a single mass or as multiple tumours often extending into the mesentery and mesenteric lymph nodes. The histological appearance of the tumour is variable. The malignant cells may resemble histiocytes with large irregular indented nuclei surrounded by moderately abundant cytoplasm. Others show a monomorphic infiltrate of large immature blast cells with prominent nucleoli. In many cases the tumour is pleomorphic with an abundance of multinucleated giant cells, some of which may show erythrophagocytosis. Intraepithelial tumour cells are present in approximately 50% of cases. The tumour is often accompanied by an inflammatory infiltrate of lymphocytes, plasma cells and eosinophils which may be so intense that the isolated malignant cells present are obscured. Early histochemical and immunohistochemical studies showed that the malignant cells contained acid phosphatase, diffusely distributed non-specific esterase and α-1 anti-trypsin, all of which are suggestive of a histiocytic origin[47,49,50]. Subsequent immunohistochemical studies showed that the tumours invariably express the antigens CD7 and HML1[48,51] (Fig. 11.5). CD7 is expressed by T cells and some null cells, and HML1 is an antibody recognizing mucosal T cells including the entire heterogeneous intraepithelial lymphocyte population, but very few cells outside the mucosae[52]. This reactivity strongly supports the suggestion that EATL is a tumour of mucosa committed T cells – possibly a tumour of intraepithelial lymphocytes. As mentioned above, detection of clonal rearrangement of the T cell receptor β-chain genes confirmed the T cell nature of the disease. A population of lymphocytes with the phenotype of the malignant cells in EATL, CD7 +, CD3 +/−, CD4 −, CD8 − has been described in normal jejunal epithelium. These cells are normally concentrated in the tips of villi, but are absent in enteropathies involving mucosal flattening such as EATL and coeliac disease[53]. The function of this population is not known.

The tumours are invariably associated with an enteropathy which is histologically indistinguishable from coeliac disease. Some patients have a history of coeliac disease, usually adult-onset, though cases complicating coeliac disease diagnosed in childhood have been described. In some cases

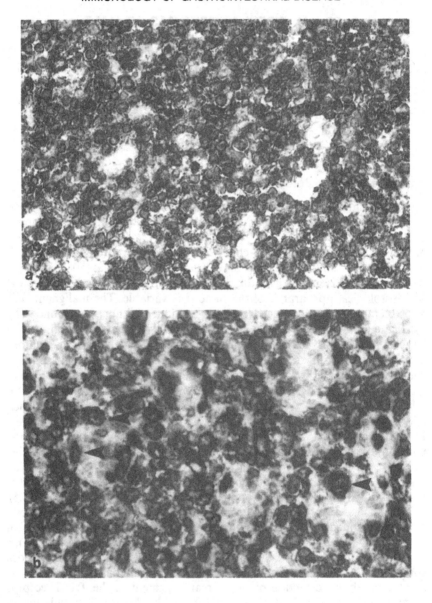

Figure 11.5 Frozen sections of enteropathy-associated T cell lymphoma stained with monoclonal antibody CD7. CD7 is expressed by T cells and some null cells. In addition to the tumour mass (a), tumour cells recognized by CD7 can be seen between the epithelial cells on the mucosal margin of the tumour (b), supporting the hypothesis that they are derived from an intraepithelial lymphocyte population. (Immunoperoxidase ×46).

there is no history of coeliac disease but the characteristic mucosal changes (villous atrophy and increase in the density of the intraepithelial lymphocyte infiltrate) are recognized in the resection specimen[54,55]. Coeliac disease and EATL have the same HLA predisposition[56]. It has been suggested, however, on the basis of an absence of antibodies to α-gliadin in these patients, that patients with EATL are not in fact suffering from coeliac disease, but from a T cell disorder that has induced malabsorption, since it is known that activated T cells can induce a coeliac-like enteropathy[57,58]. Immuno-histochemical studies of the intraepithelial lymphocyte population in patients with coeliac disease and EATL, however, have shown that these conditions can be distinguished from normal biopsies and some non-coeliac enteropathies on the basis of the sub-populations of intraepithelial lymphocytes they contain. They are, however, indistinguishable from each other using the same criteria. Both conditions contain raised percentages of intraepithelial lymphocytes with the phenotype CD3+, CD4−, CD8− compared to normal biopsies and non-coeliac enteropathies[53]. The balance of evidence suggests that the enteropathy in EATL is due to gluten sensitivity.

References

1. Isaacson, P. G. and Wright, D. H. (1984). Extranodal malignant lymphoma arising from mucosa associated lymphoid tissue. *Cancer*, **52**, 1410–16
2. Isaacson, P. G., Spencer, J. and Finn, T. (1986). Primary B cell gastric lymphoma. *Hum. Pathol.*, **17**, 72–82
3. Addis, B. J., Hyjek, E. and Isaacson, P. G. (1988). Primary pulmonary lymphoma: a reappraisal of its histogenesis and its relationship to pseudolymphoma and lymphoid interstitial pneumonia. *Histopathology*, **13**, 1–17
4. Wotherspoon, A. C., Soosay, G. N., Diss, T. C. and Isaacson, P. G. (1990). Low-grade primary B cell lymphoma of the lung. An immunohistochemical, molecular and cytogenetic study of a single case. *Am. J. Clin. Pathol.*, **94**, 655–60
5. Hyjek, E., Smith, W. J. and Isaacson, P. G. (1988). Primary B cell lymphoma of the salivary glands and its relationship to myoepithelial sialadenitis. *Hum. Pathol.*, **19**, 766–76
6. Hyjek, E. and Isaacson, P. G. (1988). Primary B cell lymphoma of the thyroid and its relationship to Hashimotos thyroiditis. *Hum. Pathol.*, **19**, 1315–26
7. Khojasteh, A., Haghshenass, M. and Haghighi, P. (1983). Immunoproliferative small intestinal disease. A third world lesion. *N. Engl. J. Med.*, **308**, 1401–5
8. Rambaud, J. C. (1983). Small intestinal lymphomas and alpha chain disease. *Clin. Gastroenterol.*, **12**, 743–66
9. Chan, J. C., Ng, C. S. and Isaacson, P. G. (1990). Relationship between high grade lymphoma and low grade B cell mucosa-associated lymphoid tissue lymphoma (MALToma) of the stomach. *Am. J. Pathol.*, **136**, 1153–64
10. Isaacson, P. G., MacLennan, K. A. and Subbuswamy, S. G. (1984). Multiple lymphomatous polyposis of the gastrointestinal tract. *Histopathology*, **8**, 641–56
11. Ladjadj, Y., Philip, T., Lenior, G. M., Tazerout, F. Z., Bendisari, K., Boukheloua, R., Biron, P., Brunat-Mentigny, M. and Abdoulola, M. (1984). Abdominal Burkitt-like lymphoma in Algeria. *Br. J. Cancer*, **49**, 503–12
12. Anaissie, E., Geha, S., Allam, C., Jabbour, J., Khakyk, M. and Salem, P. (1985). Burkitt's lymphoma in the Middle East: a study of 34 cases. *Cancer*, **56**, 2534–9
13. Isaacson, P. G. and Spencer, J. (1987). Malignant lymphoma of mucosa associated lymphoid tissue. *Histopathology*, **11**, 445–62
14. Myhre, M. J. and Isaacson, P. G. (1987). Primary B cell gastric lymphoma – as reassessment of its histogenesis. *J. Pathol.*, **152**, 1–11
15. Wright, D. H. and Isaacson, P. G. (1989). Gut-associated lymphoid tumours. In Whitehead, R. (ed.), *Gastrointestinal and Oesophageal Pathology*. Edinburgh: Churchill Livingstone, vol. 37, pp. 643–61
16. Spencer, J., Finn, T. and Isaacson, P. G. (1986). Human Peyer's patches: an immunohistochemical study. *Gut*, **27**, 405–10

17. Spencer, J., Finn, T., Pulford, K., Mason, D. Y. and Isaacson, P. G. (1985). The human gut contains a novel population of B lymphocytes which resemble marginal zone B cells. *Clin. Exp. Immunol.*, **62**, 607–12
18. Smith-Ravin, J., Spencer, J., Beverley, P. C. L. and Isaacson, P. G. (1990). Characterisation of two monoclonal antibodies (UCL4D12 and UCL3D3) that discriminate between human mantle zone and marginal zone B cells. *Clin. Exp. Immunol.*, **82**, 181–7
19. Spencer, J., Diss, T. C. and Isaacson, P. G. (1990). A study of the properties of a low-grade mucosal B cell lymphoma using a monoclonal antibody specific for the tumour immunoglobulin. *J. Pathol.*, **160**, 231–8
20. Lui, Y.-J., Oldfield, S. and MacLennan, I. C. M. (1988). Memory B cells in T cell dependent antibody responses colonise the splenic marginal zones. *Eur. J. Immunol.*, **18**, 355–62
21 Gray, D., Kumararatne, D. S., Lortan, J., Khan, M. and MacLennan, I. C. M. (1984). Relation of intrasplenic migration of marginal zone B cells to antigen localisation on follicular dendritic cells. *Immunology*, **52**, 659–69
22. Isaacson, P. G., Dogan, A., Price, S. K. and Spencer, J. (1989). Immunoproliferative small intestinal disease; an immunohistochemical study. *Am. J. Surg. Pathol.*, **13**, 1023–33
23. Isaacson, P. G., Wotherspoon, A. C., Diss, T. C. and Pan, L. X. (1991). Bcl-2 expression in lymphomas. *Lancet*, **337**, 175–6
24. Tsujimoto, Y., Finger, L. R., Yunis, J., Nowell, P. C. and Croce, C. M. (1984). Cloning of the chromosome breakpoint of neoplastic B cells with the t(14:18) chromosome translocation. *Science*, **226**, 1097–9
25. Pan, L. X., Diss, T. C., Cunningham, D. and Isaacson, P. G. (1989). The bcl-2 gene in primary B cell lymphoma of mucosa associated lymphoid tissue. *Am. J. Pathol.*, **135**, 7–11
26. Hussell, T., Spencer, J. and Isaacson, P. G. (1991). A low grade lymphoma of mucosa associated lymphoid tissue expressing immunoglobulin specific for mucosal post capillary venules. *J. Pathol.*, **163**, 172A
27. Freeman, C., Berg, J. W. and Cutler, S. J. (1972). Occurrence and prognosis of extranodal lymphomas. *Cancer*, **29**, 252–60
28. Brooks, J. and Enterline, H. T. (1983). Primary gastric lymphomas. A clinicopathological study of 58 cases with long term follow up and literature review. *Cancer*, **51**, 701–11
29. Gray, D., MacLennan, I. C. M., Bazin, H. and Khan, M. (1982). Migrant mu +, delta + and static mu +, delta − B lymphocyte subsets. *Eur. J. Immunol.*, **12**, 564–9
30. Gowans, J. L. and Knight, E. J. (1964). The route of recirculation of lymphocytes in the rat. *Proc. Roy. Soc. B*, **159**, 257–82
31. Husband, A. J. and Gowans, J. L. (1978). The origin and antigen dependent distribution of IgA containing cells in the intestine. *J. Exp. Med.*, **148**, 1146–60
32. Husband, A. J. (1982). Kinetics of extravasation and redistribution of IgA specific antibody containing cells in the intestine. *J. Immunol.*, **128**, 1355–9
33. Weingrad, D. N., Decosse, J. J., Sherlock, P., Straus, D., Leiberman, P. H. and Plippa, D. A. (1982). Primary gastrointestinal lymphoma: a 30 year review. *Cancer*, **49**, 1258–65
34. Joensuu, H., Soderstrom, K. O., Klemi, P. J. and Eerola, E. (1987). Nuclear DNA content and its prognostic value in lymphoma of the stomach. *Cancer*, **60**, 3042–8
35. Rambaud, J. C., Modigliani, R., Nguyen Phuoc, B. K., Lejeune, R., Le Carrer, M., Mehaut, M., Valleur, P., Gallian, A. and Danon, F. (1980). Non-secretory alpha-chain disease in intestinal lymphoma. *N. Engl. J. Med.*, **303**, 53
36. Ben-Ayed, F., Halphen, M., Najjar, T. *et al.* (1989). Treatment of alpha chain disease – results of a prospective study in 21 Tunisian patients by the Tunisian–French intestinal lymphoma study group. *Cancer*, **63**, 1251–6
37. Galian, A., Lecester, M. J., Scott, J., Bowgel, C., Mutuchansky, C. and Rambaud, J. C. (1977). Pathological study of alpha chain disease with special emphasis on evolution. *Cancer*, **39**, 2081–101
38. Bentaboulet, M., Mihaesco, E., Gendron, M.-C,., Brouet, J. C. and Tsapis, A. (1989). Genomic alterations in a case of alpha-chain disease leading to the generation of composite exons from the J_H region. *Eur. J. Immunol.*, **19**, 2093–8
39. Smith, W. J., Price, S. K. and Isaacson, P. G. (1987). Immunoglobulin gene rearrangement in immunoproliferative small intestinal disease (IPSID). *J. Clin. Pathol.*, **40**, 1291–7
40. Cornes, J. S. (1961). Multiple lymphomatous polyposis of the gastrointestinal tract. *Cancer*, **14**, 249–57

41. O'Briain, D. S., Kennedy, M. J. and Daly, P. A. (1989). Multiple lymphomatous polyposis of the gastrointestinal tract. A clinico-pathologically distinctive form of non-Hodgkins lymphoma of B cell centrocytic type. *Am. J. Surg. Pathol.*, **13**, 691–9
42. Bofill, M., Janossy, G., Janossa, M., Burford, G. D., Seymour, G. J., Wernet, P. and Kelemen, E. (1985). Human B cell development II. Sub-populations in the fetus. *J. Immunol.*, **134**, 1531–38
43. Spencer, J., MacDonald, T. T., Finn, T. and Isaacson, P. G. (1986). The development of gut-associated lymphoid tissue in the terminal ileum of fetal human intestine. *Clin. Exp. Immunol.*, **64**, 536–43
44. Kipps, T. J., Robbins, B. A., Tefferi, A., Meisenholder, G., Banks, P. M. and Carson, D. A. (1990). CD5 positive B cell malignancies frequently express cross reactive idiotypes associated with IgM autoantibodies. *Am. J. Pathol.*, **136**, 809–16
45. Shepherd, J. J. and Wright, D. H. (1967). Burkitt's tumour presenting as bilateral swelling of the breast. *Br. J. Surg.*, **54**, 776–80
46. Roux, M. E., McWilliams, M., Phillips-Quagliata, J. M., Weisz Carrington, P. and Lamm, M. E. (1977). Origin of IgA plasma cells in the mammary gland. *J. Exp. Med.*, **146**, 1311–22
47. Isaacson, P. G. and Wright, D. H. (1978). Malignant histiocytosis of the intestine: its relationship to malabsorption and ulcerative jejunitis. *Hum. Pathol.*, **9**, 661–77
48. Isaacson, P. G., O'Connor, N. T. J., Spencer, J. et al. (1985). Malignant histiocytosis of the intestine: a T cell lymphoma. *Lancet*, **1**, 688–91
49. Isaacson, P. G. and Wright, D. H. (1978). Intestinal lymphoma associated with malabsorption. *Lancet*, **1**, 67–70
50. Isaacson, P. G. and Wright, D. H. (1980). Malabsorption and intestinal lymphomas. In Wright, R. (ed.), *Recent Advances in Intestinal Pathology*, London: W. B. Saunders, pp. 193–212.
51. Spencer, J., Cerf-Bensussan, N., Jarry, A. et al. (1988). Enteropathy associated T cell lymphoma (malignant histiocytosis of the intestine) is recognised by a monoclonal antibody that defines a membrane molecule on human mucosal lymphocytes. *Am. J. Pathol.*, **132**, 1–5
52. Cerf-Bensussan, N., Jarry, A., Brousse, N., Lisowska-Grospierre, B., Guy-Grand, D. and Griscelli, C. (1987). A monoclonal antibody (HML1) defining a novel membrane molecule present on human intestinal lymphocytes. *Eur. J. Immunol.*, **17**, 1279–85
53. Spencer, J., MacDonald, T. T., Diss, T. C., Walker-Smith, J. A., Ciclitira, P. J. and Isaacson, P. G. (1989). Changes in intraepithelial lymphocyte sub-populations in coeliac disease and enteropathy associated T cell lymphoma (malignant histiocytosis of the intestine). *Gut*, **30**, 339–46
54. Isaacson, P. G. (1986). Malignant lymphoma. In Jewell, D. P. and Ireland, A. (eds), *Topics in Gastroenterology*. Oxford: Blackwell, vol. 14, pp. 35–43
55. Eakins, D., Fulton, T. and Haddon, D. R. (1964). Reticulum cell sarcoma of the small bowel and steatorrhoea. *Gut*, **5**, 315–23
56. O'Driscoll, B. R. C., Stevens, F. M., O'Gorman, T. A., Finnegan, P., McWeeney, J. J., Little, M. P., Connelly, C. E. and McCarthy, C. F. (1982). HLA-type of patients with coeliac disease and malignancy in the west of Ireland. *Gut*, **23**, 662–5
57. O'Farrelly, C., Feigherty, C., O'Braian, D. S., Stevens, F., Connelly, C. E., McCarthy, C. F. and Weir, D. G. (1986). Humoral response to wheat protein in patients with coeliac disease and enteropathy associated T cell lymphoma. *Br. Med. J.*, **293**, 908–10
58. MacDonald, T. T. and Spencer, J. (1988). Evidence that activated mucosal T cells play a role in the pathogenesis of enteropathy in human small intestine. *J. Exp. Med.*, **167**, 1341–9

12
The gut in HIV infection

M. ZEITZ*, R. ULLRICH and E.-O. RIECKEN

INTRODUCTION

The acquired immunodeficiency syndrome (AIDS) is caused by a human retrovirus which was originally designated by a variety of names including HTLV III (human T lymphotropic virus III) and LAV (lymphadenopathy virus)[1,2], and which is now called human immunodeficiency virus (HIV). HIV is a member of the lentivirus subfamily. A second human lentivirus, HIV-2, has been isolated from patients with AIDS, especially in Africa, which is a novel member of the human lentivirus family and not an envelope variant of original isolates of HIV[3,4]. The original isolates are now designated as HIV-1. Since the first description of AIDS cases in 1981 this disease has spread as an epidemic, and is now a major health problem all over the world. The number of patients with AIDS registered by the WHO in the middle of 1990 is more than 250 000 worldwide[5]. The estimated number of individuals infected with HIV is 6–8 million by 1990.

HIV has the ability to cause progressive deterioration of the host's immune function leading to opportunistic infections and neoplasms, the hallmarks of AIDS. A high proportion of patients infected with HIV suffers from gastrointestinal symptoms[6-8]. Although infections by opportunistic and other enteric pathogens are a major cause of these disturbances, it is important to note that even when thorough and repeated investigations are used a significant fraction of patients remains in whom neither opportunistic causes nor other intestinal pathogens can be found. This clinical finding has given rise to the hypothesis that HIV itself might cause intestinal dysfunction[9,10]. Such an 'HIV-induced' enteropathy might either be caused by direct damage of intestinal epithelial cells by HIV, or mucosal integrity could be disturbed by changes in the mucosal immune system, since a close relationship between

* Supported by a grant from the Bundesminister für Forschung und Technologie (FKZ II-048-88)

the local immune system and enterocyte growth and function has been shown in several studies[11,12] (see Chapter 8 in this volume).

In this chapter data on HIV infection of the intestinal mucosa, changes in the intestinal immune system, as well as structural and functional changes of the small intestinal mucosa in HIV infection will be discussed. Based on these data a hypothesis will be put forward that HIV itself is an intestinal pathogen causing a characteristic pattern of small intestinal damage.

GASTROINTESTINAL MANIFESTATIONS IN HIV INFECTION

Gastrointestinal symptoms such as diarrhoea, weight loss, abdominal pain, vomiting, and dysphagia are among the most common and devastating problems in HIV-infected patients. These symptoms can in part be attributed to a wide variety of opportunistic and other enteric pathogens (Table 12.1) as well as secondary malignancies like Kaposi's sarcoma and malignant lymphomas[8,13-16]. However, even repeated investigations of multiple stool samples and intestinal biopsies including electron microscopy and immunohistology fail to identify a known cause of the gastrointestinal symptoms in a significant proportion of the patients (Fig. 12.1). The percentage of patients with diarrhoea in whom no intestinal pathogen is identified varies in different

Table 12.1   Frequency of opportunistic and non-opportunistic gastro-intestinal pathogens in patients with HIV infection and gastrointestinal symptoms

Agents	Rates of detection (%)
Adenovirus	3–6
B. hominis	7–14
C. difficile	1–6
C. perfringens	1
Campylobacter sp.	2–10
Chlamydia sp.	1–3
Coronavirus	1
Cryptosporidium	5–59
Cytomegalovirus	7–45
E. histolytica	3–25
G. lamblia	2–15
Herpes simplex virus	4–29
I. belli	1–19
M. avium Complex	5–25
M. tuberculosis	1–3
Salmonella sp.	1–15
Shigella sp.	1–10
Spirochetes	1–9
Yersinia sp	1
None	15–56

Values were taken from references 10, 15–20, 106, and own unpublished results.

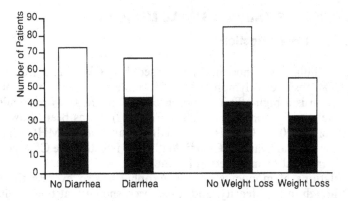

Figure 12.1 Frequency of gastrointestinal pathogens in 159 AIDS patients with and without diarrhoea or weight loss. At least three different stool samples and gastrointestinal biopsies were investigated. Diarrhoea is significantly associated with the presence of an intestinal pathogen ($p < 0.05$). However, intestinal pathogens are also present in patients without diarrhoea, and a considerable fraction of patients with diarrhoea remains, in whom no pathogen can be found. There is no significant association between weight loss and the presence of an intestinal pathogen (own unpublished results)

studies between 15% and 50%[10,15-19]. Furthermore, when analysing the presence of intestinal pathogens in stool or biopsy in relation to the presence or absence of gastrointestinal symptoms, the causative relevance of several agents detected remains questionable[20] (own results; submitted for publication, see also Fig. 12.1).

Evidence that small intestinal dysfunction with malabsorption may occur in HIV-infected patients and contribute to diarrhoea and weight loss is provided in several studies[9,10,13,21]. Laboratory parameters indicative of malabsorption, such as serum albumin, calcium, zinc, folic acid, and vitamin B_{12}, are reduced in a significant percentage of HIV-infected patients. Reduced serum concentrations are found even at early disease stages[10]. Direct tests of absorptive function were also performed in HIV-infected patients with gastrointestinal symptoms: significant fat malabsorption was found in 29–80%, xylose malaborsption in 54–100%, and vitamin B_{12} malaborsption in 75% of AIDS patients; however, the number of patients was low in these studies[9,10,13,21-24]. Lactase deficiency as measured by H_2-exhalation after oral lactose ingestion was found in about 50% of HIV-infected patients even at early stages of the disease[10]. Again, malabsorption is also recognized in the absence of an additional enteric pathogen in a considerable percentage of patients. A recent study suggests that patients with severe weight loss, high stool volumes, and severe malabsorption are more likely to harbour an additional intestinal pathogen than patients with less severe gastrointestinal symptoms, in whom even repeated investigations fail to recognize a pathogen[23].

Thus, although a wide variety of intestinal pathogens is found in HIV-infected patients with gastrointestinal symptoms, a fraction of patients remains in whom neither secondary infections nor malignancies are found; in addition, the pathogenic relevance of some abnormalities detected is doubtful.

HIV INFECTION OF THE INTESTINAL MUCOSA

Target cells of HIV infection

The severe cellular immunodeficiency caused by HIV results from virus infecting CD4-positive T lymphocytes. The molecular mechanism of this cellular tropism is a high-affinity binding of HIV to the CD4 molecule via the HIV envelope glycoprotein, gp120[25] (Fig. 12.2). It has been shown that the affinity of gp120 to CD4 is even higher than that of MHC Class II molecules, the natural ligand of CD4[25]. With HIV infection the CD4-positive T cell is either killed or impaired in function[2,26].

Subpopulations of monocytes and macrophages also express the CD4 antigen although in low density, and it has been shown that these cells can be infected with HIV[27-30]. A second mechanism by which macrophages and monocytes may be infected with HIV is the binding of antibody–HIV complexes to Fc receptors or complement receptors on these cells and subsequent phagocytosis of these complexes[31,32] (Fig. 12.2). In contrast to the CD4-positive T cell, HIV-infected macrophages and monocytes are relatively resistant to the cytopathic effect of HIV[27,33]; these cells may therefore serve as an important reservoir for the persistence of HIV in the host.

In addition, it has been shown that follicular dendritic cells are also infected with HIV *in vivo*[34-36]. HIV-infected follicular dendritic cells were observed

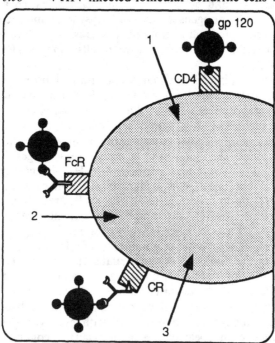

Figure 12.2 Possible mechanisms of cellular HIV infection: (1) HIV envelope antigen gp120 binds with high affinity to cell surface CD4 molecules followed by virus entry. (2) HIV–antibody complexes bind to Fc receptors on the cell surface followed by internalization of the complex. (3) HIV–antibody complexes bind to complement receptors on the cell surface

both in peripheral lymph nodes and in intestinal mucosal lymphoid follicles[37,38]. The mechanism by which these cells are infected is not completely understood, as they lack the CD4 molecule and express only the low affinity Fc receptor for IgE[35]. Since follicular dendritic cells form an extensive network of cellular processes in the centre of lymph follicles, CD4-positive T cells come into close contact with these cells and may become infected by direct cell-to-cell contact.

Presence of HIV-infected cells in the mucosa

Approximately 70% of T cells within the mucosa are targets for HIV because they bear the CD4 molecule on their surface (see below). Macrophages in the mucosa and follicular dendritic cells in mucosal lymphoid follicles may also be infected and constitute important reservoirs for HIV. Both immunohistology and *in situ* hybridization have been used to identify HIV-infected cells in the intestinal mucosa which were found in 30–50% of the investigated patients[10,37,39,40] (Table 12.2). HIV-infected mononuclear cells in the lamina propria were found in all studies and morphologically assessed as lymphocytes or macrophages; however, the definite identification of the cell type infected with HIV was not possible in these studies. In one study, binding of HIV-specific DNA probes predominantly to basal crypt cells was reported, and infected cells were identified as enterochromaffine cells, enterocytes, and goblet cells using an argentaffin stain and morphology[39]. However, in the remaining studies HIV-infected cells were either completely absent in the epithelial layer[40] or very rarely observed, and assessed rather as intraepithelial lymphocytes[10,37]. These differences might therefore be due to technical reasons rather than reflect true biological differences. Thus while intestinal epithelial cells *in vitro* are infectable by HIV[41] even in the absence of detectable CD4 expression[42], the relevance of this finding remains to be studied, since its demonstration *in vivo* is controversial; furthermore, no cytopathic alterations were documented in HIV-infected epithelial cell lines[41].

Table 12.2 Summary of different studies on the presence of HIV-infected cells in the intestinal mucosa in patients with HIV infection

	Patients/ stage	Method	HIV-detection	Infected cells	Localization
Nelson et al.[39]	10/IV	DNA Hybridization	5/10	Enterochromaffine and goblet cells, enterocytes, mononuclear cells	Cryptbase, lamina propria
Ullrich et al.[10]	11/II or III, 40/IV	Immuno-histology	20/51	Mononuclear cells	Lamina propria, two intraepithelial
Fox et al.[40]	25/IV	RNA Hybridization	7/25	Mononuclear cells	Lamina propria
Jarry et al[37]	127/IV	Immuno-histology	38/127	Mononuclear cells, (one dendritic, one epithelial cell)	Lamina propria, two intraepithelial

In conclusion, the studies available at present document HIV infection of mononuclear cells in the intestinal lamina propria, whereas the significance of HIV infection of epithelial cells is questionable.

IMMUNOPATHOGENIC MECHANISMS OF HIV INFECTION

Consequences of HIV infection for T cell function

HIV infection causes depletion of CD4-positive T cells. The exact mechanism for the cytotoxic effect of HIV is still not completely understood (Table 12.3). Several mechanisms have been discussed: intensive virus budding may be responsible for the formation of microholes in the cell membrane[43], insertion of HIV envelope glycoproteins in the T cell membrane may cause changes in membrane permeability to ions[44], and there is also evidence that binding of gp120 to intracellular CD4 induces cell death[45]. Accumulation of unintegrated viral DNA in the cytoplasm is also highly toxic for the cell[46]. The well-known phenomenon of syncytia formation after *in vitro* infection of CD4 T cells with HIV may be caused by binding of gp120 on the cell surface of infected cells to CD4 of neighbouring uninfected T cells[47,48]. Autoimmune phenomena to CD4 T cells bearing gp120 on their surface have also been described in HIV-infected patients: both antibody-dependent cytotoxicity and cellular cytotoxic mechanisms may be of relevance[49-51].

The selective killing of the CD4-positive T cell subset, which plays a central role in the immune response, will compromise the function of a variety of other cell types resulting in multiple immunological deficits of the organism[26,52]. The different subsets of the CD4-positive lymphocyte population are intimately involved in B cell function, differentiation of cytolytic T cells, suppressor T cell function, natural killer cell activity and certain macrophage/monocyte functions.

In addition to the depletion of CD4 T cells, abnormalities in CD4 T cell function have been observed at all stages of HIV infection (Table 12.3). Helper

Table 12.3 Consequences of HIV infection on T cell function

Cytotoxic effects of HIV
Formation of microholes in the cell membrane
Changes in cell membrane permeability
Accumulation of unintegrated viral DNA in the cytoplasm
Binding of HIV envelope proteins to intracellular CD4 molecules
Syncytia formation by binding of HIV antigen gp120 to surface CD4 molecules
Autoimmune processes to CD4-positive T cells bearing gp120 on the surface

Non-cytotoxic effects of HIV
Disturbed helper function of CD4 T cells for B cell differentiation
Decreased proliferation of T cells to soluble and viral antigens
Defective IL-2 and interferon-γ production by T cells
Low anti-CD3 reactivity of T cells
Impairment of signal transduction
Downregulation of the genes for CD4, CD3, CD2, and CD25
Decrease in CD29 expression ('memory' T cells)

---

activity for B cell differentiation is disturbed[53], T cell proliferative responses to soluble and viral antigens are decreased even at early stages of HIV infection[54-57], antigen-induced interferon-γ production[58] and IL-2 production[59] by T cells is low. T cell proliferation to anti-CD3 antibodies is decreased, and low anti-CD3 reactivity, independent of the number of CD4-positive T cells, seems to be of predictive value for progression to AIDS[60]. HIV infection has been reported to down-regulate cellular genes or inhibit synthesis of proteins critical for T cell function such as CD4[45,61], CD3, CD2, and CD25 (α-chain of the IL-2 receptor)[62,63]. There is also evidence for an early loss of CD29-positive memory T cells in HIV infection[64,65].

Viral antigens themselves may have stimulatory effects on T cells: HIV envelope peptides induce proliferation of T cells, and native gp120 induces increased IL-2 receptor expression in T cells[66-68]. In contrast, the response of CD4-positive T cells activated by mitogen or antigen is suppressed by HIV and HIV antigen preparations, notably gp120[66].

Thus, besides its direct cytopathic effect, HIV alters T cell function in several ways, and these functional abnormalities probably contribute substantially to the pathogenesis of the progressive immune dysfunction in HIV infection. Disturbed function of CD4-positive T cells may also be of special importance for immunoregulation at mucosal surfaces, since activated CD4-positive T cells predominate in this compartment of the immune system (see below).

Role of T cell activation in HIV replication

After entry of HIV into the target cell viral RNA is transcribed into DNA by viral reverse transcriptase. HIV-specific DNA then is partially integrated into the host genome and partially remains unintegrated in the cytoplasm. Once the HIV proviral DNA is integrated in the host's chromosomal DNA, viral replication may enter a latent phase, depending on the state of activation of the infected cell[69,70]. In resting T cells no or very low-level virus expression is observed. This may be due to a regulatory protein, rpt-1, which is selectively expressed in resting CD4 T cells, and which down-regulates both the promoter region of the IL-2 receptor α-chain gene and the expression of the HIV LTR[71]. Activation of infected lymphocytes is followed by transcription, protein synthesis, post-translational processing, assembly of viral RNA and protein and finally budding of the mature virions[69]. Recent studies indicate that factors specific to activated T cells stimulate viral transcription by binding to regions on viral DNA[72]. It has been shown that the T cell activation factor, NFκB, binds to a NFκB binding site and activates *in vitro* transcription of the HIV promoter[73].

T cell activation can be achieved *in vitro* by mitogenic, antigenic, or allogeneic stimuli; *in vivo* several concurrent infections may activate T cells and thereby induce HIV replication. Coinfections with other viruses such as herpes simplex virus, cytomegalovirus, and Epstein–Barr virus have also been shown to upregulate HIV expression[74-77]. In addition, cytokines may be important in the efficient replication of HIV[78,79]. TNF-α is an especially potent stimulator of increased HIV expression of infected cell lines *in vitro*[80-82]. Thus, efficient replication of HIV is closely associated with activation of T cells.

Characteristics of lamina propria T cells as targets for HIV

In recent years specific differences have been recognized between lamina propria T cells and T cells of other origin. Using immunohistochemical techniques on frozen tissue sections and flow cytometry on isolated lymphocytes it has been shown that intestinal lamina propria lymphocytes are predominantly of the helper/inducer phenotype (CD4-positive)[83-86]. In addition, lamina propria T cells possess a low expression of the CD45RA antigen (recognized by monoclonal antibody 2H4) and a high expression of CD45R0 (recognized by UCHL-1)[86,87]. CD45RA-low, CD45R0-high T cells have been shown to represent memory T cells, i.e. T cells which have already been in contact with antigen[88,89]. However, another marker of circulating memory T cells, CD29, is expressed only on about 50% of lamina propria T cells[86,87]. Lamina propria T cells therefore have an only partially overlapping phenotype with memory T cells. In addition, about 40% of T cells in the lamina propria express the T cell marker, HML-1, which is nearly exclusively found in the mucosa[86,90]. The specific phenotype of lamina propria T cells corresponds functionally with a specific response to antigens: in an animal model of intestinal infection and inflammation (*Chlamydia trachomatis* proctitis of non-human primates) lamina propria T cells did not proliferate when stimulated *in vitro* with specific antigen, although T cells from mesenteric lymph nodes, the spleen, or the peripheral blood did proliferate under identical conditions. However, lamina propria T cells provided help for Ig synthesis after stimulation with the same antigen[91]. Thus lamina propria T cells resemble differentiated effector cells which carry out important immunoregulatory functions in the microenvironment of the mucosa in response to enteric pathogens.

Another important finding in the context of mucosal HIV infection is that lamina propria T cells are more activated than T cells in other compartments of the immune system. Using cytofluorometric analysis of intestinal lymphocytes it was shown that lamina propria lymphocytes have increased expression of CD25, the α-chain of the IL-2 receptor, as compared to other T cells[86,92]. This result was confirmed at the molecular level: Northern blot analysis of lymphocytes isolated from different tissue sites revealed that only lamina propria lymphocytes contained clearly detectable mRNA for the IL-2 receptor without *in vitro* stimulation[92]. Other gene products associated with T cell activation were also studied: resting lamina propria T lymphocytes were similar to other T cells in that IL-2 was not detected in culture supernatants. However, after stimulation with mitogen, lamina propria lymphocytes synthesized significantly more IL-2 compared to the other populations[92]. The concept of an increased state of activation of lamina propria T cells is also supported by the finding that HML-1 is an activation antigen[86]. In summary, these results clearly demonstrate that lamina propria

T cells are more activated than T cells in other sites of the immune system; HIV infection of these cells might have specific consequences for T cell function in the intestinal mucosal immune system[93] (Fig. 12.3).

Mucosal T cells in HIV infection

Disturbances of the mucosal immune system in HIV infection have been studied so far only by immunohistological and electron microscopical techniques. A reduction in the number of CD4-positive mononuclear cells, the known target cells of the AIDS virus, in the intestinal lamina propria has been described in several studies[37,94-96]. In our own investigations only a minor reduction in the number of CD4-positive cells has been found with an increase in the number of CD8-positive cells[97,98]. Thus, as in the circulation, the CD4/CD8 ratio is decreased in the lamina propria of the intestine in AIDS (Table 12.4). Impairment of T cell function in the intestinal mucosa in HIV infection is indicated by the finding of a decreased number of CD25-positive cells (cells expressing the α-chain of the IL-2 receptor) in the lamina propria[97,98]. One important finding in most of these phenotype studies is that the reduction in the number of CD4-positive cells in the intestinal lamina propria is considerably less pronounced compared to the

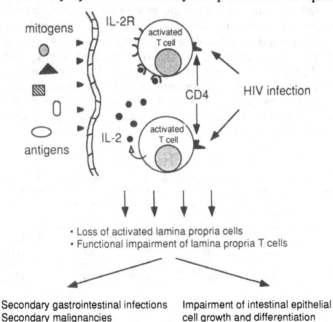

Figure 12.3 Infection by HIV of lamina propria CD4-positive T cells may lead to functional impairment of these cells. Since CD4-positive T cells play a central role in immunoregulation at mucosal surfaces, the mucosal immune barrier subsequently may be disturbed leading to opportunistic and non-opportunistic infections. Loss of activated T cells in the mucosa may also influence the growth and differentiation of intestinal epithelial cells

peripheral blood (Table 12.4). An explanation for this may be that the replication of HIV and its cytotoxic effect depend upon cellular activation and proliferation (see above). Intestinal lamina propria T cells differ from circulating T cells in both their state of activation and their inability to proliferate after stimulation with antigen. Therefore, HIV infection of intestinal CD4-positive cells may lead not to cell death, but rather to an impaired expression of surface markers essential for T cell function such as the IL-2 receptor. The loss of activated cells in HIV infection with the relative preservation of CD4-positive T cells therefore indicates mainly a functional impairment of mucosal T cells which might also be a consequence of HIV infection (see above) (Fig. 12.3).

The number of intraepithelial lymphocytes in the large and small intestinal mucosa in different stages of HIV infection has been found to be normal in most studies[99-101]; a slight increase in the number might occur in the small intestine when compared to controls[99]. Using immunohistology a decrease in CD3-positive and CD8-positive intraepithelial lymphocytes per 500 epithelial cells was found[37]. An electron microscopical study has shown that intraepithelial lymphocytes in AIDS patients possess more granules and appear activated[99]. From the studies presently available no clear conclusions can be drawn regarding changes in intraepithelial lymphocyte phenotype and function in HIV infection.

Little information exists also on mucosal secretory immunity in HIV infection: a reduction of IgA-containing plasma cells in small intestinal and colonic biopsies from patients with AIDS has been reported, and an increase of IgM-containing plasma cells, while IgG-containing cells were found to be normal[102]. In a recent study it was shown that salivary IgA_1 levels were normal in AIDS patients, whereas IgA_2 levels were markedly decreased[103]. Changes in immunoglobulin isotype expression in HIV infection might also be caused by abnormalities in mucosal T cells which regulate B cell isotype differentiation. Further studies clearly are needed to clarify the relevance of secretory mucosal immunity in AIDS.

Table 12.4 Lymphocyte subpopulations of the duodenal lamina propria in HIV infection

	Rodgers et al.[94]	Ellakany et al.[95]	Budhraja et al.[96]	Ullrich et al.[98]	Jarry et al.[37]
Number of patients	5 C, 12 HIV	10 C, 6 HIV	7 C, 14 HIV	20 C, 51 HIV	10 C, 33 HIV
T cells	60%[a]	80%[a]	80%[a]	120%[c]	115%[a]
CD4+	60%[a]	20%[a]	50%[a]	100%[c]	10%[a]
CD8+	130%[a]	200%[a]	180%[a]	160%[c]	240%[a]
CD4/CD8					
Controls	1.8[b]	2.3[b]	0.8[b]	1.9[d]	1.7[b]
HIV	0.7[b]	0.2[b]	0.2[b]	1.1[d]	0.1[b]

C = Controls; HIV = HIV-infected patients
[a] Mean of HIV-infected patients/mean of controls
[b] Mean
[c] Median of HIV-infected patients/median of controls
[d] Median

SMALL INTESTINAL STRUCTURE AND FUNCTION IN HIV INFECTION

The gut epithelium is functionally related to the mucosal immune system[11,12] (discussed in detail elsewhere in this volume); e.g. hyperregenerative adaptation of the mucosa, i.e. villous atrophy with increased proliferation of crypt cells leading to crypt hyperplasia, is found in states of mucosal T cell activation both *in vitro*[11] and *in vivo*[104]. Therefore, changes in mucosal architecture might reflect alterations in mucosal immunity. By three-dimensional morphometry of microdissected duodenal specimens partial villous atrophy was found in HIV-infected patients with gastrointestinal symptoms; however, the specific type of mucosal transformation was dependent on both the presence of secondary pathogens and mucosal HIV infection[10]. In patients with HIV-infected cells in the mucosa villous atrophy was accompanied by reduced crypt cell proliferation. If secondary infections were present, the number of mitotic figures per crypt were slightly increased but inappropriately to the villous atrophy resulting in impaired crypt hyperplasia. Thus HIV infection is associated with epithelial hypoproliferation[10,105]. In addition, the maturation of enterocytes is disturbed as indicated by decreased activities of brush-border enzymes[10,97]; e.g. lactase deficiency, the prevalence of which is about 10% in whites, was found in nearly 50% of white HIV-infected patients, and was significantly commoner in patients with mucosal HIV infection, secondary intestinal infections, or both as compared with controls. As discussed above, it is unlikely that these abnormalities in mucosal structure and function result from cytopathic HIV infection of enterocytes, since mucosal HIV infection was found restricted to mononuclear lamina propria cells in most studies. However, the findings fit into the concept of immune-mediated mucosal transformation (Fig. 12.4); crypt cell proliferation is induced by T cell activation; therefore the activated T cells present in the normal lamina propria might be involved in the maintenance of the normal mucosal architecture. The epithelial hypoproliferation seen in HIV-infected patients, which is most pronounced if mucosal HIV infection is found, thus indicates impaired activation of lamina propria T cells. In fact, this has been demonstrated by reduced expression of CD25 in the lamina propria of HIV-infected patients[98], and is in accordance with the suppressive effect of HIV on T cell activation induced by other stimuli as documented *in vitro*[66]. It is tempting to assume that enterocyte maturation is also influenced by the postulated as-yet-unidentified trophic factor(s) produced by activated lamina propria T cells. Impairment or depletion of activated regulatory T cells in the lamina propria by HIV might thus lead not only to a breakdown of the mucosal immune barrier resulting in a variety of opportunistic infections, but also to malabsorption due to mucosal atrophy or enterocyte dysfunction (see Fig. 12.3). The existence of such an HIV enteropathy is strongly supported by the presence of gastrointestinal symptoms and malabsorption in HIV-infected patients without detectable secondary abnormalities, and especially in early stages of the disease when HIV is virtually the only intestinal pathogen identifiable in a considerable proportion of patients. The intestinal abnormalities in HIV infection may thus represent a specific immunologically mediated form of an intestinal adaptation[87,97,98].

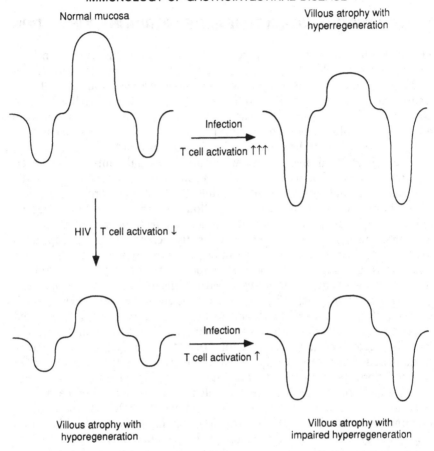

Figure 12.4 Impairment of mucosal T cell activation by HIV infection might cause enteropathy. Hyperregenerative villous atrophy is associated with, and can *in vitro* be induced by, T cell activation. The normal architecture of the mucosa is maintained by the balance between villus cell slough and crypt cell proliferation, which probably is affected by the activated T cells present in the normal lamina propria. Functional impairment or loss of these activated regulatory cells by HIV infection thus could lead to the hyporegenerative villous atrophy seen in patients with detectable HIV-infected cells in the mucosa, as well as to the inadequate crypt hyperplasia seen in patients with secondary infections

References

1. Barre, S. F., Chermann, J. C., Rey, F., Nugeyre, M. T., Chamaret, S., Gruest, J., Dauguet, C., Axler, B. C., Vezinet, B. F., Rouzioux, C., Rozenbaum, W. and Montagnier, L. (1983). Isolation of a T-lymphotropic retrovirus from a patient at risk for acquired immune deficiency syndrome (AIDS). *Science*, **220**, 868–71
2. Popovic, M., Sarngadharan, M. G., Read, E. and Gallo, R. C. (1984). Detection, isolation, and continuous production of cytopathic retroviruses (HTLV-III) from patients with AIDS and pre-AIDS. *Science*, **224**, 497–500
3. Clavel, F., Guyader, M., Guetard, D., Salle, M., Montagnier, L. and Alizon, M. (1986). Molecular cloning and polymorphism of the human immune deficiency virus type 2. *Nature*, **324**, 691–5

4. Franchini, G., Collalti, E., Arya, S. K., Fenyo, E. M., Biberfeld, G., Zagury, J. F., Kanki, P. J., Wong, S. F. and Gallo, R. C. (1987). Genetic analysis of a new subgroup of human and simian T-lymphotropic retroviruses: HTLV-IV, LAV-2, SBL-6669, and STLV-IIIAGM. *Aids Res. Hum. Retroviruses*, **3**, 11–17

5. Statistics from the World Health Organization and the Centers for Disease Control (1990). *AIDS*, **4**, 1305–10

6. Janoff, E. N. and Smith, P. D. (1988). Perspectives on gastrointestinal infections in AIDS. *Gastroenterol. Clin. N. Am.*, **17**, 451–63

7. Smith, P. D. and Janoff, E. N. (1988). Infectious diarrhea in human immunodeficiency virus infection. *Gastroenterol. Clin. N. Am.*, **17**, 587–98

8. Riecken, E. O., Zeitz, M. and Ullrich, R. (1990). Non-opportunistic causes of diarrhoea in HIV infection. *Bailliere's Clin. Gastroenterol.*, **4**, 385–403

9. Kotler, D. P., Gaetz, H. P., Lange, M., Klein, E. B. and Holt, P. R. (1984). Enteropathy associated with the acquired immunodeficiency syndrome. *Ann. Intern. Med.*, **101**, 421–8

10. Ullrich, R., Zeitz, M., Heise, W., L'age, M., Höffken, G. and Riecken, E. O. (1989). Small intestinal structure and function in patients infected with human immunodeficiency virus (HIV): Evidence for HIV-induced enteropathy. *Ann. Intern. Med.*, **111**, 15–21

11. MacDonald, T. T. and Spencer, J. (1988). Evidence that activated mucosal T cells play a role in the pathogenesis of enteropathy in human small intestine. *J. Exp. Med.*, **167**, 1341–9

12. Riecken, E. O., Stallmach, A., Zeitz, M., Schulzke, J. D., Menge, H. and Gregor, M. (1989). Growth and transformation of the small intestinal mucosa – importance of connective tissue, gut associated lymphoid tissue and gastrointestinal regulatory peptides. *Gut*, **30**, 1630–40

13. Dworkin, B., Wormser, G. P., Rosenthal, W. S., Heier, S. K., Braunstein, M., Weiss, L., Jankowski, R., Levy, D. and Weiselberg, S. (1985). Gastrointestinal manifestations of the acquired immunodeficiency syndrome: a review of 22 cases. *Am. J. Gastroenterol.*, **80**, 774–8

14. Friedman, S. L., Wright, T. L. and Altman, D. F. (1985). Gastrointestinal Kaposi's sarcoma in patients with acquired immunodeficiency syndrome. *Gastroenterology*, **89**, 102–8

15. René, E., Marche, C., Regnier, B., Saimot, A. G., Vilde, J. L., Perrone, C., Michon, C., Wolf, M., Chevalier, T., Vallot, T., Brun-Vesinet, F., Pangon, P., Deluol, A. M., Camus, F., Roze, C., Pignon, J. P., Mignon, M. and Bonfils, S. (1989). Intestinal infections in patients with acquired immunodeficiency syndrome. *Dig. Dis. Sci.*, **34**, 773–80

16. Smith, P. D., Lane, H. C., Gill, V. G., Manischewitz, J. F., Quinnan, G. V., Fauci, A. S. and Masur, H. (1988). Intestinal infections in patients with the acquired immunodeficiency syndrome (AIDS). Etiology and response to therapy. *Ann. Intern. Med.*, **108**, 328–33

17. Colebunders, R., Lusakumuni, K., Nelson, A. M., Gigase, P., Lebughe, I., vanMarck, E., Kapita, B., Francis, H., Salaun, J. J., Quinn, T. C. and Piot, P. (1988). Persistent diarrhoea in Zairian AIDS patients: an endoscopic and histological study. *Gut*, **29**, 1687–91

18. Connolly, G. M., Shanson, D., Hawkins, D. A., Webster, J. N. and Gazzard, B. G. (1989). Non-cryptosporidial diarrhoea in human immunodeficiency virus (HIV) infected patients. *Gut*, **30**, 195–200

19. Heise, W., Mostertz, P., Skörde, J. and L'age, M. (1988). Gastrointestinale Befunde bei der HIV-Infektion. *Dtsch. Med. Wochenschr.*, **113**, 1588–93

20. Laughon, B. E., Druckman, D. A., Vernon, A., Quinn, T. C., Polk, B. F., Modlin, J. F., Yolken, R. H. and Bartlett, J. G. (1988). Prevalence of enteric pathogens in homosexual men with and without acquired immunodeficiency syndrome. *Gastroenterology*, **94**, 984–93

21. Gillin, J. S., Shike, M., Alcock, N., Urmacher, C., Krown, S., Kurtz, R. C., Lightdale, C. J. and Winawer, S. J. (1985). Malabsorption and mucosal abnormalities of the small intestine in the acquired immunodeficiency syndrome. *Ann. Intern. Med.*, **102**, 619–22

22. Harriman, G. R., Smith, P. D., Horne, M. K., Fox, C. H., Koenig, S., Lack, E. E., Lane, H. C. and Fauci, A. S. (1989). Vitamin B_{12} malabsorption in patients with acquired immunodeficiency syndrome. *Arch. Intern. Med.*, **149**, 2039–41

23. Conolly, G. M., Forbes, A. and Gazzard, B. G. (1990). Investigation of seemingly pathogen-negative diarrhoea in patients infected with HIV1. *Gut*, **31**, 886–9

24. Kotler, D. P., Francisco, A., Clayton, F., Scholes, J. V. and Orenstein, J. M. (1990). Small intestinal injury and parasitic disease in AIDS. *Ann. Intern. Med.*, **113**, 444–9

25. McDougal, J. S., Kennedy, M. S., Sligh, J. M., Cort, S. P., Mawle, A. and Nicholson, J. K. (1986). Binding of HTLV-III/LAV to T4+ T cells by a complex of the 110K viral protein and the T4 molecule. *Science*, **231**, 382–5

26. Rosenberg, Z. F. and Fauci, A. S. (1989). The immunopathogenesis of HIV infection. *Adv. Immunol.*, **47**, 377–431
27. Ho, D. D., Rota, T. R. and Hirsch, M. S. (1986). Infection of monocyte/macrophages by human T lymphotropic virus type III. *J. Clin. Invest.*, **77**, 1712–5
28. Stewart, S. J., Fujimoto, J. and Levy, R. (1986). Human T lymphocytes and monocytes bear the same Leu-3(T4) antigen. *J. Immunol.*, **136**, 3773–8
29. Gartner, S., Markovits, P., Markovitz, D. M., Kaplan, M. H., Gallo, R. C. and Popovic, M. (1986). The role of mononuclear phagocytes in HTLV-III/LAV infection. *Science*, **233**, 215–9
30. Crowe, S., Mills, J. and McGrath, M. S. (1987). Quantitative immunocytofluorographic analysis of CD4 surface antigen expression and HIV infection of human peripheral blood monocyte/macrophages. *Aids Res. Hum. Retroviruses*, **3**, 135–45
31. Bolognesi, D. P. (1989). AIDS. Do antibodies enhance the infection of cells by HIV? [news]. *Nature*, **340**, 431–2
32. Takeda, A., Tuazon, C. U. and Ennis, F. A. (1988). Antibody-enhanced infection by HIV-1 via Fc receptor-mediated entry. *Science*, **242**, 580–3
33. Nicholson, J. K., Cross, G. D., Callaway, C. S. and McDougal, J. S. (1986). In vitro infection of human monocytes with human T lymphotropic virus type III/lymphadenopathy-associated virus (HTLV-III/LAV). *J. Immunol.*, **137**, 323–9
34. Tenner-Racz, K., Racz, P., Bofill, M., Schulz-Meyer, A., Dietrich, M., Kern, P., Weber, J., Pinching, A. J., Veronese-Dimarzo, F., Popovic, M., Klatzmann, D., Gluckman, J. C. and Janossy, G. (1986). HTLV-III/LAV viral antigens in lymph nodes of homosexual men with persistent generalized lymphadenopathy and AIDS. *Am. J. Pathol.*, **123**, 9–15
35. Schriever, F., Freedman, A. S., Freeman, G., Messner, E., Lee, G., Daley, J. and Nadler, L. M. (1989). Isolated human follicular dendritic cells display a unique antigenic phenotype. *J. Exp. Med.*, **169**, 2043–58
36. Biberfeld, P., Chayt, K. J., Marselle, L. M., Biberfeld, G., Gallo, R. C. and Harper, M. E. (1986). HTLV-III expression in infected lymph nodes and relevance to pathogenesis of lymphadenopathy. *Am. J. Pathol.*, **125**, 436–42
37. Jarry, A., Cortez, A., René, E., Muzeau, F. and Brousse, N. (1990). Infected cells and immune cells in the gastrointestinal tract of AIDS patients. An immunohistochemical study of 127 cases. *Histopathology*, **16**, 133–40
38. Racz, P. (1990). Pathomorphologie des intestinalen Immunsystems. Presented at the 3rd German AIDS-Congress, 17–24 November, Hamburg
39. Nelson, J. A., Wiley, C. A., Reynolds-Kohler, C., Reese, C. E., Margaretten, W. and Levy, J. A. (1988). Human immunodeficiency virus detected in bowel epithelium from patients with gastrointestinal symptoms. *Lancet*, **1**, 259–62
40. Fox, C. H., Kotler, D., Tierney, A., Wilson, C. S. and Fauci, A. S. (1989). Detection of HIV-1 RNA in the lamina propria of patients with AIDS and gastrointestinal disease. *J. Infect. Dis.*, **159**, 467–71
41. Adachi, A., Koenig, S., Gendelmann, H. E., Daugherty, D., Gattoni, C. S., Fauci, A. S. and Martin, M. (1987). Productive, persistent infection of human colorectal cell lines with human immunodeficiency virus. *J. Virol.*, **61**, 209–13
42. Bourinbaiar, A. S. and Phillips, D. M. (1990). HIV transmission across intact epithelia. VIIIth International Congress of Virology
43. Leonard, R., Zagury, D., Desportes, I., Bernard, J., Zagury, J. F. and Gallo, R. C. (1988). Cytopathic effect of human immunodeficiency virus in T4 cells is linked to the last stage of virus infection. *Proc. Natl. Acad. Sci. USA*, **85**, 3570–4
44. Lynn, W. S., Tweedale, A. and Cloyd, M. W. (1988). Human immunodeficiency virus (HIV-1) cytotoxicity: perturbation of the cell membrane and depression of phospholipid synthesis. *Virology*, **163**, 43–51
45. Hoxie, J. A., Alpers, J. D., Rackowski, J. L., Huebner, K., Haggarty, B. S., Cedarbaum, A. J. and Reed, J. C. (1986). Alterations in T4 (CD4) protein and mRNA synthesis in cells infected with HIV. *Science*, **234**, 1123–7
46. Shaw, G. M., Hahn, B. H., Arya, S. K., Groopman, J. E., Gallo, R. C. and Wong, S. F. (1984). Molecular characterization of human T-cell leukemia (lymphotropic) virus type III in the acquired immune deficiency syndrome. *Science*, **226**, 1165–71
47. Lifson, J. D., Feinberg, M. B., Reyes, G. R., Rabin, L., Banapour, B., Chakrabarti, S., Moss, B., Wong, S. F., Steimer, K. S. and Engleman, E. G. (1986). Induction of CD4-dependent

cell fusion by the HTLV-III/LAV envelope glycoprotein. *Nature*, **323**, 725-8
48. Lifson, J. D., Reyes, G. R., McGrath, M. S., Stein, B. S. and Engleman, E. G. (1986). AIDS retrovirus induced cytopathology: giant cell formation and involvement of CD4 antigen. *Science*, **232**, 1123-7
49. Katz, J. D., Nishanian, P., Mitsuyasu, R. and Bonavida, B. (1988). Antibody-dependent cellular cytotoxicity (ADCC)-mediated destruction of human immunodeficiency virus (HIV)-coated CD4+ T lymphocytes by acquired immunodeficiency syndrome (AIDS) effector cells. *J. Clin. Immunol.*, **8**, 453-8
50. Lyerly, H. K., Matthews, T. J., Langlois, A. J., Bolognesi, D. P. and Weinhold, K. J. (1987). Human T-cell lymphotropic virus IIIB glycoprotein (gp120) bound to CD4 determinants on normal lymphocytes and expressed by infected cells serves as target for immune attack. *Proc. Natl. Acad. Sci. USA*, **84**, 4601-5
51. Lanzavecchia, A., Roosnek, E., Gregory, T., Berman, P. and Abrignani, S. (1988). T cells can present antigens such as HIV gp120 targeted to their own surface molecules. *Nature*, **334**, 530-2
52. Lane, H. C. and Fauci, A. S. (1985). Immunologic abnormalities in the acquired immunodeficiency syndrome. *Annu. Rev. Immunol.*, **3**, 477-500
53. Lane, H. C., Masur, H., Edgar, L. C., Whalen, G., Rook, A. H. and Fauci, A. S. (1983). Abnormalities of B-cell activation and immunoregulation in patients with the acquired immunodeficiency syndrome. *N. Engl. J. Med.*, **309**, 453-8
54. Lane, H. C., Depper, J. M., Greene, W. C., Whalen, G., Waldmann, T. A. and Fauci, A. S. (1985). Qualitative analysis of immune function in patients with the acquired immunodeficiency syndrome. Evidence for a selective defect in soluble antigen recognition. *N. Engl. J. Med.*, **313**, 79-84
55. Shearer, G. M., Bernstein, D. C., Tung, K. S., Via, C. S., Redfield, R., Salahuddin, S. Z. and Gallo, R. C. (1986). A model for the selective loss of major histocompatibility complex self-restricted T cell immune responses during the development of acquired immune deficiency syndrome (AIDS). *J. Immunol.*, **137**, 2514-21
56. Giorgi, J. V., Fahey, J. L., Smith, D. C., Hultin, L. E., Cheng, H. L., Mitsuyasu, R. T. and Detels, R. (1987). Early effects of HIV on CD4 lymphocytes in vivo. *J. Immunol.*, **138**, 3725-30
57. Hoy, J. F., Lewis, D. E. and Miller, G. G. (1988). Functional versus phenotypic analysis of T cells in subjects seropositive for the human immunodeficiency virus: a prospective study of in vitro responses to *Cryptococcus neoformans*. *J. Infect. Dis.*, **158**, 1071-8
58. Murray, H. W., Scavuzzo, D. A., Kelly, C. D., Rubin, B. Y. and Roberts, R. B. (1988). T4+ cell production of interferon gamma and the clinical spectrum of patients at risk for and with acquired immunodeficiency syndrome [see comments]. *Arch. Intern. Med.*, **148**, 1613-16
59. Antonen, J. and Krohn, K. (1986). Interleukin 2 production in HTLV-III/LAV infection: evidence of defective antigen-induced, but normal mitogen-induced IL-2 production. *Clin. Exp. Immunol.*, **65**, 489-96
60. Schellekens, P. T., Roos, M. T., De, W. F., Lange, J. M. and Miedema, F. (1990). Low T-cell responsiveness to activation via CD3/TCR is a prognostic marker for acquired immunodeficiency syndrome (AIDS) in human immunodeficiency virus-1 (HIV-1)-infected men. *J. Clin. Immunol.*, **10**, 121-7
61. Yuille, M. A., Hugunin, M., John, P., Peer, L., Sacks, L. V., Poiesz, B. J., Tomar, R. H. and Silverstone, A. E. (1988). HIV-1 infection abolishes CD4 biosynthesis but not CD4 mRNA. *J. Acquir. Immune Defic. Syndr.*, **1**, 131-7
62. Stevenson, M., Zhang, X. H. and Volsky, D. J. (1987). Downregulation of cell surface molecules during noncytopathic infection of T cells with human immunodeficiency virus. *J. Virol.*, **61**, 3741-8
63. Prince, H. E., Kleinman, S. H., Maino, V. C. and Jackson, A. L. (1988). In vitro activation of T lymphocytes from human immunodeficiency virus (HIV)-seropositive blood donors. I. Soluble interleukin 2 receptor (IL2R) production parallels cellular IL2R expression and DNA synthesis. *J. Clin. Immunol.*, **8**, 114-20
64. Van Noesel, C. J., Gruters, R. A., Terpstra, F. G., Schellekens, P. T., van Lier, R. A. and Miedema, F. (1990). Functional and phenotypic evidence for a selective loss of memory T cells in asymptomatic human immunodeficiency virus-infected men. *J. Clin. Invest.*, **86**, 293-9
65. De Paoli, P., Battistin, S., Crovatto, M., Modolo, M. L., Carbone, A., Tirelli, U. and Santini, G. (1988). Immunologic abnormalities related to antigenaemia during HIV-1 infection.

Clin. Exp. Immunol., **74**, 317–20
66. Nair, M. P., Pottathil, R., Heimer, E. P. and Schwartz, S. A. (1988). Immunoregulatory activities of human immunodeficiency virus (HIV) proteins: effect of HIV recombinant and synthetic peptides on immunoglobulin synthesis and proliferative responses by normal lymphocytes. *Proc. Natl. Acad. Sci. USA*, **85**, 6498–502
67. Kornfeld, H., Cruikshank, W. W., Pyle, S. W., Berman, J. S. and Center, D. M. (1988). Lymphocyte activation by HIV-1 envelope glycoprotein. *Nature*, **335**, 445–8
68. Pahwa, S., Pahwa, R., Saxinger, C., Gallo, R. C. and Good, R. A. (1985). Influence of the human T-lymphotropic virus/lymphadenopathy-associated virus on functions of human lymphocytes: evidence for immunosuppressive effects and polyclonal B-cell activation by banded viral preparations. *Proc. Natl. Acad. Sci. USA*, **82**, 8198–202
69. Ho, D. D., Pomerantz, R. J. and Kaplan, J. C. (1987). Pathogenesis of infection with human immunodeficiency virus. *N. Engl. J. Med.*, **317**, 278–86
70. Farzadegan, H., Polis, M. A., Wolinsky, S. M., Rinaldo, C. J., Sninsky, J. J., Kwok, S., Griffith, R. L., Kaslow, R. A., Phair, J. P., Polk, B. F., *et al.* (1988). Loss of human immunodeficiency virus type 1 (HIV-1) antibodies with evidence of viral infection in asymptomatic homosexual men. A report from the Multicenter AIDS Cohort Study. *Ann. Intern. Med.*, **108**, 785–90
71. Patarca, R., Freeman, G. J., Schwartz, J., Singh, R. P., Kong, Q. T., Murphy, E., Anderson, Y., Sheng, F. Y. W., Singh, P., Johnson, K. A., Guarnagia, S. M., Durfee, T., Blattner, F. and Cantor, H. (1988). rpt-1, an intracellular protein from helper/inducer T cells that regulates gene expression of interleukin 2 receptor and human immunodeficiency virus type 1 [published erratum appears in *Proc. Natl. Acad. Sci. USA*, 1988, **85**(14), 5224]. *Proc. Natl. Acad. Sci. USA*, **85**, 2733–7
72. Nabel, G. and Baltimore, D. (1987). An inducible transcription factor activates expression of human immunodeficiency virus in T cells. *Nature*, **326**, 711–13
73. Kawakami, K., Scheidereit, C. and Roeder, R. G. (1988). Identification and purification of a human immunoglobulin-enhancer-binding protein (NF-kappa B) that activates transcription from a human immunodeficiency virus type 1 promoter in vitro. *Proc. Natl. Acad. Sci. USA*, **85**, 4700–4
74. Gendelman, H. E., Phelps, W., Feigenhaum, L., Ostrove, J. M., Adachi, A., Howley, P. M., Khoury, G., Ginsberg, H. S. and Martin, M. A. (1986). Transactivation of the human immunodeficiency virus long terminal repeat sequence by DNA viruses. *Proc. Natl. Acad. Sci. USA*, **83**, 9759–63
75. Davis, M. G., Kenney, S. C., Kamine, J., Pagano, J. S. and Huang, E. S. (1987). Immediate-early gene region of human cytomegalovirus trans-activates the promoter of human immunodeficiency virus. *Proc. Natl. Acad. Sci. USA*, **84**, 8642–6
76. Kenney, S., Kamine, J., Markovitz, D., Fenrick, R. and Pagano, J. (1988). An Epstein-Barr virus immediate–early gene product trans-activates gene expression from the human immunodeficiency virus long terminal repeat. *Proc. Natl. Acad. Sci. USA*, **85**, 1652–6
77. Rando, R. F., Pellett, P. E., Luciw, P. A., Bohan, C. A. and Srinivasan, A. (1987). Transactivation of human immunodeficiency virus by herpesviruses. *Oncogene*, **1**, 13–8
78. Folks, T. M., Justement, J., Kinter, A., Dinarello, C. A. and Fauci, A. S. (1987). Cytokine-induced expression of HIV-1 in a chronically infected promonocyte cell line. *Science*, **238**, 800–2
79. Rosenberg, Z. F. and Fauci, A. S. (1990). Immunopathogenic mechanisms of HIV infection: cytokine induction of HIV expression. *Immunol. Today*, **11**, 176–80
80. Clouse, K. A., Powell, D., Washington, I., Poli, G., Strebel, K., Farrar, W., Barstad, P., Kovacs, J., Fauci, A. S. and Folks, T. M. (1989). Monokine regulation of human immunodeficiency virus-1 expression in a chronically infected human T cell clone. *J. Immunol.*, **142**, 431–8
81. Duh, E. J., Maury, W. J., Folks, T. M., Fauci, A. S. and Rabson, A. B. (1989). Tumor necrosis factor alpha activates human immunodeficiency virus type 1 through induction of nuclear factor binding to the NF-kappa B sites in the long terminal repeat. *Proc. Natl. Acad. Sci. USA*, **86**, 5974–8
82. Folks, T. M., Clouse, K. A., Justement, J., Rabson, A., Duh, E., Kehrl, J. H. and Fauci, A. S. (1989). Tumor necrosis factor alpha induces expression of human immunodeficiency virus in a chronically infected T-cell clone. *Proc. Natl. Acad. Sci. USA*, **86**, 2365–8

83. Selby, W. S., Jannossy, G., Bofill, M. and Jewell, D. P. (1984). Intestinal lymphocyte subpopulations in inflammatory bowel disease: an analysis by immunohistological and cell isolation techniques. *Gut*, **25**, 32–40

84. James, S. P., Fiocchi, C., Graeff, A. S. and Strober, W. (1986). Phenotypic analysis of lamina propria lymphocytes: Predominance of helper-inducer and cytolytic T-cell phenotypes and deficiency of suppressor–inducer phenotypes in Crohn's disease and control patients. *Gastroenterology*, **91**, 1483–9

85. James, S. P., Graeff, A. S. and Zeitz, M. (1987). Predominance of helper-inducer T cells in mesenteric lymph node and intestinal lamina propria lymphocytes of normal non-human primates. *Cell. Immunol.*, **107**, 372–83

86. Schieferdecker, H. L., Ullrich, R., Weiss-Breckwoldt, A. N., Schwarting, R., Stein, H., Riecken, E. O. and Zeitz, M. (1990). The HML-1 antigen of intestinal lymphocytes is an activation antigen. *J. Immunol.*, **144**, 2541–9

87. Zeitz, M., Schieferdecker, H. L., James, S. P. and Riecken, E. O. (1990). Special functional features of T-lymphocyte subpopulations in the effector compartment of the intestinal mucosa and their relation to mucosal transformation. *Digestion*, **46** (Suppl. 2), 280–9

88. Sanders, M. E., Makgoba, M. W., Sharrow, S. O., Stephany, D., Springer, T. A., Young, H. A. and Shaw, S. (1988). Human memory T lymphocytes express increased levels of three cell adhesion molecules (LFA-3, CD2 and LFA-1) and three other molecules (UCHL1, CDw29 and Pgp-1) and have enhanced IFN-production. *J. Immunol.*, **140**, 1401–7

89. Sanders, M. E., Makgoba, M. and Shaw, S. (1988). Human naive and memory T cells: reinterpretation of helper–inducer and suppressor–inducer subsets. *Immunol. Today*, **9**, 195–9

90. Cerf-Bensussan, N., Jarry, A., Brousse, N., Liskowska-Grospierre, B., Guy-Grand, D. and Griscelli, C. (1987). A monoclonal antibody (HML-1) defining a novel membrane molecule present on human intestinal lymphocytes. *Eur. J. Immunol.*, **17**, 1279–85

91. Zeitz, M., Quinn, T. C., Graeff, A. S. and James, S. P. (1988). Mucosal T cells provide helper function but do not proliferate when stimulated by specific antigen in lymphogranuloma venereum proctitis in nonhuman primates. *Gastroenterology*, **94**, 353–66

92. Zeitz, M., Greene, W. C., Peffer, N. J. and James, S. P. (1988). Lymphocytes isolated from the intestinal lamina propria of normal nonhuman primates have increased expression of genes associated with T cell activation. *Gastroenterology*, **94**, 647–55

93. Zeitz, M., James, S. P., Ullrich, R. and Riecken, E. O. (1989). Characteristics of intestinal T lymphocytes as potential target cells of HIV. In Classen, M. and Dancygier, H. (eds), *AIDS in Gastroenterology and Hepatology*. Gräfelfing: Demeter Verlag, pp. 14–17

94. Rodgers, V,. D., Fassett, R. and Kagnoff, M. F. (1986). Abnormalities in intestinal mucosal T cells in homosexual populations including those with the lymphadenopathy syndrome and acquired immunodeficiency syndrome. *Gastroenterology*, **90**, 552–8

95. Ellakany, S., Whiteside, T. L., Schade, R. R. and vanThiel, D. H. (1987). Analysis of intestinal lymphocyte subpopulations in patients with acquired immunodeficiency syndrome (AIDS) and AIDS-related complex. *Am. J. Clin. Pathol.*, **87**, 356–64

96. Budhraja, M., Levendoglu, H., Kocka, F., Mangkornkanok, M. and Sherer, R. (1987). Duodenal mucosal T cell subpopulation and bacterial cultures in acquired immune deficiency syndrome. *Am. J. Gastroenterol.*, **82**, 427–31

97. Zeitz, M., Ullrich, R. and Riecken, E. O. (1990). The role of the gut-associated lymphoid tissue in the pathogenesis of the acquired immunodeficiency syndrome (HIV-infection). In MacDonald, T. T., Challacombe, S. J., Bland, P. W., Stokes, C. R., Heatley, R. V. and Mowat, A. M. (eds), *Advances in Mucosal Immunology. Proceedings of the Fifth International Congress of Mucosal Immunology*. Dordrecht: Kluwer, pp. 655–9

98. Ullrich, R., Zeitz, M., Heise, W., L'age, M., Ziegler, K., Bergs, C. and Riecken, E. O. (1990). Mucosal atrophy is associated with loss of activated T cells in the duodenal mucosa of human immunodeficiency virus (HIV)-infected patients. *Digestion*, **46** (Suppl. 2), 302–7

99. Weber, J. R., Jr. and Dobbins, W. O. (1986). The intestinal and rectal epithelial lymphocyte in AIDS. *Am. J. Surg. Pathol.*, **10**, 627–39

100. Batman, P. A., Miller, A. R. O., Forster, S. M., Harris, J. R., Pinching, A. J. and Griffin, G. E. (1989). Jejunal enteropathy associated with human immunodeficiency virus infection: quantitative histology. *J. Clin. Pathol.*, **42**, 275–81

101. Cummins, A. G., LaBrooy, J. T., Stanley, D. P., Rowland, R. and Shearman, D. J. C. (1990). A quantitative histological study of enteropathy associated with HIV infection. In

MacDonald, T. T., Challacombe, S. J., Bland, P. W., Stokes, C. R., Heatley, R. V. and Mowat, A. M. (eds), *Advances in Mucosal Immunology. Proceedings of the Fifth International Congress of Mucosal Immunology.* Dordrecht: Kluwer, pp. 669–70
102. Kotler, D. P., Scholes, J. V. and Tierney, A. R. (1987). Intestinal plasma cell alterations in the acquired immunodeficiency syndrome. *Dig. Dis. Sci.,* **32**, 129–38
103. Jackson, S. (1990). Secretory and serum IgA are inversely altered in AIDS patients. In MacDonald, T. T., Challacombe, S. J., Bland, P. W., Stokes, C. R., Heatley, R. V. and Mowat, A. M. (eds), *Advances in Mucosal Immunology. Proceedings of the Fifth International Congress of Mucosal Immunology.* Dordrecht: Kluwer, pp. 665–8
104. Griffiths, C. E., Barrison, I. G., Leonard, J. N., Caun, K., Valdimarsson, H. and Fry, L. (1988). Preferential activation of CD4 T lymphocytes in the lamina propria of gluten-sensitive enteropathy. *Clin. Exp. Immunol.,* **72**, 280–3
105. Cummins, A. G., LaBrooy, J. T., Stanley, D. *et al.* (1990). Quantitative histological study of enteropathy associated with HIV infection. *Gut,* **31**, 317–21
106. Quinn, T. C. (1989). Protozoon infections in the gastrointestinal tract of homosexual men and patients with the acquired immunodeficiency syndrome. In Classen, M. and Dancygier, H. (eds), *AIDS in Gastroenterology and Hepatology.* Gräfelfing: Demeter Verlag, pp. 36–8

13
Immunity to enterotoxin-producing bacteria

A.-M. SVENNERHOLM and J. HOLMGREN

BACKGROUND

Enteric infection associated with diarrhoeal disease is a major health problem, particularly in developing countries where these infections cause at least 1 billion episodes of diarrhoea and 5–10 million deaths each year[1-3]. Although a wide variety of bacteria, viruses and parasites may cause diarrhoea through many different pathogenic mechanisms, the most common cause is bacteria that give rise to disease through production of enterotoxins. It has been estimated that such bacteria account for almost 50% of all diarrhoeal episodes.

Vibrio cholerae O1 is the prototype for the group of enterotoxin-producing bacteria. Other members include enterotoxigenic *Escherichia coli* (ETEC), some but not all non-O1 *V. cholerae*, *V. parahaemolyticus*, *Aeromonas hydrophila* and a number of Gram-negative genera which occasionally may produce enterotoxins, e.g. *Salmonella*, *Citrobacter*, *Klebsiella* and *Campylobacter*.

The disease caused by enterotoxin-producing bacteria is characterized by watery stools without blood and mucus. In the most severe cases the diarrhoea may result in moderate to severe dehydration that is sometimes fatal; the mortality rate in non-treated severe cholera may be as high as 50–60%. In some instances the diarrhoea is accompanied by nausea, vomiting, abdominal cramps, anorexia and fever[3]. Most cases of entertoxin-induced disease can be successfully treated by oral rehydration therapy although parenteral administration of water and electrolytes may be necessary in severely dehydrated patients[4].

V. cholerae O1 is most often associated with severe and sometimes life-threatening disease with purging of up to 25 litres of water and electrolytes per day; more than 150 000 people die from cholera each year. ETEC is the most common cause of diarrhoea in developing countries (~25% of all cases) and in travellers to these areas (~30–50% of all cases). The clinical spectrum of ETEC diarrhoea is variable, ranging from mild to cholera-like life-threatening disease[1-3].

The only vaccine that has been available for immunoprophylaxis against enterotoxin-induced diarrhoeas is the parenteral killed whole-cell cholera vaccine which has only afforded up to 50% protection for 3–6 months[4]. Recently, however, a new oral cholera vaccine based on a combination of cholera B subunit and killed whole cells has been developed and shown to afford 60–70% protection for at least 3 years[5]; efforts are now underway to introduce the use of this vaccine in several countries. For immunoprophylaxis against other enterotoxin-induced infections no vaccine is yet available, although the oral B subunit–whole cell cholera vaccine was shown to afford substantial, though rather short-lasting, protection also against diarrhoea caused by ETEC producing cholera-like, heat-labile enterotoxin[6].

There are several approaches to develop new vaccines for immunoprophylaxis against entertoxin-induced diarrhoeal diseases. Such vaccines should be designed to induce immune responses interfering with the major pathogenic events of the various infections. This review will outline present knowledge on the immune mechanisms operating against enterotoxigenic bacteria based on studies in experimental animals infected with such organisms or immunized with toxin antigens, as well as in humans convalescing from natural disease or given toxoid-containing vaccines.

PATHOGENIC MECHANISMS IN ENTEROTOXIN-INDUCED DIARRHOEAL DISEASE

Bacterial colonization

The major pathogenic mechanisms of enterotoxigenic bacteria include colonization of the small intestine and elaboration of one or more enterotoxins that through various mechanisms may induce water and electrolyte secretion resulting in diarrhoea. The colonization is dependent on receptor–ligand interactions between bacteria and host cells which usually are specific for the species, phenotype and epithelial cell type of the host. All enterotoxin-producing bacteria seem to possess distinct attachment factors, so-called adhesins or colonization factors, that are either fimbrial or outer-membrane proteins in nature[7,8]. The host receptors, on the other hand, usually consist of oligosaccharides or glycoconjugates on the epithelial cell surface or in the mucus layer[9]. Analogous carbohydrates have been found in human secretions, e.g. in milk, and have been proposed to have a protective function against cholera and maybe also against entertoxin-induced *E. coli* diarrhoea[10,11].

In *V. cholerae* the toxin-coregulated pilus (TCP) has been shown to be of importance for colonization of the intestine[12]. Other adhesins such as the mannose-binding pilus antigen associated with the El Tor biotype[10,13,13a] may also play a role. In ETEC, various species-associated colonization factor fimbriae have been identified. A majority of human ETEC isolates express either of three distinct colonization factors antigens (CFAs), i.e. CFA/I, CFA/II or CFA/IV[8]. Whereas CFA/I is a homogeneous protein consisting of ~100 identical subunits of 15 kD each, CFA/II consists of three subcomponents, i.e. the coli surface antigens CS1, CS2 and CS3 and CFA/IV of CS4, CS5 and CS6; all of these CS factors consist of 15–20 kD subunits[8]. Usually CS3 is expressed alone or together with CS1 and CS2, and CS6 is found together with CS4 or CS5. Recently a number of additional putative colonization factors, e.g. PCFO159, PCFO166, CS7, CS17 and CFA/III have been described[14]. ETEC is also a common cause of diarrhoea in piglets and calves and specific fimbriae, e.g. K88, K99, 987P and F41 have been identified in a majority of porcine strains whereas ETEC isolated from calves usually express K99 and sometimes F41[15]. The adhesins in enterotoxigenic organisms other than *V. cholerae* O1 and ETEC have not yet been characterized.

Enterotoxin production

The intestine-colonizing bacteria, without invading the intestinal epithelium, produce one or more protein enterotoxins which bind to specific receptors on the mucosal cells. Through a cytotonic (rather than cytotoxic) action associated with increased formation of cyclic AMP and/or cyclic GMP in the epithelium, the enterotoxins stimulate excessive electrolyte and fluid secretion primarily from the small intestinal crypt cells[16,17]. The prototype enterotoxin is cholera toxin (CT) that is produced by *V. cholerae* O1 bacteria. Through extensive characterization during the 1970s CT became probably the best-defined of all bacterial toxins. Much of the knowledge that has accumulated from studies of CT has also been applicable to many other enterotoxins[16]. CT is built from two different types of polypeptide, i.e. five identical B subunits that are spontaneously associated in a ring into which a single toxic-active A subunit is non-covalently inserted[16]. The B subunit pentamer is responsible for the binding of the CT molecule to specific ganglioside GM1 receptors in the small intestinal epithelial cells, whereas the A subunit transverses the cell membrane and through a well-defined enzymic reaction increases the adenylate cyclase activity and thereby causes a much-enhanced formation of cyclic AMP in the cells. This process is associated with decreased uptake of NaCl (by villous cells) and enhanced secretion of Cl^- and HCO_3^- (by crypt cells) resulting in increased outpouring of water and electrolytes.

ETEC may produce a heat-labile enterotoxin (LT), a heat-stable entertoxin (ST) or both toxins[3]. LT is structurally, functionally and immunologically closely related though not identical to CT. Thus, similar to CT, LT consists of five copies of B subunit and one copy of A subunit, and both of these subunits crossreact immunologically with the corresponding CT subunits although there are also specific A and B subunit epitopes on both toxins[18]. *E. coli* LT also binds to ganglioside GM1 receptors, but (different from CT) also binds to one or more glycoprotein receptors[19]. Several bacteria other than vibrios and *E. coli* may produce CT- or LT-like enterotoxins. In an early study of enteropathogens in Ethiopian children with diarrhoea, Wadström *et al.*[20] identified a number of different species of bacteria that produced enterotoxins. Recently Swedish travellers to Southeast Asia were also found to be infected with non-*E. coli* strains, e.g. *Morganella morganii* and *Citrobacter freundii*, that produced enterotoxins reacting with a monoclonal antibody against *E. coli* LT[21].

E. coli ST has very distinct properties from LT and CT. In human ETEC strains the methanol-soluble STa is the only heat-stable enterotoxin produced whereas porcine ETEC may produce either or both of STa and a methanol-insoluble heat-stable toxin[17] designated STb. STa is a small molecule consisting of 18 (STp) or 19 (STh) amino acids each. The two subtypes of STa only differ in a few amino acids and crossreact immunologically, whereas STb is a 71-amino acid protein without any sequence homology with STa. STa is not immunogenic unless coupled to a carrier protein, e.g. bovine serum albumin (BSA), CTB or CFAs[22,23]. Accordingly, STa that is released during infection does not induce any ST antibody responses; it is also still unknown whether anti-ST immunity induced by an artificial STa–carrier protein conjugate could protect against disease caused by ST-producing *E. coli* in humans.

STa-like enterotoxins may also be produced by *Yersinia enterocolitica*, *V. cholerae* non-O1 or *V. mimicus*. All these STs are composed of 17–30 amino acids and have several amino acid sequences in common; like STa they all induce fluid secretion in the gut by stimulating the epithelial cells to increased formation of cyclic GMP[17,24]. In recent studies we have shown that other Gram-negative species, e.g. *Klebsiella pneumoniae*, *Pseudomonas aeruginosa* and *Citrobacter freundii*, may also produce enterotoxins that react with antibodies against *E. coli* STa[21], but the role of these enterotoxin-producing organisms in diarrhoeal disease remains to be clarified.

IMMUNE MECHANISMS AGAINST ENTEROTOXIN-PRODUCING BACTERIA

Since neither the bacteria nor their enterotoxins penetrate beyond the intestinal epithelium during infection, protective immunity against enterotoxin-induced diarrhoeal disease is thought to depend solely on preventive mechanisms operating against colonization or toxin action in the gut lumen, in the mucus layer or on the epithelium surface.

Non-specific protection

A number of non-specific defence mechanisms may act as a first line of defence to prevent enterotoxin-producing bacteria from colonizing the small intestine[25–28]. These factors include the acid milieu in the stomach to which enterotoxin-producing microorganisms are usually very sensitive, intestinal peristalsis which is effective in preventing bacterial colonization and intestinal secretions that wash the intestinal surface and also contain a number of proteolytic enzymes. They possibly also include host-derived antibiotic factors, the normal flora which competes with more pathogenic microorganisms for essential metabolites, and the mucus layer that functions as a mechanical as well as chemical barrier. For example, neutralization of gastric acidity by bicarbonate or cimetidine before ingestion of bacteria has resulted in a drastic decrease in the infectious dose required to induce clinical cholera in human volunteers[27].

The possibility of non-specifically interfering with the enterotoxin action of *V. cholerae* O1 has been evaluated by repeatedly providing large quantities of the specific CT receptor, i.e. the ganglioside GM1, to patients with manifest cholera[29]. Although this treatment afforded some decrease in intestinal fluid secretion, the logistic problem of maintaining effective receptor competition in a rapidly renewing organ such as the intestine is enormous, making the approach of receptor prophylaxis in the intestine relatively inefficient. The possibility of blocking the intestinal GM1 receptors by peroral administration of large quantities of isolated cholera B subunit has also been attempted. However, this treatment had only a limited effect against cholera during the initial days after administration, i.e. before a local antitoxic immune response was induced[30].

SIgA

The best known entity providing specific immune protection for the gut is the secretory IgA (SIgA) system[31]. In non-invasive enteric infections like those caused by enterotoxin-producing bacteria, SIgA appears to be the main – although perhaps not the only – protective molecule[31,32]. Systemic immunity may play only a limited role, although circulating antibodies may diffuse from the capillaries in the intestinal mucosa and act on the mucosal surface. However, such circulating antibodies are predominantly of IgG isotype and consequently very sensitive to proteolytic degradation by intestinal enzymes.

The resistance of SIgA to intestinal proteases[31] makes antibodies of this istotype uniquely well suited to protect intestinal mucosal surfaces. SIgA antibodies which may appear within a week after onset of infection, and even more rapidly after reimmunization, i.e. within as little as 3 days[33], function as a second line of defence against enterotoxin-induced diarrhoeas. The antibodies act through immune exclusion, i.e. by preventing the bacteria and their secreted enterotoxins from binding to, and further acting on, the intestinal epithelial cells[31,32]. Recently, SIgA was also shown to mediate antibody-dependent T-cell-mediated cytotoxicity in experimental systems in the gut[34]; to interfere with the utilization of necessary growth factors for bacterial pathogens in the intestinal environment, e.g. iron; and to facilite antigen uptake by Peyer's patches[26,35]. The intestinal SIgA response to antigen exposure is of relatively short duration, lasting for only weeks to a few months. However, in studies of cholera immune responses the SIgA system has been shown to exhibit potent immunological memory for several years, that could rapidly and efficiently be stimulated by renewed antigen exposure[36-38].

Cell-mediated immunity

Cell-mediated immune reactions such as MHC-restricted cellular cytotoxicity, natural killer cell activity and antibody-dependent cytotoxicity (ADCC) are probably of little importance in preventing non-invasive infections like those caused by entertoxin-producing bacteria. Recently, however, evidence has accumulated that interferon-γ (IFN-γ) producing T cells in the gut mucosa might also play a role in intestinal immune defence. Such cells are present in very large numbers in the human duodenal mucosa, and there they may undergo significant expansion following intestinal antigenic exposure[39]. IFN-γ may enhance IgA production, increase the expression of MHC antigen as well as secretory component receptors on the enterocyte surface and probably also allow antigen presentation by different mucosal cells including enterocytes. It may also interfere with tight junction permeability between intestinal epithelial cells[40] as well as with active electrolyte secretion by enterocytes *in vitro*, thereby preventing enterotoxin-induced fluid secretion[41].

STUDIES OF IMMUNE RESPONSES IN ANIMALS

The classical animal model for studying enterotoxin-induced fluid secretion in the gut is the ligated small bowel loop technique[42]. This method has been used in different species, e.g. rabbits, rats or mice, to assess the protective effect of antibacterial as well as antitoxic antibodies either in active or passive immunization studies. Using this model we could show that immunization with cholera toxin or its B subunits (CTB) or with whole vibrios or isolated lipopolysaccharides (LPS) resulted in significant protection in rabbits against experimental cholera[43,44]. Furthermore, combined immunization with toxin and bacterial antigens induced a protective effect that was considerably better than the sum of the effects induced by each antigen component alone, i.e. antibacterial and antitoxic immunities cooperated synergistically in protecting against cholera. In subsequent studies similar synergistic cooperation has been observed between antibodies against the different ETEC colonization factor antigens and anti-LT antibodies for protection against LT-producing ETEC carrying the homologous CFAs[44].

Antitoxic immunity

Studies in rats and mice have shown a direct correlation between protection against cholera toxin-induced fluid secretion and intestinal synthesis of SIgA antibodies, and also between protection and the number of antitoxin-producing cells in the intestine[32,45]. These results, together with the nature of cholera disease, suggest that locally formed SIgA antibodies are of major importance for providing antitoxic immunity in the gut.

Neutralization of heat-labile entertoxins is primarily provided by antibodies against the B subunit portion of the toxin molecule. Thus, antibodies against CTB have been found to be equally effective as antibodies against holotoxin in protecting against CT-induced fluid accumulation in the gut[25]. The neutralization does not necessarily require direct steric blocking of the GM1 binding site of the B subunit, but may also result from antibody-mediated conformational changes induced via other epitopes. Antibodies against the A subunit portion of CT have been essentially inefficient in neutralizing this toxin, whereas some monoclonal antibodies against LTA subunit have had neutralizing capacity[46]. Cholera A subunit, on the other hand, seems to have strong immunomodulating properties in various species. Thus, whereas isolated CTB is very inefficient in inducing anti-enterotoxin immune responses in mice or rabbits after peroral administration, feeding of CT may result in strong local antitoxin antibody formation[45,47]. Indeed, CT may also potentiate immune responses to non-related protein antigens up to 50-fold as determined by the increase in antibody-producing cells in lamina propria when the antigen was given perorally together with CT[45]. The strong adjuvant action of CT found in many systems most probably has a multifactorial background. Thus, CT has been found to increase the uptake of antigens across intestinal epithelial cells, to markedly stimulate antigen-presenting cells (via production of interleukin-1), to induce isotype switching leading to increased expression of IgA in B cells and to inhibit preferentially suppressor T-cell populations[45,48].

Antibodies against CTB may also cross-protect against *E. coli* LT disease, and vice-versa anti-LT antibodies may be effective against experimental cholera, although immunity against the homologous toxin is usually somewhat better[46]. In a recent study we have shown that active immunization with CTB was as effective as administration of LTB in inducing protection against challenge with various strains of LT producing *E. coli* (Svennerholm A.-M., unpublished).

For immune protection against ST-producing *E. coli*, antisera raised against native STa coupled to a carrier protein have been effective in neutralizing this toxin as studied in rabbit ligated loops or in infant mice[49]. However, immunization with non-toxic ST peptides, either derived by protein synthesis or by the use of synthetic oligonucleotides[50,51] have failed to induce ST neutralizing immunity.

Anti-colonization immunity

To evelute anticolonization immunity in animals non-ligated intestine models are preferable. By using the reversible intestinal tie adult rabbit diarrhoea (RITARD) model[52] de la Cabada *et al.*[53] observed decreased fluid accumulation in intestine after immunization with very high doses of purified CFA/I. In subsequent experiments using this model we could show that CFA/I, as well as the different CS components of CFA/II and CFA/IV, when present on whole bacteria, are colonizing factors and protective antigens[54,55]. At present, we are evaluating the colonizing ability and protective immunogenicity of some of the 'new' putative colonization factors in ETEC (Svennerholm *et al.*, to be published). These studies have shown that, e.g., PCFO159, CS7 and CS17 are colonizing factors in rabbit intestine and that only those PCFs that promote ETEC colonization give rise to strong immune responses after intestinal infection.

In previous studies it was shown that *V. cholerae* LPS is the predominant antigen affording antibacterial immunity against experimental cholera, but that other antigens may contribute to such protective immunity[56]. Based on studies in mice it has recently been suggested that the toxin-coregulated pilus (TCP) of *V. cholerae* O1 is also a protective antigen. TCP can probably induce anticolonization immunity that may enhance anti-LPS antibodies in protecting against cholera[57]. However, the relative importance of TCP immunity remains to be shown. Recent studies have also revealed that *V. cholerae* O1 may express a number of antigens during growth *in vivo* that cannot be identified on corresponding bacteria grown under various conditions *in vitro*[58]. We are at present evaluating if antibodies against such *in vivo* antigens may play a role in immune protection against cholera.

ANTIBODY RESPONSES IN HUMANS

Clinical cholera is probably the optimal immunization for inducing protective immunity against subsequent infection with *V. cholerae* O1 bacteria. This is probably due to the capacity of the natural infection to induce high levels of specific SIgA antibodies as well as immunological memory for such antibody formation locally in the intestine[32,33]. In addition to the locally produced SIgA antibodies, intestinal secretions may also contain specific antibodies of IgG and IgM classes that have diffused from the circulation. However, antibodies of the latter isotypes are considerably more sensitive to degradation by proteolytic enzymes than SIgA antibodies and, therefore, probably less important in protecting against mucosal pathogens like *V. cholerae* or ETEC. Hence, evaluation of mucosal immune responses to infections with enterotoxin-producing bacteria or vaccines against such organisms should be focused on determination of SIgA antibodies.

Methods for determination of SIgA antibodies against enterotoxin-producing bacteria

Determination of intestinal antibody responses in humans has been subject to considerable problems both with regard to collection of clinical specimens and to lack of suitable antibody detection methods. Analyses of stool specimens not only include difficulties in extracting the coproantibodies but also in the considerable proteolytic degradation of immunoglobulins during passage through the entire intestine. Intestinal aspirates only contain antibodies formed in the duodenum and proximal jejunum, and determination of antibody-producing cells in intestinal biopsies is an invasive procedure. To avoid some of these problems we have used the intestinal lavage method by which the volunteers drink an isotonic salt solution until a watery diarrhoea ensues; the liquid stool is collected, enzyme-inactivated and concentrated by freeze-drying. Although laborious, this method allows collection of specimens containing antibodies produced from the entire small intestine; the lavages can then be assayed for specific antibody contents e.g. by different enzyme-linked immunosorbent assay (ELISA) techniques[33,59].

Based on the knowledge of a common mucosal immune system[35] we have also evaluated whether immune responses in the intestine may be reflected in other more easily available secretions such as milk, saliva and serum. Unfortunately, however, we could not identify any non-intestinal secretion that satisfactorily allowed such indirect determinations. However, serum IgG, and particularly IgA antibody responses, induced by oral antigen stimulation reflected the intestinal SIgA responses relatively well[60].

As an alternative to determining SIgA antibodies in intestinal fluid the number of antibody-secreting cells (ASC), either circulating in the blood or in intestinal biopsies, may be assayed using the recently developed enzyme-linked immunospot (ELISPOT) method[39,61]. By this approach, suspensions of lymphoid cells are incubated in tissue culture medium in antigen-coated wells and the specific antibodies formed are determined by conventional ELISA steps. Single antibody-secreting cells of different isotypes could then be recognized as coloured spots appearing on the antigen-coated surface. By using this method human lymphoid cells secreting specific antibodies of different isotypes and with different specificities could be detected.

Antibody responses induced by natural disease or asymptomatic infection

Clinical cholera has been shown to give rise to high levels of SIgA antibodies not only against CT but also against the cell wall LPS locally in the intestine[33]. Significant SIgA antibody responses often also appear in milk and saliva, and most convalescents develop significant antitoxic IgG and IgA titre rises as well as vibriocidal antibody responses in serum. The cholera antibody levels observed have usually been significantly higher in the convalescents than in healthy persons living in the same area and subjected to repeated natural exposure to *V. cholerae* organisms[62].

Significant antibody responses to repeated natural exposure are suggested by the observation of increased levels of vibriocidal antibody titres in serum with age in persons living in cholera-endemic areas[63]. Antitoxic serum antibody levels, on the other hand, do not show the same increase with age, probably due to high infection rates with LT-producing *E. coli*, predominantly in early childhood. Thus, anti-LT titres in serum seem to peak in children below 4 years of age and decrease thereafter[64]. In a study of convalescents from entertoxin-induced *E. coli* diarrhoea we have also shown significant antibody responses in intestinal lavage fluid as well as in serum against the most important protective antigens of these organisms, i.e. different CFAs, the O-antigen of the infecting strain and LT[59].

Studies in human volunteers have also demonstrated that adult Americans experimentally infected with *V. cholerae* or ETEC respond with high levels of specific antitoxic as well as antibacterial antibodies in jejunal fluids and in serum[65,66]. Comparison of antitoxic immune responses in convalescents from cholera and ETEC disease showed that antitoxin titres in serum developed both against CT and *E. coli* LT, but that the titre against the homologous toxin was always higher than that against the heterologous toxin[67].

In addition to eliciting an SIgA antibody response which is usually of short duration, lasting for 1 or a few months after onset of disease, mucosal infection may also induce long-lasting immunological memory. Induction of such a memory may explain why protective immunity after mucosal infection can be seen in the absence of significant mucosal levels of SIgA antibodies. As support for this assumption we have found that oral administration of relatively low doses of cholera antigens to cholera convalescents resulted in considerably higher and earlier-appearing SIgA antibody responses in intestinal secretions than observed in similarly immunized healthy controls[33]. Furthermore, infection with E. coli that produces LT which crossreacts immunologically with CT, could prime the intestine to respond with an anamnestic IgA response to a subsequent oral vaccination with cholera toxoid[68].

Acquired immunity to enterotoxin-producing bacteria

Infection with enterotoxin-producing organisms and the diarrhoeal diseases that may occur in early childhood, may result in partial or complete immunity against illness or even infection. This is supported by the findings of a reverse disease-to-infection rate with age both in cholera and ETEC disease in children in endemic areas[3,63]. Thus, both diseases predominate in children with a peak of cholera in the age group between 2 and 9 years, and of ETEC disease in children below 2 years of age. In a recent study in Mexico a dramatic drop in ETEC disease rate with age was found in children between 1 and 5 years, although the infection rate was almost the same in the various age groups[69].

Further support for acquired immunity in cholera is the observation in Bangladesh of a very low re-infection rate, suggesting approximately 90% protection against a second episode of cholera in endemic areas[70]. Human volunteers suffering from symptomatic cholera were also effectively protected against reinfection for several years after the initial cholera episode[65]. However, there is some evidence that the degree of protective immunity induced by cholera disease is biotype-related. Thus, studies in human volunteers have suggested that whereas cholera induced by vibrios of the classical biotype affords 100% protection for several years, disease caused by V. cholerae O1 of the El Tor biotype gives rise to only 80–90% protection. Furthermore, Clemens et al.[71] recently demonstrated that symptomatic cholera reinfections in Bangladesh were only seen in patients who had previously suffered from cholera disease due to El Tor, but not to classical vibrios.

ETEC is a considerably more heterogeneous group than V. cholerae with numerous serotypes, colonization factors and enterotoxins. By comparing the relative proportion of the different toxin types of ETEC associated with first versus second episodes of diarrhoea in Bangladesh there was no evidence of protection induced by enterotoxin[72]. Similarly it has been shown in Mexico that children infected with ETEC had no less disease-to-infection rate on the second as compared to the initial infection with LT producing E. coli[73]. However, there was a reduced risk of diarrhoea in infants reinfected with

ETEC producing the same as compared with different CFAs. Further support for a protective role of CFA immunity is studies in human volunteers showing that infection with ETEC afforded significant protection against reinfection with a heterologous strain carrying homologous CFA[66].

Studies of the diarrhoea incidence in breastfed children also suggest the protective effect of antitoxic as well as antibacterial antibodies against enterotoxin-producing bacteria. Specific SIgA antibodies against the most prevalent enteropathogens are usually found in the milk of lactating mothers. The protective role of these antibodies has been difficult to assess, e.g. by comparing diarrhoea morbidity in breastfed and bottlefed children, due to several confounding factors. In a study in Bangladesh, however, strong evidence for the protective effect of SIgA antibodies against cholera was achieved[74]. Thus, children who drank milk that contained high levels of anticholera toxin and/or antibacterial SIgA antibodies attracted symptomatic cholera in significantly lower numbers than children who drank milk with low levels of such antibodies.

DEVELOPMENT OF CANDIDATE VACCINES AGAINST CHOLERA AND ETEC DIARRHOEA

Effective vaccines against enterotoxin-induced diarrhoeal diseases should obviously induce antibacterial as well as antitoxic immune responses that may enhance each other synergistically. Based on this assumption we have constructed a new improved cholera vaccine, and recently also a prototype ETEC vaccine, that each contain an enterotoxoid in combination with inactivated bacteria expressing the most important protective antigens of *V. cholerae* and ETEC bacteria, respectively.

In order to be efficacious, vaccines against non-invasive enteric infections must be able to stimulate the local gut mucosal immune system. Such stimulation is usually better achieved by giving the vaccines by the oral rather than the parenteral route. Oral vaccines are in general also easier to produce and administer, since they do not require any medically trained personnel or any medical supplies. However, important factors in the development of effective enteric vaccines include not only the route of antigen administration but also the number of immunizations, immunization intervals, etc.

The other important determinant of an efficacious vaccine is the nature of the antigen encountered. Effective mucosal immunogens should not be degraded in the intestine; they should bind to or penetrate into the epithelium, thus facilitating uptake in the Peyer's patches, and they should ideally also have adjuvant immunomodulating activity, e.g. CT. Examples of such mucosal immunogens are different bacterial toxins and fimbrial adhesins that bind in a ligand–receptor-specific manner to mucosal surfaces. Certain particulate antigens, including some types of killed bacteria, have also been found to be useful mucosal immunogens. These aspects have been taken into consideration when designing the vaccines against cholera- and ETEC-induced diarrhoea.

Oral cholera vaccines

Conventional parenteral cholera vaccines have only afforded up to 50% protection against cholera for 3-6 months[32]. Since cholera remains an important cause of illness and death in many developing countries much research has been devoted to the development of an improved oral cholera vaccine that could stimulate intestinal immunity more efficiently. Against this background we have developed an oral cholera vaccine consisting of the non-toxic, yet strongly immunogenic B-subunit of CT in combination with heat- and formalin-killed cholera vibrios[32,44,75]. This B-subunit-whole cell (B-WC) cholera vaccine, which is taken as a drink in a bicarbonate–citrate solution, has in extensive clinical trials, including a large field trial in Bangladesh, proved to be safe and to provide long-term protection[5].

In initial studies in Swedish volunteers the vaccine was shown to be completely safe and to induce strong serum antibody responses against the toxoid as well as the bacterial component. Subsequent studies in Bangladesh revealed that two peroral doses of vaccine were considerably more efficient than combinations of peroral and parenteral or repeated parenteral immunizations in inducing antitoxic IgA antibody responses locally in the gut[76].

We also evaluated to what extent immunization with the vaccine could mimic clinical cholera in inducing intestinal antitoxic and antibacterial SIgA antibody responses. These studies revealed that two peroral doses of B-WC vaccine were equally efficient as clinical cholera in inducing these antibody responses in intestinal lavage fluid[33]. The vaccination also induced an immunological memory that could be boosted by a dose that was too low to elicit an immune response in itself. The memory induced was of long duration, since immunization of Swedish volunteers who had received a priming immunization with B-WC vaccine 5 years earlier responded considerably better to a single booster dose with the same vaccine than previously non-immunized Swedes of similar ages[37]. Furthermore, Bangladeshi volunteers previously given two doses of cholera B-subunit responded already on day 3 after a single booster dose given 15 months later, whereas no such early responses were seen in previously non-immunized controls[36]. Peroral immunization with either the complete B-WC vaccine or the WC component alone also induced significant protection in American volunteers against challenge with a dose of live cholera vibrios that caused disease in 100% of concurrently tested unvaccinated controls[77].

On the basis of these studies a large double-blind placebo control field trial in rural Bangladesh with over 90 000 participants was initiated. As shown in Table 13.1 the results of the study have established that both the B-WC vaccine and the WC component alone confer long-lasting protection against cholera[5]. During the initial 6 months of study the combined vaccine conferred 85% protection against cholera, and this protection was similar in all age groups. This protection was significantly higher than that induced by the WC component alone, being around 60% during the first 6 months[78]. Thereafter, however, the efficacy was similar, ~60%, for both vaccines for the 3-year follow-up period[5]. The protective effect was considerably higher in those volunteers that were more than 5 years old when vaccination began

(Table 13.1). The protection induced by the vaccines was the same against severe as mild disease, and was of similar magnitude after two or three peroral doses of vaccine.

The combined B-WC vaccine also provided highly significant (67%) protection against diarrhoea caused by LT-producing *E. coli* for a couple of months after vaccination[6]. Surprisingly, the protective effect was comparable against *E. coli* producing LT alone as against *E. coli* producing LT in combination with ST. Furthermore, both the B-WC and the WC alone vaccines were capable of reducing the overall diarrhoea morbidity among the vaccinees. Thus, there was a 50% reduction in admission for life-threatening diarrhoea in the vaccinated as compared with the placebo group over the 3-year follow-up period[5].

These promising results with the B-WC vaccine will hopefully lead to the vaccine being licensed in several countries shortly. Further developmental work is also going on to prepare a second-generation B-WC vaccine. A recombinant non-toxic *V. cholerae* strain that produces isolated B subunit in very high concentrations has been constructed[79] allowing simplified production of the B component of the vaccine. Furthermore, the recombinant vaccine strain may be cultured to allow expression of TCP, which might enhance antibacterial immunity compared to that attained within the field trial; former B-WC preparations lacked this adhesin in immunogenic form. Since significantly better protection against cholera caused by vibrios of the classical than of the El Tor biotype was observed in the field trial[5] attempts should also be made to improve El Tor immunity. Recently, we have identified an immunogenic El Tor-associated fimbriae that may provide additional antibacterial immunity against *V. cholerae* El Tor[13a].

Progress has also been made towards the development of a live attenuated cholera vaccine. By recombinant DNA techniques *V. cholerae* O1 mutant

Table 13.1 Randomized placebo-controlled field trial of the oral B subunit-whole cell (B-WC) and whole-cell (WC) cholera vaccines alone given in three (or two) doses in the field trial in Bangladesh[5,78]

	Vaccine efficacy (%)	
	B-WC	WC
After 6 months of follow-up		
All ages	85	58
Persons ≥6 years	77	62
Children 2–5 years	92	53
After 3 years of follow-up		
All ages	50	52
Persons ≥6 years	63	68
Children 2–5 years	26	23
Recipients of only two doses, all ages	64	39
Overall protection after two or three doses, all ages		
(including estimate for adult men)[a]	62	60

[a] Only children and women >15 years were recruited for the trial [5]

strains have been prepared in which the genes encoding cholera toxin have been deleted[80]. The high frequency of diarrhoea observed after immunization with the initial candidate vaccine strains, precluded their use as potential vaccines. However, a recently developed strain, CVD 103-HgR, that has been prepared by deleting the A-subunit gene from *V. cholerae* O1 bacteria, has been well tolerated[81]. A single dose led to significant antibacterial antibody responses in 96% of the volunteers and significant antitoxic immune responses in 88% of them. The vaccine also induced significant protective immunity against challenge with biotype-heterologous *V. cholerae* O1 El Tor bacteria[81]. Studies to evaluate this vaccine strain in cholera endemic areas have been initiated.

VACCINES AGAINST ETEC DIARRHOEA

Infection with ETEC is the most important cause of diarrhoea both in children in developing countries and among travellers to these areas[3]. Although ETEC seem to account for more than 1 billion diarrhoeal episodes and 1 million deaths annually among children in developing countries, no vaccine for use in humans is yet available. Based on recent knowledge about virulence factors and protective antigens in ETEC several groups have worked intensively on the development of a new ETEC vaccine for use in humans. Such a vaccine should be given orally, and ideally evoke both anticolonization and antitoxic IgA antibody responses in the gut.

Based on these premises the following inactivated or live ETEC vaccine candidates may be considered: (1) purified CFAs and enterotoxoid, (2) live bacteria expressing the major CFAs and producing enterotoxoid or (3) killed CFA-positive *E. coli* in combination with enterotoxoid. Vaccines consisting of purified fimbriae may probably be too expensive to prepare; furthermore, isolated CFAs have been shown to be very sensitive to proteolytic degradation in the human gastrointestinal tract[28,82]. Since the different CFAs are normally not expressed in the same strain, and it has not yet been possible to clone the genes for different CFAs into the same host organism, a live CFA vaccine has probably to consist of a mixture of different strains.

With such live vaccines there is a risk of overgrowth of one of the included vaccine strains with suppression of the others. Alternatively, a colonizing host organism, e.g. the attenuated live typhoid vaccine strain, Ty21a, may be used as a carrier for the expression of foreign genes encoding e.g. CFAs and B subunit[66]. However, it has still not been possible to express more than one CFA in the same culture of Ty21a. Therefore, a vaccine consisting of killed ETEC bacteria expressing the most prevalent CFAs and given together with a suitable enterotoxoid is the most promising vaccine candidate within reach. Inactivation could be achieved either by colicin E2 treatment[83] or by mild formalin treatment[84].

A prototype CFA–ETEC-toxoid vaccine

The vaccine we have developed consists of a mixture of killed *E. coli* expressing CFA/I and the different CS components of CFA/II and CFA/IV and of enterotoxoid CTB[84,85]. Strains that belong to common ETEC O-groups, and that express the different fimbriae in high concentrations, have been selected. The bacteria have been inactivated by mild formalin treatment which results in complete killing of the bacteria without significant losses in the antigenicity of the different CFAs or O antigens. Furthermore the CFA antigens of these inactivated bacteria have been stable during storage for long periods, and even after incubation in human gastrointestinal secretions[84].

The prototype ETEC vaccine has recently been evaluated for safety and immunogenicity in adult Swedish volunteers. This has included an evaluation of the capacity of the vaccine to induce local SIgA antibody responses against the most important antigens, i.e. the different CFAs expressed by the vaccine strains and CTB, in intestinal lavage fluid. Antibody responses in serum[85], as well as production of specific antibodies by peripheral blood lymphocytes, have also been assessed.

Hitherto approximately 50 volunteers have received two or three oral doses with 10^{11} formalin-killed E. coli organisms and 1 mg of CTB in buffered bicarbonate solution 2 weeks apart. Immunization with the prototype vaccine did not result in any significant adverse local or systemic reactions. Intestinal lavages collected immediately before and then 7–9 days after the second and third immunization from 11 of the volunteers, were examined for specific ELISA IgA titres divided by the total IgA content of each specimen. Significant IgA antibody responses were observed against CFA/I, CFA/II as well as CTB in most of the vaccines. The frequency of responses was comparable to that previously observed[59] in adult Bangladeshis convalescing from infection with CFA-positive E. coli. Also the magnitudes of the intestinal antibody responses against the CFAs were comparable to those previously seen in the convalescents, whereas the anti-LT responses were somewhat higher after vaccination than after E. coli LT disease[85]. These results suggest that it is possible to induce substantial CFA antibody responses locally in the intestine by an inactivated vaccine. Such responses have previously been difficult to induce by oral immunization with isolated fimbriae[28].

The ETEC prototype vaccine also gave rise to significant rises in antibody-secreting cells (ASCs) with specificity for CFA/I, CFA/II and CTB in 85–100% of the volunteers (Wennerås, C., Svennerholm, A.-M. and Czerkinsky, C., to be published). The responses were predominantly in cells producing IgA antibodies supporting an intestinal origin. Significant serum antibody responses against CTB were also observed in most of the volunteers, whereas the responses against CFAs were relatively modest[85].

In subsequent studies we plan to evaluate the vaccine for protective efficacy against ETEC disease both in travellers and in children in endemic areas. Due to the extremely high incidence of ETEC infections in many groups of travellers (up to 5% of them may develop ETEC diarrhoea each week during their initial stay in a highly ETEC endemic area), such protective efficacy trials could probably be performed using a relatively small number of volunteers. Hopefully, an effective ETEC vaccine will soon be available.

The experience with the ETEC vaccine suggests that not only cholera B-subunit but also other antigens that bind to specific receptors in the intestinal mucosa such as the CFAs may be very effective in eliciting significant intestinal SIgA antibody responses. Against this background, enteric vaccines based on antigens or vaccine components binding in a receptor–ligand manner to the intestinal epithelium have the potential of providing protective immunity against the non-invasive enteropathogens, live *V. cholerae* and ETEC.

Acknowledgements

Financial support for the studies described on cholera and ETEC vaccines has been provided by the Swedish Medical Research Council, the Swedish Agency for Research Cooperation with Developing Countries (SAREC), the CDD Programme of the World Health Organisation and the International Centre for Diarrhoeal Disease Research, Dhaka, Bangladesh.

References

1. Farthing, M. J. G. and Keusch, G. T. (eds) (1989). *Enteric Infection. Mechanisms, Manifestations and Management*. London: Chapman & Hall
2. Guerrant, R. L. (1985). Microbial toxins and diarrhoeal disease: introduction and overview. In Evered, D. and Whelan, J. (eds), *Microbial Toxins and Diarrhoeal Disease*. Ciba Foundation Symposium 112. London: Pitman, pp. 1–13
3. Black, R. E. (1986). The epidemiology of cholera and enterotoxigenic *E. coli* diarrheal disease. In Holmgren, J., Lindberg, A. and Möllby, R. (eds), *Development of Vaccines and Drugs against Diarrhea*. 11th Nobel Conference, Stockholm. Lund: Studentlitteratur, pp. 23–32
4. Holmgren, J., Lindberg, A. and Möllby, R. (eds) (1986). *Development of Vaccines and Drugs against Diarrhea*. Lund: Studentlitteratur
5. Clemens, J. D., Sack, D. A., Harris, J. R., Van Loon, F., Chakraborty, J., Ahmed, F., Rao, M. R., Kan, M. R., Yunus, M. D., Huda, N., Stanton, B. F., Kay, B. A., Walter, S., Eeckels, R., Svennerholm, A.-M. and Holmgren, J. (1990). Field trial of oral cholera vaccines in Bangladesh: Results from three-year follow-up. *Lancet*, **355**, 270–3
6. Clemens, J. D., Sack, D. A., Harris, J. R., Chakraborty, J., Neogy, P. K., Stanton, B., Huda, N., Khan, M. U., Kay, B. A., Khan, M. R., Ansaruzzaman, M., Yunus, M., Rao, M. R., Svennerholm, A.-M. and Holmgren, J. (1990). Cross-protection by B subunit-whole cell cholera vaccine against diarrhea associated with heat-labile toxin-producing enterotoxigenic *Escherichia coli*: results of a large-scale field trial. *J. Infect. Dis.*, **158**, 372–7
7. Duguid, J. P. and Old, D. C. (1980). Adhesive properties of Enterobactericeae. In Beachy, E. H. (ed.), *Bacterial Adherence, Receptors and Recognition*, Series B. London: Chapman & Hall, pp. 185–217
8. Evans, D. J. Jr and Evans, D. G. (1989). Determinants of microbial attachment and their genetic control. In Farthing, M. J. G. and Keusch, G. T. (eds), *Enteric Infection. Mechanisms, Manifestations and Management*. London: Chapman & Hall, pp. 15–30
9. Warner, L. and Kim, Y. S. (1989). Intestinal receptors for microbial attachment. In Farthing, M. J. G. and Keusch, G. T. (eds), *Enteric Infection. Mechanisms, Manifestations and Management*. London: Chapman & Hall, pp. 31–40
10. Holmgren, J., Svennerholm, A.-M., Lindblad, M. (1983). Receptor-like glycocompounds in human milk that inhibit classical and El Tor *Vibrio cholerae* cell adherence (hemagglutination). *Infect. Immun.*, **39**, 147–54
11. Holmgren, J., Ahrén, C. and Svennerholm, A.-M. (1981). Nonimmunoglobulin fraction of human milk inhibits bacterial adhesion (hemagglutination) and entertotoxin binding of *Escherichia coli* and *Vibrio cholerae*. *Infect. Immun.*, **33**, 136–41
12. Taylor, R. K., Miller, V. L., Furlong, D. B. and Mekalanos, J. J. (1987). Use of phoA gene fusions to identify a pilus colonization factor coordinately regulated with cholera toxin. *Proc. Natl. Acad. Sci. USA*, **84**, 2833–7
13. Hall, R. H., Vial, P. A., Kaper, J. B., Mekalanos, J. J. and Levine, M. M. (1988). Morphological studies on fimbriae expressed by *Vibrio cholerae* O1. *Microb. Pathogen.*, **4**, 257–65

13a. Jonson, G., Holmgren, J. and Svennerholm, A.-M. (1991). Identification of a mannose-binding pilus on *V. cholerae* El Tor. *Microb. Pathogen.* (in press)
14. McConnell, M. M. (1991). Newly characterized putative colonization factors of human enterotoxigenic *Escherichia coli*. In Wadström, T., Svennerholm, A.-M., Wolf-Watz, H. and Mäkälä, H. (eds), *Molecular Pathogenesis of Gastrointestinal Infection*. London: Plenum (In press)
15. Nagy, B. (1986). Vaccines against toxigenic *Escherichia coli* disease in animals. In Holmgren, J., Lindberg, A. and Möllby, R. (eds), *Development of Vaccines and Drugs against Diarrhea*. 11th Nobel Conference, Stockholm. Lund: Studentlitteratur, pp. 53–61
16. Holmgren, J. (1985). Toxins affecting intestinal transport processes. In Sussman, M. (ed.), *The Virulence of* Escherichia coli. London: Academic Press, pp. 177–91
17. Rao, M. C. (1985). Toxins which activate guanylate cyclase: heat-stable enterotoxins. In Evered, D. and Whelan, J. (eds), *Microbial Toxins and Diarrhoeal Disease*. Ciba Foundation Symposium 112. London: Pitman, pp. 74–93
18. Clements, J. D. and Finkelstein, R. A. (1978). Immunological cross-reactivity between a heat-labile entertoxin(s) of *Escherichia coli* and subunits of *Vibrio cholerae* enterotoxin. *Infect. Immun.*, **21**, 1036–9
19. Holmgren, J., Fredman, P., Lindblad, M., Svennerholm, A.-M. and Svennerholm, L. (1982). Rabbit intestinal glycoprotein receptor for *Escherichia coli* heat-labile enterotoxin lacking affinity for cholera toxin. *Infect. Immun.*, **38**, 424–33
20. Wadström, T., Aust-Kettis, A., Habte, D., Holmgren, J., Meuwisse, G., Möllby, R. and Söderlind, O. (1976). Enterotoxin-producing bacteria and parasites in stools of Ethiopian children with diarrhoeal disease. *Arch. Childh. Dis.*, **51**, 865–70
21. Åhrén, C., Jertborn, M., Herclik, L., Kaijser, B. and Svennerholm, A.-M. (1990). Infection with bacterial enteropathogens in Swedish travellers to South-East Asia – a prospective study. *Epidemiol. Infect.*, **105**, 325–33
22. Frantz, J. C. and Robertson, D. C. (1981). Immunological properties of *Escherichia coli* heat-stable enterotoxins: development of a radioimmunoassay specific for heat-stable enterotoxins with suckling mouse activity. *Infect. Immun.*, **33**, 193–8
23. Svennerholm, A.-M., Wikström, M., Lindblad, M. and Holmgren, J. (1986). Monoclonal antibodies against *E. coli* heat-stable toxin (STa) and their use in a diagnostic ST ganglioside GM1-enzyme-linked immunosorbent assay. *J. Clin. Microbiol.*, **24**, 585–90
24. Takao, T., Shimonishi, Y., Kobayashi, O., Nishinura, M., Arita, T., Takeda, T., Honda, S. and Miwatani, T. (1985). Amino acid sequence of heat-stable enterotoxin produced by *Vibrio cholerae* non-O1. *FEBS Lett.*, **193**, 250–4
25. Holmgren, J. and Lycke, N. (1986). Immune mechanisms of enteric infections. In Holmgren, J., Lindberg, A. and Möllby, R. (eds), *Development of Vaccines and Drugs against Diarrhea*. 11th Nobel Conference, Stockholm. Lund, Sweden: Studentlitteratur, pp. 9–22
26. Lee, J.-Y., Boman, A., Chuanxin, S., Andersson, M., Jörnvall, H., Mutt, V. and Boman, H. G. (1989). Antibacterial peptides from pig intestine: isolation of a mammalian cecropin. *Proc. Natl. Acad. Sci. USA*, **86**, 9159–62
27. Cash, R., Music, S., Libonati, J., Snyder, M., Wenzel, R. and Hornick, B. (1974). Response of man to infection with *V. cholerae*. I. Clinical, serologic and bacteriologic responses to a known inoculum. *J. Infect. Dis.*, **129**, 45–52
28. Levine, M. M., Morris, J. G., Losonsky, G., Boedeker, E. and Rowe, B. (1986). Fimbriae (pili) adhesins as vaccines. In Lark, D. (ed), *Protein–Carbohydrate Interactions in Biological Systems*. London: Academic Press, pp. 143–145
29. Stoll, B. J., Holmgren, J., Bardhan, P. K., Huq, I., Greenough, W. B., Fredman, P. and Svennerholm, L. (1980). Binding of intraluminal toxin in cholera: trial of GM1 ganglioside charcoal. *Lancet*, **2**, 888–91
30. Glass, R. I., Holmgren, J., Khan, M. R., Hossain, K. M. B., Huq, M. I. and Greenough, W. B. (1984). A randomized, controlled trial of the toxin-blocking effects of B subunit in family members of patients with cholera. *J. Infect. Dis.*, **149**, 495–500
31. Mestecky, J. and McGhee, J. R. (1987). Immunoglobulin A (IgA): molecular and cellular interactions involved in IgA biosynthesis and immune response. *Adv. Immunol.*, **40**, 153–245
32. Holmgren, J. and Svennerholm, A.-M. (1983). Cholera and the immune response. *Progr. Allergy*, **33**, 106–19
33. Svennerholm, A.-M., Jertborn, M., Gothefors, L., Karim, A. M. M. M., Sack, D. A. and

Holmgren, J. (1984). Mucosal antitoxic and antibacterial immunity after cholera disease and after immunization with a combined B subunit-whole cell vaccine. *J. Infect. Dis.*, 149, 884–93

34. Tagliabue, A., Boraschi, D., Villa, D. F., Keren, D. R., Lowell, G. H., Rappuoli, R. and Nencioni, L. (1984). IgA-dependent cell-mediated activity against enteropathogenic bacteria: distribution, specificity, and characterization of the effector cells. *J. Immunol.*, 133, 988–92

35. Brandtzaeg, P., Bjerke, K., Haltsensen, T. S., Hvatum, M., Kett, K., Krajci, P., Kvale, D., Müller, F., Wilsson, D., Roynum, T. O., Scott, H., Sollid, L. M., Thrane, P. and Valnes, K. (1990). Local immunity: the human mucosa in health and disease. In MacDonald, T., Challacombe, J., Bland, W. *et al.* (eds), *Advances in Mucosal Immunology*. London: Kluwer, pp. 1–12

36. Svennerholm, A.-M., Gothefors, L., Sack, D. A., Bardhan, P. K. and Holmgren, J. (1984). Local and systemic antibody responses and immunological memory in humans after immunization with cholera B subunit by different routes. *Bull. WHO*, 62, 909–18

37. Jertborn, M., Svennerholm, A.-M. and Holmgren, J. (1988). Five-year immunologic memory in Swedish volunteers after oral cholera vaccination. *J. Infect. Dis.*, 157, 374–7

38. Lycke, N. and Holmgren, J. (1989). Adoptive transfer of gut mucosal antitoxin memory by isolated B cells 1 year after oral immunization with cholera toxin. *Infect. Immun.*, 57, 1137–41

39. Quiding, M., Nordström, I., Kilander, A., Andersson, G., Hanson, L.-A., Holmgren, J. and Czerkinsky, C. (1991). Intestinal immune responses in humans. Oral cholera vaccination induces strong intestinal antibody responses, gamma-interferon production, and evokes local immunological memory. *J. Clin. Invest.*, 88, 143–8

40. Madara, J. L. and Stafford, J. (1989). Interferon-gamma directly affects barrier function of cultured intestinal epithelial monolayers. *J. Clin. Invest.*, 83, 724

41. Holmgren, J., Fryklund, J. and Larsson, H. (1989). Gamma-interferon-mediated down-regulation of electrolyte secretion by intestinal epithelial cells: a local immune mechanism? *Scand. J. Immunol.*, 30, 499–503

42. De, S. N. and Chatterje, D. N. (1953). An experimental study of the mechanism of action of Vibrio cholerae on the intestinal mucous membrane. *J. Pathol. Bacteriol.*, 46, 559–62

43. Svennerholm, A.-M. and Holmgren, J. (1976). Synergistic protective effect in rabbits of immunization with *Vibrio cholerae* lipopolysaccharide and toxin/toxoid. *Infect. Immun.*, 13, 735–40

44. Svennerholm, A.-M., Åhrén, C., Lopez-Vidal, Y., Lycke, N. and Holmgren, J. (1986). Development of enteric vaccines based on synergism between antitoxin and anti-colonization immunity. In Lark, D. (ed.), *Protein–Carbohydrate Interactions in Biological Systems*. London: Academic Press, pp. 147–54

45. Lycke, N. and Svennerholm, A.-M. (1990). Presentation of immunogens at the gut and other mucosal surfaces. In Woodrow, G. C. and Levine, M. M. (eds), *New Generation Vaccines*, Basel: Marcel Dekker, pp. 207–27

46. Svennerholm, A.-M., Wikström, M., Lindblad, M. and Holmgren, J. (1986). Monoclonal antibodies to *Escherichia coli* heat-labile enterotoxins: neutralising activity and differentiation of human and porcine LTs and cholera toxin. *Med. Biol.*, 64, 23–30

47. Pierce, N. F. (1978). The role of antigen form and function in the primary and secondary intestinal immune responses to cholera toxoid and toxin in rats. *J. Exp. Med.*, 148, 195–206

48. Lycke, N., Karlsson, U., Sjölander, A. and Magnusson, K.-E. (1991). The adjuvant action of cholera toxin is associated with an increased intestinal permeability for luminal antigens. *Scand. J. Immunol.*, 33, 691–8

49. Takeda, T., Takeda, Y., Aimoto, S., Takao, T., Ikemura, H., Shimonishi, Y. and Miwatani, T. (1983). Neutralization of activity of two different heat-stable enterotoxins (STh and STp) of enterotoxigenic *Eswcherichia coli* by homologous and heterologous antisera. *FEMS Microbiol. Lett.*, 20, 357–9

50. Svennerholm, A.-M., Lindblad, M., Svennerholm, B. and Holmgren, J. (1988). Synthesis of nontoxic, antibody-binding *Escherichia coli* heat-stable enterotoxin (ST_a) peptides. *FEMS Microbiol. Lett.*, 55, 23–8

51. Sanchez, J., Svennerholm, A.-M. and Holmgren, J. (1988). Genetic fusion of a non-toxic heat-stable enterotoxin-related decapeptide antigen to cholera toxin B-subunit. *FEBS Lett.*, 241, 110–14

52. Spira, W. M., Sack, R. B. and Froelich, J. L. (1981). Simple adult rabbit model for *Vibrio cholerae* and enterotoxigenic *Escherichia coli* diarrhea. *Infect. Immun.*, 32, 739–47

53. De la Cabada, F. J., Evans, D. J. and Evans, D. G. (1981). Immune protection against enterotoxigenic *Escherichia coli* diarrhea in rabbits by peroral administration of purified colonization factor antigen I (CFA/I). *FEMS Microbiol. Lett.*, **II**, 303–7

54. Åhrén, C. M. and Svennerholm, A.-M. (1985). Experimental enterotoxin-induced *Escherichia coli* diarrhea and protection induced by previous infection with bacteria of the same adhesin or enterotoxin type. *Infect. Immun.*, **50**, 255–61

55. Svennerholm, A.-M., Wennerås, C., Holmgren, J., McConnell, M. M. and Rowe, B. (1990). Roles of different coli surface antigens of colonization factor antigen II in colonization by and protective immunogenicity of enterotoxigenic *Escherichia coli* in rabbits. *Infect. Immun.*, **58**, 341–6

56. Svennerholm, A.-M. (1980). The nature of protective immunity in cholera. In Ouchterlony, Ö. and Holmgren, J. (eds), *Cholera and Related Diarrheal Diseases*. 43rd Nobel Symposium, Stockholm 1978. Basel: Karger, pp. 171–84

57. Sun, D., Tillman, D. M., Marion, T. N. and Taylor, R. K. (1990). Production and characterization of monoclonal antibodies to the toxin coregulated pilus (TCP) of *Vibrio cholerae* that protect against experimental cholera in infant mice. *Serodiagn. Immunother. Infect. Dis.*, **4**, 73–81

58. Jonson, G., Svennerholm, A.-M. and Holmgren, J. (1989). *Vibrio cholerae* expresses cell surface antigens during intestinal infection which are not expressed during *in vitro* culture. *Infect. Immun.*, **57**, 1809–15

59. Stoll, B. J., Svennerholm, A.-M., Gotehfors, L., Barua, D., Huda, S. and Holmgren, J. (1986). Local and systemic antibody responses to naturally acquired enterotoxigenic *Escherichia coli* diarrhea in an endemic area. *J. Infect. Dis.*, **153**, 527–37

60. Jertborn, M., Svennerholm, A.-M. and Holmgren, J. (1986). Saliva, breast milk and serum antibody responses as indirect measures of intestinal immunity after oral cholera vaccination or natural disease. *J. Clin. Microbiol.*, **24**, 203–9

61. Czerkinsky, C., Svennerholm, A.-M., Quiding, M., Jonsson, R. and Holmgren, J. (1991). Antibody-producing cells in peripheral blood and salivary glands after oral cholera vaccination in humans. *Infect. Immun.*, **59**, 996–1001

62. Glass, R. I., Svennerholm, A.-M., Khan, M. R., Huda, S., Huq, I. and Holmgren, J. (1985). Seroepidemiological studies of El Tor cholera in Bangladesh: association of serum antibody levels with protection. *J. Infect. Dis.*, **151**, 236–42

63. Mosley, W. J. (1969). Vaccines and somatic antigens. The role of immunity in cholera. A review of epidemiological and serological studies. *Tex. Rep. Biol. Med.* (Suppl. 1), 227–41

64. Clemens, J. D., Svennerholm, A.-M., Harris, J. R., Huda, S., Rao, M., Neogy, P. K., Khan, M. R., Ansaruzzaman, M., Rahaman, S., Ahmed, F., Sack, D. A., Kay, B., Van Loon, F. and Holmgren, J. (1990). Seroepidemiologic evaluation of anti-toxic and anti-colonization factor immunity against infections by LT-producing *Escherichia coli* in rural Bangladesh. *J. Infect. Dis.*, **162**, 448–53

65. Levine, M. M., Kaper, J. B., Black, R. E. and Clements, M. L. (1983). New knowledge on pathogenesis of bacterial enteric infections as applied to vaccine development. *Microbiol. Rev.*, **47**, 510–50

66. Levine, M. M. (1990). Vaccines against enterotoxigenic *Escherichia coli* infections. In Woodrow, G. C. and Levine, M. M. (eds), *New Generation Vaccines*. Basel: Marcel Dekker, pp. 649–60

67. Svennerholm, A.-M., Holmgren, J., Black, R. and Levine, M. (1983). Serologic differentiation between antitoxin responses to infection with *Vibrio cholerae* and enterotoxin-producing *Escherichia coli*. *J. Infect. Dis.*, **147**, 514–21

68. Holmgren, J., Svennerholm, A.-M., Gothefors, L., Jertborn, M. and Stoll, B. (1988). Enterotoxigenic *Escherichia coli* diarrhea in an endemic area prepares the intestine for an anamestic immunoglobulin antitoxin response to oral cholera B subunit vaccination. *Infect. Immun.*, **56**, 230–3

69. López-Vidal, Y., Calva, J. J., Trujillo, A., De Léon, A. P., Ramos, A., Svennerhom, A.-M. and Ruiz-Palacios, G. M. (1990). Enterotoxins and adhesins of enterotoxigenic *Escherichia coli*: are they risk factors for acute diarrhea in the community? *J. Infect. Dis.*, **162**, 442–7

70. Glass, R. I., Becker, S., Huq, M. I., Stoll, B. J., Khan, M. U., Merson, M. H., Lee, J. V. and Black, R. E. (1982). Endemic cholera in rural Bangladesh, 1966–1980. *Am. J. Epidemiol.*, **116**, 959–70

71. Clemens, J. D., Van Loon, F., Sack, D. A., Rao, M. R., Ahmed, F., Chakraborty, J., Kay, B. A., Khan, M. R., Yunus, M. D., Harris, J. R., Svennerholm, A.-M. and Holmgren, J. (1991). Biotype as a determinant of the natural immunizing effect of *V. cholerae* 01: implications for vaccine development. *Lancet*, **337**, 883–4

72. Black, R. E. (1990). Overview of diarrheal diseases and strategies for their control. In Sack, D. A. and Freij, L. (eds), *Prospects for Public Health Benefits in Developing Countries from New Vaccines against Enteric Infections*. SAREC Report 1990. Stockholm: SAREC, pp. 115–20

73. Cravioto, A., Reyes, R. E., Trujillo, F., Uribe, F., Navarro, A., De La Roca, J. M., Hernandez, J. M., Perez, G. and Vzquez, V. (1990). Risk of diarrhea during the first year of life associated with initial and subsequent colonization by specific enteropathogens. *Am. J. Epidemiol.*, **131**, 886–901

74. Glass, R., Svennerholm, A.-M., Stoll, B. J., Khan, M. R., Hossain, K. M. B., Huq, M. I. and Holmgren, J. (1983). Protection against cholera in breast-fed children by antibodies in breast milk. *N. Engl. J. Med.*, **308**, 1389–92

75. Holmgren, J., Clemens, J., Sack, D. A. and Svennerholm, A.-M. (1989). New cholera vaccines. *Vaccine*, **7**, 94–6

76. Svennerholm, A.-M., Sack, D. A., Holmgren, J. and Bardhan, P. K. (1982). Intestinal antibody responses after immunization with cholera B subunit. *Lancet*, **1**, 305–8

77. Black, R. E., Levine, M. M., Clements, M. L., Young, C. R., Svennerholm, A.-M. and Holmgren, J. (1987). Protective efficacy in man of killed whole vibrio oral cholera vaccine with and without the B subunit of cholera toxin. *Infect. Immun.*, **55**, 1116–20

78. Clemens, J. D., Sack, D. A., Harris, J. R., Chakraborty, J., Khan, M. R., Stanton, B. F., Kay, B. A., Khan, M. U., Yunus, M. D., Atkinson, W., Svennerholm, A.-M. and Holmgren, J. (1986). Field trial of oral cholera vaccines in Bangladesh. *Lancet*, **1**, 124–7

79. Sanchez, J. and Holmgren, J. (1989). Recombinant system for overexpression of cholera toxin B subunit in *Vibrio cholerae* as a basis for vaccine development, *Proc. Natl. Acad. Sci., USA*, **86**, 481–5

80. Kaper, J. B. (1990). Attenuated *Vibrio cholerae* strains prepared by recombinant DNA techniques used as live oral vaccines. In Woodrow, G. C. and Levine, M. M. (eds), *New Generation Vaccines*, Basel.: Marcel Dekker, pp. 304–10

81. Levine, M. M., Herrington, D., Losonsky, G., Tall, B., Kaper, J. B., Ketley, J., Tacket, C. and Cryz, S. (1988). Safety, immunogenicity, and efficacy of recombinant live oral cholera vaccines, CVD103 and CVD193-HgR. *Lancet*, **2**, 467–70

82. Schmidt, M., Kelley, E. P., Tseng, L. Y. and Boedeker, E. C. (1985). Towards an oral *E. coli* pilus vaccine for travellers' diarrhea: susceptibility to proteolytic digestion. *Gastroenterology*, **82**, 1575–80

83. Evans, D. J., Evans, D. G., Opekun, A. R. and Graham, D. Y. (1988). Immunoprotective oral whole cell vaccine for enterotoxigenic *Escherichia coli* diarrhea prepared by in situ destruction of chromosomal and plasmid DNA with colicin E2. *FEMS Microbiol. Immunol.*, **47**, 9–14

84. Svennerholm, A.-M., Holmgren, J. and Sack, D. A. (1989). Development of oral vaccines against enterotoxinogenic *Escherichia coli* diarrhoea. *Vaccine*, **7**, 196–8

85. Svennerholm, A.-M., Åhrén, C., Wennerås, C. and Holmgren, J. (1991). Development of an oral vaccine against enterotoxigenic *Escherichia coli* diarrhea. In Wadström, T. *et al.* (eds), *Molecular Pathogenesis of Gastrointestinal Infections*. London: Plenum (In press)

14
Host responses to *Helicobacter (Campylobacter) pylori* infection

R. V. HEATLEY

INTRODUCTION

Spiral organisms have been recognized within the mammalian stomach for almost 100 years. There had, however, been interest in the association between bacteria and peptic ulcers even before that time. Although there have been occasional references over the years since this time, suggesting that a relationship may exist between various microorganisms and human peptic ulcer disease, until recent years few would have seriously credited any significant pathogenic role for bacteria in this condition[1]. In 1983 and early 1984, however, three separate groups almost simultaneously reported their observations relating to the association between a newly recognized spiral organism and chronic gastritis, and this has focused attention firmly on the role this agent may have in peptic ulcer disease[1].

The organism discovered at that time was initially thought to resemble other *Campylobacter* organisms and was known as *Campylobacter*-like organism (or CLO). This name has subsequently changed to *Campylobacter pyloridis* and then *C. pylori*. It has been recognized subsequently, however, that this organism is in fact representative of a new genus, and the current internationally accepted terminology refers to this bacterium as *Helicobacter pylori*.

CLINICAL SIGNIFICANCE

Helicobacter pylori has been found associated only with human gastric epithelium, although there is some limited evidence of animal infection. In the human stomach the organism lies closely adjacent to the gastric epithelial cells and often deep in the gastric pits underlying the surface mucus layer.

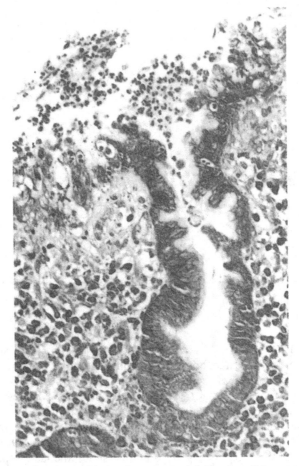

Figure 14.1 Active chronic gastritis showing polymorph infiltration of the upper foveolar and surface epithelium in an area of *H. pylori* colonization. The organisms are seen at the surface and as dark granules within polymorphs in the exudate (modified Giemsa stain). Courtesy Dr M. Dixon

The organism does not usually occur in entirely normal stomachs. The presence of this bacterium is closely associated with active inflammation and the organism is found in the stomach in the majority of those suffering from chronic active gastritis and also duodenal ulcer disease[2]. *H. pylori* can colonize the duodenum in patients who have developed metaplastic gastric epithelium in this site. This finding may explain the close association between the presence of this organism and active duodenitis and duodenal ulcer disease[3].

Eradication of *H. pylori* is by no means easy, and no single antibacterial agent or ulcer-healing drug is effective. The most successful forms of therapy are combinations that include bismuth salts and at least two antibiotics, namely amoxycillin, ampicillin or tetracycline and metronidazole. Although short-term clearance can be fairly readily achieved with such a regime, recurrence is common and long-term eradication is less readily achievable.

The importance of *H. pylori* infection and its relevance to gastroduodenal disease has come to light only recently, and is currently being actively explored. This organism appears to play a major pathogenic role in chronic active gastritis and probably also peptic ulcer disease.

It is for these reasons that so much active interest has focused on this fascinating infection of an organ, that for all practical purposes has otherwise always been regarded as sterile. Infection rates vary throughout the world, depending on the population groups studied, but in most Western countries approximately half the population is affected by 50 years of age. The incidence of infection can, however, vary dramatically between differing populations. Why prevalence rates vary so considerably is unknown, as is the full extent of the host responses to this fastidious organism, which is only currently being fully explored.

H. PYLORI AND GASTRITIS

The strong association between *H. pylori* and type B, non-autoimmune chronic gastritis has now concentrated attention on mucosal immune mechanisms in the stomach which previously had focused almost entirely on type A, autoimmune gastritis. Many abnormalities of humoral and cell-mediated immunity have been documented in this condition, although their contribution to the pathogenesis of pernicious anaemia remains unclear[4].

Type B, non-autoimmune chronic gastritis is a histological entity, maximal in the antrum, consisting of a chronic cellular infiltrate of plasma cells, T lymphocytes and macrophages, with or without an active component of neutrophils and also, on occasion, mucosal atrophy. Presumably this mucosal response results from the presence of *H. pylori* organisms and the immunological stimuli of antigenic material associated with these bacteria.

H. PYLORI ANTIGENS

The total protein profile of *H. pylori* differs considerably from that of *Campylobacter* organisms, which they otherwise resemble closely. Although *H. pylori* isolates are very similar[5,6], outer membrane preparation profiles show some variability between strains[7,8]. Studies on lipopolysaccharide (LPS) profiles demonstrate considerable heterogeneity. Immunofluorescence, co-agglutination and immunoblotting studies, using rabbit hyperimmune sera, identify several distinct 'strains'[7,9]. Immunoblotting studies using LPS preparations from six strains also reveal different patterns. The distribution of the strains into these patterns is not the same as that based on protein profiles, which suggests considerable antigen diversity amongst *H. pylori* strains[7]. Knowledge of such variations is of particular importance in the choice of antigen for serological and local antibody studies.

Western blotting and radioimmunoprecipitation techniques have been used to investigate antigen specificity of systemic responses[7,8]. Unlike *Campylobacter* organisms, *H. pylori* does not appear to express a single surface-exposed major outer membrane protein. Immunoblotting studies demonstate several major protein antigens that are detected by most sera. These include two urease-associated proteins (63 and 56 kD), a putative flagellin (54 kD), 110–120 kD and 48 kD surface proteins, and a 31 kD outer membrane protein[8,10-14]. Unfortunately, a number of these proteins share antigenic determinants with some *Campylobacter* species[7,8,12]. A particularly interesting protein (110–120 kD) has been identified which appears to be *H. pylori*-specific[12,13]. Antibodies to this protein have been reported in over 80% of sera from *H. pylori*-positive subjects[12]. Those *H. pylori*-positive subjects who are serologically negative for the protein appear to be colonized with *H. pylori* strains that do not express this protein[12]. More recently, attention has focused on the cell-bound urease enzyme of *H. pylori*. Recent studies using molecular cloning suggest that the $66 + 31$ kD antigens may be part of the high molecular weight urease enzyme which has been characterized[15].

H. pylori is thus an immunogenic organism with the putative urease proteins being among the immunodominant antigens. To determine *H. pylori* antibodies by enzyme-linked immunosorbent assay (ELISA), a complex antigenic preparation is required because of the antigenic variation and cross-reacting antigenic determinants found in *H. pylori*. At present, whole bacterial preparations, crude sonicates, ultracentrifuged sonicates, and acid extracts are employed. The latter two preparations (with similar protein profiles) have improved specificity over the whole-cell antigen preparations and in the future cloned species-specific antigens should be available[16,17].

SYSTEMIC IMMUNE RESPONSE

A variety of techniques have been employed to identify antibodies against *H. pylori*, including agglutination methods, complement fixation and enzyme-linked immunosorbent assays[6]. The latter is the most sensitive and convenient technique, although the choice of antigen is critical. In *H. pylori*-associated gastritis, both the immunoglobulin IgG and IgA titres are raised, although the best predictive value is obtained with the IgG assay[6]. Systemic IgM responses are not generally seen, which is not surprising in view of the chronicity of infection. In *H. pylori*-associated gastritis the activity or severity of the gastric inflammation fails to correlate with the titre of the systemic response. The systemic response is long-standing if accompanied by continuous colonization. With successful eradication the antibody levels would be expected to fall. The systemic IgG and IgA titres have been shown to fall, suggesting that serial antibody titres may have some value in monitoring treatment[18]. Recolonization is associated with a return of the inflammatory reaction, but as yet there is no information regarding the details of reinfection immunity, either at the systemic or local level. Studies on subclass response are limited, but significant increases in IgG1, IgG2 and IgG4 with no increase in IgG3 have been documented.

The systemic humoral response, although a good marker for colonization, probably has little role in defence, since *H. pylori* is a non-invasive organism. In an *H. pylori* ingestion study, Morris and Nicholson[19] followed the development of the systemic immune response. An IgM response was first seen with seroconversion occurring by day 18 after ingestion. IgG and IgA seroconversion occurred together after day 60, at which time the IgM response was down to baseline levels.

In practice, serology has been mainly used as an epidemiological tool, for which it is well suited[20,21]. In routine clinical practice, serology has yet to find a role, although it may soon become useful with the introduction of commercially produced kits[22]. Moreover, it has been suggested that it may prove a cost-effective screening test for young dyspeptic patients[23].

LOCAL HUMORAL RESPONSE

Initial studies on local *H. pylori* humoral responses concentrated on identifying organism-specific antibodies in gastric juice. Measurable titres of

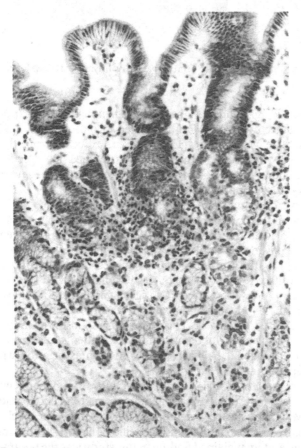

Figure 14.2 'Early' chronic gastritis showing predominantly midzonal infiltration by lymphocytes and polymorphs centred on the pit–isthmus region. There is no increase of cells in the superficial lamina propria. Courtesy Dr M. Dixon

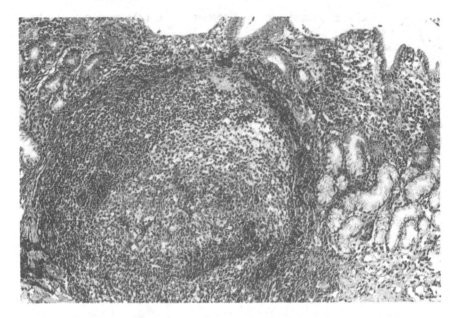

Figure 14.3 *Helicobacter pylori*-positive chronic gastritis with lymphoid follicle formation. Courtesy Dr M. Dixon

H. pylori-specific IgA and IgM have been demonstrated in approximately one-third of subjects with *H. pylori*-associated chronic gastritis[24]. The absence of a demonstrable gastric juice IgG response is expected, since this antibody would be rapidly degraded in the acidic gastric juice. No specific IgA, IgM or IgG antibodies were found in the juice of the *H. pylori*-negative, histologically normal patients[24].

Short-term organ culture studies have demonstrated that only *H. pylori*-positive biopsies produce *H. pylori*-specific IgG, IgA and IgM antibodies[25]. Class-specific plasma cell counts were assessed in the same patients and the density of the plasma cell infiltrate was found to correlate with the specific immunoglobulin titre[26]. The data thus suggest that a proportion of the plasma cell infiltrate, which characterizes chronic gastritis, is involved in the local humoral response to *H. pylori* antigens. Similar studies have also been carried out in the duodenum and demonstrate a duodenal humoral response in *H. pylori*-infected patients[27]. The duodenal response was most marked in those patients with active duodenitis, and these patients have previously been shown to have duodenal *H. pylori* colonization in association with areas of gastric metaplasia[3].

Antibody coating of *H. pylori* in tissue sections from patients with chronic gastritis has been investigated using an immunoperoxidase technique[28]. IgG, IgA and IgM coating has been demonstrated. It is, however, unclear whether this coating is by specific binding or non-specific Fc binding of immunoglobulins. An interesting and unexplained finding in this study was the failure of bacteria deep in the gastric pits to be coated, despite being in a location where a high concentration of IgA might be expected.

The studies on local humoral immunity so far carried out have demonstrated a specific response to *H. pylori*. The functional effects of this response are as yet unknown. *In vitro* studies have demonstrated *H. pylori* to be sensitive to antibody-dependent complement-mediated bactericidal activity of serum[29]. In the presence of serum opsonins, the bacteria were phagocytosed and effectively killed by neutrophils. Another potential mechanism of complement activation would be through lipid A, the lipid moiety of LPS that has been demonstrated to be present in *H. pylori*. Phagocytosis of bacteria has certainly been shown in the stomach, but the contribution of local complement and local antibody response to this is unclear[30]. In type B non-autoimmune gastritis an IgG autoantibody to gastrin-secreting cells has been demonstrated in 8% of patients[31]. There is, however, no evidence that this antibody is cytotoxic. The possibility of crossreacting antibodies between *H. pylori* and gastric tissue has been suggested by *H. pylori*-specific monoclonal antibodies. At least two groups have described monoclonal antibodies raised against *H. pylori* which crossreact with human gastric epithelium.

LOCAL CELL-MEDIATED IMMUNITY

It has become widely recognized that *H. pylori* infection is associated particularly with a neutrophilic response (active gastritis)[32]. In active gastritis the neutrophils appear predominantly between epithelial cells, being most numerous in the deep portion of the gastric pit[28]. Relatively few neutrophils

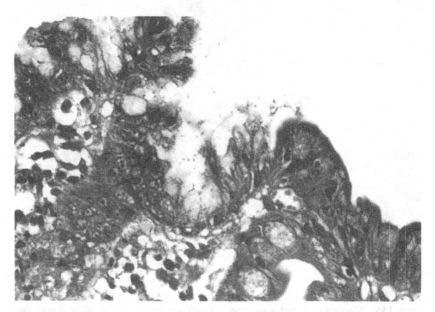

Figure 14.4 Chronic gastritis with intestinal metaplasia. The heavy colonization of the normal gastric epithelium ends abruptly with the change to intestinal type epithelium composed of absorptive cells and goblet cells (modified Giemsa stain). Courtesy Dr M. Dixon

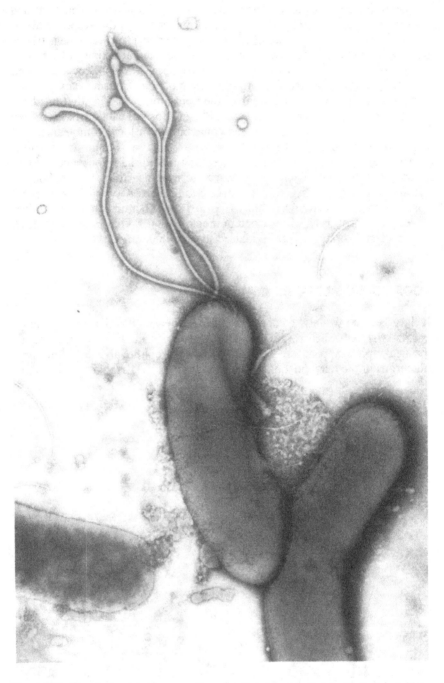

Figure 14.5 Negatively stained preparation of cultured human isolate of *H. pylori*. Note sheathed flagellar filaments originating from one of the dome-shaped ends of the organism. The flagellar bulbs are particularly well shown. Magnification ×31 000. Courtesy of Drs A. Curry and D. M. Jones

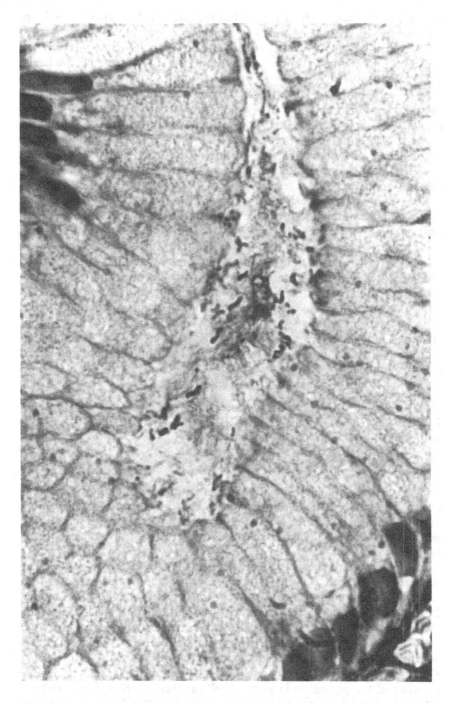

Figure 14.6   Antral mucosa stained for IgA. *H. pylori* strongly positive for IgA are present on the surface, while those in the gastric pit are weakly positive. Original magnification ×320. Courtesy of Dr J. Wyatt

are seen in the gastric gland lumen, but phagocytosed *H. pylori* have been documented[30]. Treatment studies in which the neutrophil response remits after eradication of *H. pylori* suggest that this response is focused on the organisms rather than the organisms favouring the environment of an actively inflamed mucosa[33].

In *H-pylori*-associated gastritis T cells are increased in both the epithelial compartment and lamina propria. Studies on T cell subsets give conflicting results, with some workers reporting the majority of epithelial T cells to be of the suppressor/cytotoxic phenotype and others reporting an increase in the T-helper phenotype[35,36]. In the latter study the T-helper cells from patients with gastritis showed increased expression of CD7, a T cell stimulation marker.

Recent studies on type B gastritis have demonstrated that the inflamed mucosa, unlike normal gastric mucosa, becomes HLA-DR positive. It is thus possible that gastric epithelial cells are capable of antigen recognition and presentation[35,37].

There is little information regarding the role of macrophages, which are generally greatly increased in number in type B gastritis. Tumour necrosis factor-α (TNF-α) is a cytokine produced mainly by activated macrophages and monocytes which has multiple modulatory effects on immune activation. We have shown secretion of TNF-α from antral mucosa is considerably enhanced in *H. pylori*-infected individuals. Furthermore, local secretion was increased most in those patients who had evidence of neutrophil migration into the epithelium (active gastritis)[38].

POSSIBLE PATHOGENETIC MECHANISMS IN GASTRIC INFLAMMATION

Bacterial adherence

One of the major characteristics differentiating enteropathic from non-enteropathic *Escherichia coli* is the ability of the former to adhere to receptors on the epithelial surface[39]. Such adherence protects the bacteria from peristalsis and results in high concentrations of toxins locally at the epithelial cell surface.

The adherence of *H. pylori* to gastric epithelium by pedestals very similar to those found with *E. coli* has been reported[40]. Such pedestals are seen relatively uncommonly; however, other ultrastructural changes are common. Intracellular oedema occurs together with intracellular mucin depletion. Where bacteria are numerous, often in the intercellular regions, microvilli are depleted or absent, together with the organized cores of microfilaments which normally contribute to the cytoskeleton of the apical cytoplasm[40]. Disruption of the intercellular junctions has been demonstrated, as has the presence of the organisms in parietal cell canaliculi[41]. *H. pylori* have been seen in neutrophil phagocytic vacuoles and recently they have been reported to be covered by epithelial microvilli and/or engulfed within phagocytotic vacuoles or in close contact with foci of cell necrosis containing cytoplasmic

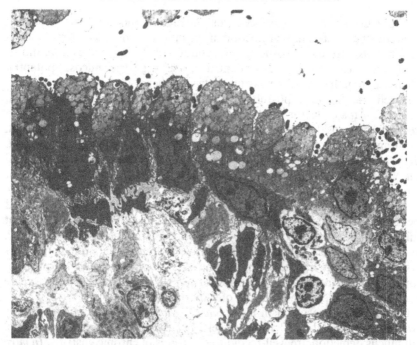

Figure 14.7 Transmission electron micrograph of an antral biopsy from a patient with active gastritis. Numerous *H. pylori* are shown on the surface and adjacent to the epithelial cells. Magnification ×2050. Courtesy of Mr H. Steer

debris[30,42]. Within these areas partially autolysed organisms have been seen. Following elimination of *H. pylori* by bismuth salts the ultrastructural changes regress[40]. Although these ultrastructural abnormalities strongly implicate *H. pylori* as a pathogenic organism, they tell us little of the underlying cytopathic mechanism.

Biochemical factors

One well-recognized method for gut bacteria to exert a cytopathic effect is via toxin production. Mattsby-Baltzer and Goodwin have presented data showing that *H. pylori* lipopolysaccharide contains lipid A, a class of substance responsible for the endotoxic properties of a wide range of Gram-negative bacteria[43].

Leunk *et al.* have studied the effect of broth culture filtrates on mammalian cell lines[44]. They found that 45% of the bacterial strains tested produced cytopathic effects. These effects were abolished by rabbit antisera (against whole or sonicated *H. pylori*) but not by antiserum against a lipopolysaccharide fraction.

H. pylori has a wide range of enzymes, a number of which may play a role in pathogenesis[6]. The most notable is urease, the activity of which is so marked as to enable colonization to be diagnosed by a urea breath test or a biopsy urease test. It has been postulated that the ammonia produced envelops the bacterium, protecting it from acidic damage. Ammonia is certainly toxic to cells in tissue culture, and recent animal studies have shown ammonia to cause a dose-dependent decrease in gastric mucosal potential difference, together with increasing gastric epithelial damage[45,46].

Hazell and Lee have postulated that the urease activity at the epithelial surface is a major factor in pathogenesis, with the rapid hydrolysis of urea creating a mucosal urea gradient and a transmucous ammonia gradient, resulting in an increase of epithelial surface pH[47]. This in turn, they suggest, might affect mucosal charge gradient, paracellular permeability and epithelial cell Na^+/K^+-ATPase, leading to back-diffusion of H^+ ions and concomitant hypochlorhydria. This may then, in extreme circumstances, result in gastric ulcer formation. There is little direct evidence to support this hypothesis, and the finding of gastric urease-positive spirals in other animals without inflammation is against the urease being of prime pathogenic importance[48]. As this enzyme is seen in all the spirals colonizing mammalian upper gastrointestinal mucus-secreting epithelia, it would appear to play an important role in bacterial colonization or survival. Studies using urease blockers may help define the role of this enzyme.

One important mechanism by which *H. pylori* might be pathogenic is by direct alteration of the gastric mucus gel. Increased cell turnover and epithelial cell mucus depletion are well-recognized features of chronic gastritis. *In vitro* studies of gastric mucus glycoprotein synthesis and secretion suggest an increased turnover of mucus glycoprotein in *H. pylori*-associated chronic

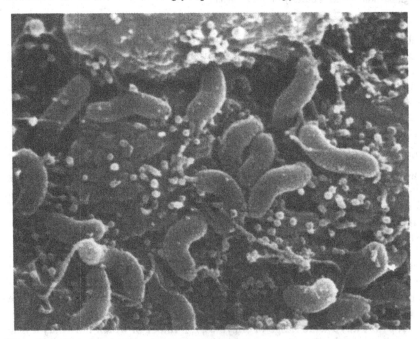

Figure 14.8 Scanning electron micrograph showing *H. pylori* colonization of an antral biopsy in a patient with *H. pylori* antral gastritis. Magnification ×11 250. Courtesy of Mr H. Steer

gastritis[49]. Whether this is purely secondary to the increased epithelial cell turnover found in chronic gastritis is unclear. *H. pylori* has been demonstrated to have proteolytic enzymes capable of degrading porcine gastric mucus[50]. Interestingly, the optimum pH for this reaction is pH 7. The same group has also reported that the mucus in peptic ulcer patients is less viscous than in normals, has a higher proportion of low-molecular-weight mucin, less mucin polymer and a diminished ability to retard H^+ diffusion[51,52].

If, as seems likely, *H. pylori* compromises the mucus–bicarbonate barrier, the gastric epithelium would then become exposed to aggressive luminal factors, long suspected to be involved in causing gastric mucosal damage, including acid, pepsin, bile and perhaps also drugs. These agents, singly or in combination, may then be the factors resulting in mucosal inflammation.

CONCLUSIONS

There is now little doubt that *H. pylori* is causally related to chronic active gastritis. It probably also has a role in the pathogenesis of peptic ulcer disease and perhaps also in gastric cancer. We have as yet, unfortunately, little information regarding the mechanisms of pathogenicity of this organism. It appears likely that the local mucosal barrier is compromised by this bacterium but this is not known for certain. Furthermore, the inflammatory response seen in Type B chronic gastritis is presumably directed, at least in part, at *H. pylori* antigens. This chronic immune response may well be damaging, but other bacterial factors could also adversely affect the normal mucosal defences. Differing pathogenic mechanisms may have changing significance at various phases of colonization and in individual patients. Different bacterial strains may also have variable pathogenic potential. In contrast to chronic gastritis, *H. pylori* colonization (and associated inflammation) in duodenal ulceration appears to be a necessary prerequisite upon which focal ulceration may subsequently occur intermittently, presumably due to the interplay of other poorly understood factors.

The local immune response is in itself of considerable interest since *H. pylori* colonization persists for long periods of time, despite the continuing inflammatory response of the host. Studies to date have demonstrated a specific local humoral response, development of epithelial HLA-DR expression and an alteration of T cell subsets in patients with *H. pylori* colonization. Data concerning colonization in patients with different types of immuno-deficiency are limited. HIV-infected patients have been found to have a lower frequency of colonization than age-matched controls by histology. Whether this is a true reduction due to their altered immunity, or a result of treatment, is unclear.

H. pylori gastrointestinal colonization is unique to humans. During infection a specialized epithelial niche is infected, without competition from other bacteria, and this then results in a long-standing infection in association with chronic inflammation, presumably lasting for years. We must assume that the bacteria gain benefit from the associated chronic inflammation. As the system is not complicated by other bacteria it provides a good model for studying bacteria–epithelial interactions. Such knowledge may be particularly relevant in the wider understanding of epithelial microbial ecology, bacterial pathogenicity and gut defence mechanisms.

References

1. Rathbone, B. J. and Heatley, R. V. (1989). The historical associations between bacteria and peptic-ulcer disease. In Rathbone, B. J. and Heatley, R. V. (eds), *Campylobacter Pylori and Gastroduodenal Disease*. Oxford: Blackwell Scientific Publications, pp. 1–4
2. Rathbone, B. J., Wyatt, J. I. and Heatley, R. V. (1986). *Campylobacter pyloridis* – a new factor in peptic ulcer disease? *Gut*, **27**, 635–41
3. Wyatt, J. I., Rathbone, B. J., Dixon, M. F. and Heatley, R. V. (1987). *Campylobacter pyloridis* and acid induced gastric metaplasia in the pathogenesis of duodenitis. *J. Clin. Pathol.*, **40**, 841–8
4. Rathbone, B. J. and Heatley, R. V. (1986). Gastritis. In Losowsky, M. S. and Heatley, R. V. (eds), *Gut Defences in Clinical Practice*. Edinburgh and London: Churchill Livingstone, pp. 228–42
5. Pearson, A. D., Bamforth, J., Booth, D. *et al.* (1984). Polyacrylamide gel electrophoresis of spiral bacteria from the gastric antrum. *Lancet*, **1**, 1349–50
6. Megraud, F., Bonnet, M., Garnier, M., *et al.* (1985). Characterization of *Campylobacter pyloridis* by culture, enzymatic profile and protein content. *J. Clin. Microbiol.*, **22**, 1007–10
7. Perez-Perez, G. I. and Blaser, M. J. (1987). Conservation and diversity of *Campylobacter pyloridis* major antigens. *Infect. Immun.*, **55**, 1256–63
8. Newell, D. G. (1987). Identification of the outer membrane proteins of *Campylobacter pyloridis* and antigenic cross-reactivity between *C. pyloridis* and *C. jejuni*. *J. Gen. Microbiol.*, **133**, 163–70
9. Danielsson, D., Blomberg, B., Jarnerot, G. *et al.* (1988). Heterogeneity of *C. pylori* as demonstrated by co-agglutination testing with rabbit antibodies. *Scand. J. Gastroenterol.*, **23**(S142), 58–63
10. Newell, D. G. (1987). Human antibody responses to the surface protein antigens of *Campylobacter pyloridis*. *Serodiagn. Immunother.*, **1**, 209–17
11. Dunn, B. E., Perez-Perez, G. I. and Blaser, M. J. (1989). Two-dimensional gel electrophoresis and immunoblotting of *Campylobacter pylori* proteins. *Infect. Immun.*, **57**, 1825–33
12. Kist, M., Apel, I. and Jacobs, E. (1988). Protein antigens of *Campylobacter pylori*: the problem of species specificity. In Menge, H., Gregor, M., Tytgat, G. N. J., *et al.* (eds), *Campylobacter pylori*. Berlin: Springer-Verlag, pp. 19–26
13. von Wulffen, H. (1988). Systemic immune responses to *Campylobacter pylori* colonization. In Menge, H., Gregor, M., Tytgat, G. N. J., *et al.* (eds), *Campylobacter pylori*. Berlin: Springer-Verlag, pp. 157–63
14. von Wulffen, H., Grote, H. J., Gaterman, S., *et al.* (1988). Immunoblot analysis of immune response to *Campylobacter pylori* and its clinical associations. *J. Clin. Pathol.*, **41**, 653–9
15. Mobley, H. L. T., Cortesia, M. J., Rosenthal, L. E. and Jones, B. D. (1988). Characterization of urease from *Campylobacter pylori*. *J. Clin. Microbiol.*, **26**, 831–6
16. Newell, D. G. and Rathbone, B. J. (1989). The serodiagnosis of *Campylobacter pylori* infections. *Serodiagn. Immunother.*, **3**, 1–6
17. Hirschl, A. M., Pletschette, M., Hirschl, M., *et al.* (1988). Comparison of different antigen preparations in the evaluation of the immune response against *Campylobacter pylori*. *Eur. J. Clin. Microbiol.*, **7**, 570–5
18. Vaira, D., Holton, J., Cairns, S. R., Faizon, M., Polydoran, A., Dowsett, J. F. and Salmon, R. R. (1988). Antibody titre to *Campylobacter pylori* after treatment for gastritis. *Br. Med. J.*, **297**, 397
19. Morris, A. and Nicholson, G. (1987). Ingestion of *Campylobacter pyloridis* causes gastritis and raised fasting gastric pH. *Am. J. Gastroenterol.*, **82**, 192–9
20. Dwyer, B., Nanxiong, S., Kaldor, J., Tee, W., Lambert, J., Luppino, M. and Flannery, G. (1988). Antibody response to *Campylobacter pylori* in an ethnic group lacking peptic ulceration. *Scand. J. Infect. Dis.*, **20**, 63–8

21. Dwyer, B., Kaldor, J., Tee, W., Marakowski, E. and Raias, K. (1988). Antibody response to *Campylobacter pylori* in diverse ethnic groups. *Scand. J. Infect. Dis.*, **20**, 349–50
22. Crabtree, J. E., Shallcross, T. M., Heatley, R. V. and Wyatt, J. I. (1991). Evaluation of a commercial ELISA for serodiagnosis of *Helicobacter pylori* infection. *J. Clin. Pathol.* (In press)
23. Sobala, G., Rathbone, B. J., Wyatt, J. I., Dixon, M., Heatley, R. V. and Axon, A. T. R. (1989). Investigating young patients with dyspepsia. *Lancet*, **1**, 50–1
24. Rathbone, B. J., Wyatt, J. I., Worsley, B. W., Shires, S. E., Trejdosiewicz, L. K., Heatley, R. V. and Losowsky, M. S. (1986). Systemic and local antibody responses to gastric *Campylobacter pyloridis* in non-ulcer dyspepsia. *Gut*, **27**, 642–7
25. Rathbone, B. J., Wyatt, J. I., Tompkins, D., Heatley, R. V. and Losowsky, M. S. (1986). *In vitro* production of *Campylobacter pyloridis* specific antibodies by gastric mucosal biopsies. *Gut*, **27**, A607
26. Wyatt, J. I. and Rathbone, B. J. (1988). Immune response of the gastric mucosa to *Campylobacter pylori*. *Scand. J. Gastroenterol.*, **23** (Suppl. 142), 44–9
27. Crabtree, J. E., Rathbone, B. J., Shallcross, T. M., Heatley, R. V. and Losowsky, M. S. (1988). Duodenal secretion of *Campylobacter pylori* specific antibodies in patients with gastritis and duodenitis. *Gut*, **29**, A1438
28. Wyatt, J. I., Rathbone, B. J. and Heatley, R. V. (1987). Local immune response to gastric *Campylobacter* in non-ulcer dyspepsia. *J. Clin. Pathol.*, **39**, 863–70
29. Pruul, H., Lee, P. C., Goodwin, C. S., *et al.* (1987). Interaction of *Campylobacter pyloridis* with human immune defence mechanisms. *J. Med. Microbiol.*, **23**, 233–8
30. Shousha, S., Bull, T. B. and Parkins, R. A. (1984). Gastric spiral bacteria. *Lancet*, **2**, 101
31. Vandelli, C., Bottazzo, G. F., Doniach, D., *et al.* (1979). Auto-antibodies to gastrin-producing cells in antral (type B) chronic gastritis. *N. Engl. J. Med.*, **300**, 1406–10
32. Warren, J. R. (1983). Unidentified curved bacilli on gastric epithelium in active chronic gastritis. *Lancet*, **1**, 1273.
33. Rauws, E. A. J., Langenberg, W., Houtoff, H. J., *et al.* (1988). *Campylobacter pyloridis*-associated chronic active gastritis. A prospective study of its prevalence and the effects of antibacterial and antiulcer treatment. *Gastroenterology*, **94**, 33–40
34. Engstrand, L., Scheynius, A., Grimelius, L., *et al.* (1988). Induced expression of class II transplantation antigens on gastric epithelial cells in patients with *Campylobacter pylori*-positive gastric biopsies. *Gastroenterology*, **94**, A115
35. Papadimitriou, C. S., Ioachim-Velogianni, E. E., Tsianos, E. B., *et al.* (1988). Epithelial HLA-DR expression and lymphocyte subsets in gastric mucosa in type B chronic gastritis. *Virchows Arch.*, **A413**, 197–204
36. Rathbone, B. J., Wyatt, J. I., Trejdosiewicz, L. K., *et al.* (1988). Mucosal T cell subsets in normal gastric antrum and *C. pylori*-associated chronic gastritis. *Gut*, **29**, A1438
37. Engstrand, L., Scheynius, A., Pahlson, C., *et al.* (1989). Association of *Campylobacter pylori* with induced expression of class II transplantation antigens on gastric epithelial cells. *Infect. Immun.*, **57**, 827–32
38. Crabtree, J. E., Shallcross, T. M., Wyatt, J. I. and Heatley, R. V. (1990). Tumour necrosis factor alpha secretion by *Helicobacter pylori* colonised gastric mucosa. *Gut*, **31**, A600
39. Old, D. C. (1985). Bacterial adherence. *Med. Lab. Sci.*, **42**, 78–85
40. Goodwin, C. S., Armstrong, J. A. and Marshall, B. J. (1986). *Campylobacter pyloridis*, gastritis and peptic ulceration. *J. Clin. Pathol.*, **39**, 353–65
41. Chen, X. G., Correa, P., Offerhaus, J., Rodriguez, E., Janney, F., Hoffmann, E., Fox, J. and Hunter, F. (1986). Diavolitsis. Ultrastructure of the gastric mucosa harboring *Campylobacter*-like organisms. *Am. J. Clin. Pathol.*, **86**, 575–82
42. Tricottet, V., Bruneval, P., Vire, O. and Camilleri, J. P. (1986). *Campylobacter*-like organisms and surface epithelium abnormalities in active, chronic gastritis in humans: an ultrastructural study. *Ultrastruct. Pathol.*, **10**, 113–22
43. Mattsby-Baltzer, I. and Goodwin, C. S. (1988). Lipid A in *C. pylori*. In Kaijser, B. and Falsen, E. (eds), *Campylobacter IV*. University of Göteborg, Göteborg. Abstract No. 232.
44. Leunk, R. D., Johnson, P. T., David, B. D., Kraft, W. G. and Morgan, D. R. (1988). Identification of cytotoxic activity produced by *Campylobacter pyloridis*. In Kaijser, B. and Falsen, E. (eds), *Campylobacter IV*. University of Göteborg, Göteborg. Abstract No. 97
45. Murakami, M., Yoo, J. K., Mizuno, M., Saita, H., Inada, M. and Miyake, T. (1987). Effects of ammonia, urea and urease on the rat gastric mucosa. *Gastroenterology*, **92**, 1544

46. Murakami, M., Yoo, J. K., Mizuno, M., Saita, H., Inada, M. and Miyake, T. (1987). Role of gastric ammonia, urea and urease in gastric mucosal lesions in azotemia. *Gastroenterology*, **92**, 1545
47. Hazell, S. L. and Lee, A. (1986). *Campylobacter pyloridis*, urease, hydrogen ion back diffusion and gastric ulcers. *Lancet*, **2**, 15–17
48. Tompkins, D. S., Wyatt, J. I., Rathbone, B. J. and West, A. P. (1988). The characterization and pathological significance of gastric *Campylobacter*-like organisms in the ferret: a model for chronic gastritis? *Epidem. Inf.*, **101**, 269–78
49. Crabtree, J. E., Rathbone, B. J., Wyatt, J. I., Heatley, R. V. and Losowsky, M. S. (1987). *In vitro* mucus glycoprotein synthesis and secretion by gastric mucosa colonized with *Campylobacter pyloridis*. *Gut*, **28**, A1409
50. Slomiany, B. L., Bilski, J., Sarosiek, J., Murty, V. L. N., Dworkin, B., Van Horn, K., Zielenski, J. and Slomiany, A. (1987). *Campylobacter pyloridis* degrades mucin and undermines gastric mucosal integrity. *Biochem. Biophys. Res. Commun.*, **144**, 307–14
51. Slomiany, B. L., Bilski, J., Murty, V. L. N., Sarosiek, J., Dworkin, B., Van Horn, K. and Slomiany, A. (1987). *Campylobacter pyloridis* degrades mucin and undermines gastric mucosal integrity. *Gastroenterology*, **92**, 1645
52. Sarosiek, J., Gabryelewicz, A. and Slomiany, B. L. (1987). Changes in the macromolecular organization and physical properties of gastric mucus with peptic ulcer. *Gastroenterology*, **92**, 1615

15
The immunology of giardiasis

M. F. HEYWORTH

Protozoan parasites of the genus *Giardia* infect the small intestinal lumen of mammals and other vertebrates. Although *Giardia* taxonomy has not been completely standardized, three main species of *Giardia* are currently recognized, namely, *Giardia lamblia* (essentially synonymous with *G. duodenalis* and *G. intestinalis*), *G. muris* (a parasite of rodents), and *G. agilis* (which infects the gastrointestinal tract of amphibians)[1-3]. In addition, a *Giardia* species termed *G. psittaci* has been isolated from the intestine of budgerigars.[4] *Giardia lamblia* is the cause of human giardiasis.

The life-cycle of *Giardia* species is relatively simple, with two distinct stages (trophozoite and cyst). Trophozoites are motile organisms with flagella and an adhesive disc which enables them to become attached to the luminal surface of intestinal epithelial cells[5,6]. Figure 15.1 shows *G. muris* trophozoites that were incubated with trophozoite-specific mouse monoclonal antibodies followed by fluorescein-conjugated antibody directed against mouse immunoglobulin. Trophozoites encyst within the intestinal lumen[8], and the resulting cysts are excreted in the faeces. *Giardia* cysts are thick-walled, ellipsoidal structures that remain viable outside the host[9]. After cysts have

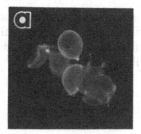
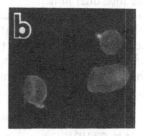

Figure 15.1 Fluorescence photomicrographs of *Giardia muris* trophozoites incubated with *G. muris*-specific mouse monoclonal antibodies (mAbs), followed by fluorescein-conjugated anti-mouse Ig. Designations and isotypes of the mAbs were as follows: (**a**) 1A3.1, IgG$_3\kappa$; (**b**) 1B1.1, IgMκ. The trophozoites were obtained from *G. muris*-infected nude mice. Figure modified from ref. 7

been ingested by a new host, trophozoites emerge from the cysts in response to gastric acid[10], and then colonize the small intestinal lumen.

Human infection with *G. lamblia* can be asymptomatic, but can also cause clinical problems. These include watery diarrhoea, and malabsorption with steatorrhoea and weight loss[11-13]. Although the mechanisms responsible for diarrhoea and malabsorption in giardiasis are poorly understood, various studies have provided some insight into these processes. Work with *G. lamblia*-infected human subjects, *Giardia*-infected rodents, and *in vitro* systems suggests that the following factors contribute to diarrhoea and malabsorption in giardiasis: (a) shortening of duodenal villi, (b) shortening of microvilli on small intestinal epithelial cells, (c) deficiency of disaccharidases on the small intestinal epithelium, and (d) uptake of bile salts in the intestinal lumen by *Giardia* trophozoites[14-19]. Exactly how *Giardia* trophozoites cause intestinal epithelial abnormalities is not known[17].

Interest in the immunological aspects of giardiasis was sparked in the 1970s, following the observation that this infection is particularly severe and persistent in individuals who are immunodeficient. Since that time, numerous clinical and basic studies have been carried out in an attempt to understand the immunological responses to *Giardia* species. During the past decade, considerable progress has been made in understanding these responses. Worldwide emergence of the human acquired immunodeficiency syndrome (AIDS) has provided impetus for this work. Although giardiasis does not rank with *Pneumocystis carinii* pneumonia, cryptosporidiosis, or toxoplasmosis as a 'major' AIDS-associated opportunistic infection, giardiasis has been described in patients with AIDS[20,21]. Unlike several genera of microorganisms that cause opportunistic infection in AIDS, *Giardia* species have a relatively simple life-cycle and their ability to induce symptoms does not depend on invasion of host tissues. Accordingly, the host immunological response to *Giardia* species is easier to study than the response to other clinically relevant protozoa with a more complex life-cycle that includes invasion of host cells or tissues. Information gained from studies of *Giardia*-directed immunity can assist in the design of projects aimed at exploring immunological responses to other protozoa, such as cryptosporidia, whose life-cycle is complex. In addition, it is worth noting that studies with rodent models of giardiasis have provided insight into the normal 'mechanics' of immune responses to antigens in the intestinal lumen.

In this chapter, human studies, experimental animal work, and molecular studies of *Giardia* trophozoites are discussed, with respect to the light that these investigations shed on the understanding of *Giardia*-specific immunity. Topics that are considered include the role of antibody and of T lymphocytes in the clearance of *Giardia* infections.

HUMAN STUDIES

As noted above, immunodeficiency predisposes to chronic giardiasis. Table 15.1 lists the human immunodeficiency states that are associated with

Table 15.1 Human immunodeficiency states associated with giardiasis

Example or cause of immunodeficiency	Comments	References
'Common variable' hypogammaglobulinaemia (deficiency of IgG, IgA, ±IgM)[a]	Intestinal plasma cells diminished in number or absent; associated with chronic giardiasis	11, 22–24
X-linked immunoglobulin deficiency	Associated with chronic giardiasis	25, 26
Radiotherapy/cytotoxic chemotherapy	Bone marrow transplant recipients and/or patients with malignancy	27, 28
Acquired immunodeficiency syndrome (AIDS) due to human immunodeficiency virus (HIV)	Giardia-specific serum antibody levels lower than in HIV-negative Giardia-infected persons	20, 21

[a] With or without intestinal nodular lymphoid hyperplasia

this infection. One conclusion that can be drawn from this table is that immunoglobulin deficiency appears to be a sufficient condition for the development of chronic *G. lamblia* infection in human subjects. By extension, it can be argued that clearance of *G. lamblia* infection, in immunocompetent persons, depends on *Giardia*-specific antibody. As discussed below, studies in experimental animals support the view that clearance of *Giardia* infections is antibody-dependent.

Besides the immunodeficiency states listed in Table 15.1, other situations that appear to be associated with giardiasis include cystic fibrosis and lactation[29,30]. If lactation does predispose to giardiasis, this predisposition might reflect diversion of IgA-producing cells from the maternal intestine to the mammary glands. Conceivably, *Giardia*-specific IgA would then be secreted preferentially into the milk, rather than into the maternal intestinal lumen. A relevant experimental finding is that latent *G. muris* infection in adult female mice becomes reactivated during pregnancy and lactation[31].

Direct evidence that human subjects mount antibody responses to *G. lamblia* has come from studies of sera and secretions. Antibodies against *G. lamblia* have been demonstrated in human sera by immunofluorescence microscopy (using *Giardia* cysts or trophozoites incubated with the sera followed by fluorescent anti-human immunoglobulin), and by enzyme-linked immunosorbent assay (ELISA)[32–34]. Trophozoite-specific antibodies of the IgG, IgM, and IgA isotypes have been detected in human sera[35,36]. Available evidence suggests that serum levels of trophozoite-specific IgM decline more rapidly than serum levels of trophozoite-specific IgG, after an episode of *G. lamblia* infection[35,37]. Examining human sera for *Giardia*-specific antibodies is not a reliable diagnostic test for current *Giardia* infection, but may provide a retrospective guide to the prevalence of former infection in a population[38–40].

In one published study, the time-course of *Giardia*-specific antibody responses was examined in human volunteers who were experimentally infected with *G. lamblia* (by enteric inoculation of cultured trophozoites)[41]. Trophozoite-specific IgM, IgG, and IgA were detectable in sera obtained from some of these individuals at 2 weeks after trophozoite inoculation. In this study, trophozoite-specific IgA was detected in jejunal fluid from infected volunteers, using an ELISA technique[41]. Earlier work showed IgA coating of *G. lamblia* trophozoites on human jejunal biopsy specimens, but it was not clear from that study whether the IgA on the organisms was *Giardia*-specific[42]. *Giardia*-specific IgA has been detected in human milk, and an inverse correlation has been observed between *Giardia*-specific IgA titre in maternal milk and prevalence of *G. lamblia* infection in suckling human infants[43,44]. This finding supports the view that such IgA helps to protect infants against giardiasis.

There is circumstantial evidence that human subjects can acquire protective immunity to giardiasis. Thus, the prevalence of *G. lamblia* infection in Bangladesh is significantly higher in young children than in older individuals[45]. Similarly, during an outbreak of giardiasis in Colorado, a higher incidence of gastrointestinal symptoms was seen in short-term than in long-term residents of the area[46].

Recent work has shed some light on the identity of trophozoite antigens that are recognized by *Giardia*-specific antibodies in human sera. In two studies, these antibodies have been shown to react mainly with one or more trophozoite proteins of molecular weight (MW) 30–34 kD[21,47]. [125]I labelling of intact trophozoites, followed by gel electrophoresis of trophozoite proteins and gel autoradiography, suggests that at least one of these antigens is present on trophozoite surfaces[47]. Two other reports provide evidence that *Giardia*-specific human serum antibodies largely recognize trophozoite surface proteins of MW 72 kD or 88 kD, respectively[48,49]. The divergent nature of these findings might, theoretically, be explained by antigenic heterogeneity of *G. lamblia* trophozoites, or by the existence of trophozoite antigens consisting of non-covalently attached subunits.

ANIMAL STUDIES

Rodent models of giardiasis have helped to advance the understanding of *Giardia*-specific immune responses. Most of the relevant work has been carried out using mice infected with *G. muris*, but *Giardia*-infected rats, and *G. lamblia*-infected gerbils have also been studied[50-52]. Interestingly, *Giardia* infections do not cause overt illness in rodents, although impaired weight gain in *G. muris*-infected mice has been reported[50]. The main value of rodent models of giardiasis lies in the opportunities which they provide for (a) direct examination of intestinal immune responses, and (b) experimental induction of immunodeficiency by administration of immunosuppressive drugs or monoclonal antibodies (mAbs). Because experimental work of this type is not logistically feasible in human subjects, most of the available information about *Giardia*-specific intestinal immunity has come from rodent studies.

About 15 years ago, it was shown that immunocompetent mice would become infected with *G. muris* after being fed with cysts of this parasite[50]. It was also found that immunocompetent mice would stop excreting *G. muris* cysts a few weeks after the onset of infection, and that feeding of additional cysts did not re-establish *G. muris* infection in mice that had previously cleared it[50,53]. These observations were interpreted as evidence that *G. muris* infection leads to the development of *Giardia*-specific protective immunity in mice.

Various genetic and experimentally induced immunodeficiency states impair the ability of rodents to clear *Giardia* infections (Table 15.2). In the 1970s, it was shown that athymic nude mice are unable to clear *G. muris* infection[54,55]. This observation led to the realization that *Giardia*-specific protective immunity in mice is T-cell-dependent, but did not identify the T-cell subset (helper or cytotoxic) important in generating protection. To address this question, the present author treated immunocompetent BALB/c mice with mAbs that specifically recognize either mouse helper T cells or cytotoxic T cells. Respectively, these mAbs bind to the murine CD4 (L3T4) or CD8 (Ly-2) antigen. Treatment of mice with the mAbs leads to depletion of the relevant T-lymphocyte subset from blood and from lymphoid organs, including Peyer's patches[62,65-67]. Mice selectively depleted of CD4+ T lymphocytes, and infected with *G. muris* cysts, develop abnormally prolonged *Giardia* infection (Fig. 15.2)[62,63]. In contrast, selective depletion of CD8+ T lymphocytes does not inhibit the capacity of mice to clear the infection[62]. These results indicate that clearance of *G. muris* infection, by immunocompetent mice, is dependent on helper T cells and not on cytotoxic T cells.

As a result of infection with *G. muris*, immunocompetent mice generate a trophozoite-specific intestinal IgA response, whereas helper T-cell depleted mice (and nude mice) do not[56,63]. Similarly, mice treated from birth onwards with rabbit antiserum directed against mouse IgM lack the ability to clear *G. muris* infection or to develop an intestinal IgA response against *G. muris* trophozoites[64].

The findings discussed above suggest, but do not prove, that trophozoite-specific intestinal IgA is required for the physiological clearance of murine *Giardia* infections.

Table 15.2 Genetic and experimentally induced immunodeficiency states that prolong *Giardia* infections in rodents, or increase the parasite burden

Example or cause of immunodeficiency	Comments	References
Nude (athymic) mice	Deficiency of T lymphocytes; impaired antibody response to *G. muris*	54–56
X-linked immunodeficient (*xid*) mice	Deficiency of B lymphocytes	57
Corticosteroid treatment (mice, gerbils)		58–60
Cyclosporin A treatment (mice)		61
Irradiation (mice)		59
Selective depletion of helper (CD4+) T lymphocytes (mice)	Mice treated with anti-CD4 monoclonal antibody. Impaired antibody response to *G. muris*	62, 63
Treatment with anti-IgM antibody (mice)	Impaired antibody response to *G. muris*	64

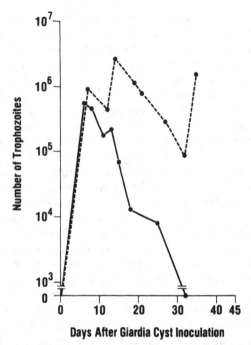

Figure 15.2 Time-course of *Giardia muris* infection in BALB/c mice that were either immunologically normal (solid line), or treated with anti-CD4 monoclonal antibody to deplete helper T lymphocytes (dashed line). Each point shows the mean number of *G. muris* trophozoites obtained from three mice, except for the last point on the dashed line, which shows the mean number of trophozoites obtained from four mice. Both groups of mice were infected with *G. muris* cysts on Day 0. Figure modified from ref. 63

Various methods have been used to demonstrate *Giardia*-specific antibodies in rodent sera and secretions. Immunofluorescence microscopy of trophozoites obtained from infected rodents is a subjective technique, but has provided evidence that *Giardia*-specific IgA becomes bound to trophozoites in the intestine of immunocompetent animals[51,56,63]. This technique initially suggested that IgG also binds to *G. muris* trophozoites in the intestine of infected mice[56], but later work using the same method did not confirm the existence of a *Giardia*-specific IgG response in the mouse intestine[63]. Trophozoite-specific IgA has been detected in intestinal secretions of *G. muris*-infected immunocompetent mice by radioimmunoassay, ELISA, and flow cytometry[64,68-71]. In these assays, sonicated or intact *G. muris* trophozoites from nude mice were used as antigen, to detect *Giardia*-specific intestinal IgA from immunocompetent mice. Use of *Giardia*-infected nude mice as the source of trophozoites was dictated by the fact that *G. muris* cannot yet be cultured *in vitro*, unlike *G. lamblia* (M. F. Heyworth, unpublished observations)[72,73]. Trophozoite-specific IgG is not detectable in the intestinal secretions of *G. muris*-infected immunocompetent mice[69,71], and there is no evidence of an intestinal IgM response to *G. muris* in such animals[56].

The present author has used flow cytometry to show that *Giardia*-specific antibodies, in sera and intestinal secretions from *G. muris*-infected mice, are directed against trophozoite surfaces. Before using this technique to detect these antibodies in mouse sera and intestinal secretions, it was validated by carrying out flow cytometry of *G. muris* trophozoites that had been incubated with *Giardia*-specific mouse mAbs followed by fluorescein-conjugated antibody against mouse immunoglobulin (Fig. 15.3)[7]. Results of flow cytometry experiments that demonstrate *G. muris*-specific antibodies in mouse sera and intestinal secretions are shown in Figs 15.4–15.6. In Fig. 15.6 it can be seen that *G. muris* infection leads to the appearance of trophozoite-specific IgG and IgA in serum of immunocompetent mice. This finding contrasts with the exclusive presence of trophozoite-specific IgA in intestinal secretions (Fig. 15.5).

Other investigators have demonstrated trophozoite-specific IgA in bile and milk from *Giardia*-infected rodents[51,74].

There is evidence that trophozoite-specific antibodies can protect rodents against *Giardia* infection, and can facilitate clearance of an established infection in such animals. Incubation of *G. muris* trophozoites with *Giardia*-specific IgA reduces their infectivity for mice[75], and intraduodenal or intraperitoneal administration of trophozoite-specific antibodies to *Giardia*-infected rodents diminishes intestinal trophozoite and faecal cyst counts[76,77]. Furthermore, suckling of neonatal mice with milk containing *Giardia*-specific IgA temporarily protects them against *G. muris* infection[74].

Immunoprecipitation experiments have shown that antibodies in sera of *G. muris*-infected BALB/c mice recognize one or more trophozoite proteins

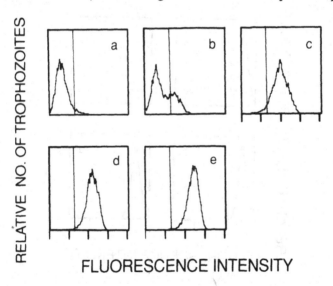

Figure 15.3 Flow cytometry profiles of *Giardia muris* trophozoites incubated without (panel a), or with (b–e), *G. muris*-specific mouse monoclonal antibodies (mAbs), followed in each case by fluorescein-conjugated anti-mouse Ig. The *Giardia*-specific mAbs were designated as follows: (b) 2B5.3, (c) 3C7.2, (d) 1A3.1, (e) 1B1.1. Respectively, the immunoglobulin isotypes of these four mAbs were $IgG_{2b}\kappa$, $IgG_1\kappa$, $IgG_3\kappa$, and $IgM\kappa$[7]. Fluorescein staining (fluorescence) intensity is shown on a logarithmic scale. Data in Figs 15.3–15.6 were generated using trophozoites from *G. muris*-infected nude mice

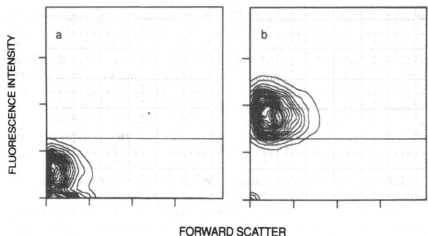

FORWARD SCATTER

Figure 15.4 Flow cytometry contour plots of *Giardia muris* trophozoites that were incubated with intestinal secretions obtained from (**a**) uninfected, or (**b**) *G. muris*-infected, BALB/c mice. After exposure to BALB/c mouse intestinal secretions, the trophozoites were incubated with fluorescein-conjugated antibody directed against mouse IgA. Fluorescein staining (fluorescence) intensity is shown on a logarithmic scale, and forward scatter (an indication of trophozoite size or aggregation) on a linear scale. Panel **b** shows binding of *Giardia*-specific IgA to trophozoite surfaces. Intestinal secretions used to generate this panel were obtained 28 days after the start of *G. muris* infection

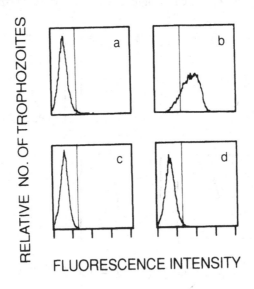

FLUORESCENCE INTENSITY

Figure 15.5 Flow cytometry profiles of *Giardia muris* trophozoites that were incubated with intestinal secretions from uninfected (panels **a, c**), or *G. muris*-infected (**b, d**), BALB/c mice. Intestinal secretions used to generate panels **b** and **d** were obtained 28 days after the start of *G. muris* infection. After exposure to BALB/c mouse intestinal secretions, the trophozoites were incubated with fluorescein-conjugated antibody directed against mouse IgA (**a, b**) or against mouse IgG (**c, d**). Fluorescein staining (fluorescence) intensity is shown on a logarithmic scale. Figure modified from ref. 71

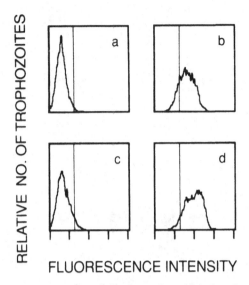

Figure 15.6 Flow cytometry profiles of *Giardia muris* trophozoites that were incubated with sera from uninfected (panels **a**, **c**), or *G. muris*-infected (**b**, **d**), BALB/c mice. Sera from *Giardia*-infected mice (panels **b** and **d**) were obtained 35 days after the start of *G. muris* infection. After exposure to mouse sera, the trophozoites were incubated with fluorescein-conjugated antibody directed against mouse IgA (**a**, **b**) or against mouse IgG (**c**, **d**). Fluorescein staining (fluorescence) intensity is shown on a logarithmic scale

of approximate MW 30 kD[78]. By means of Western blotting, the present author has found that, in addition, intestinal IgA from such mice binds to one or more trophozoite proteins of this MW[71]. Intestinal IgA from non-infected BALB/c mice does not bind to the 30 kD trophozoite protein(s); this observation indicates that the 30 kD band seen on Western blotting with intestinal secretions represents binding of trophozoite-specific IgA (Fig. 15.7)[71]. Using Western blotting, the author has found that intestinal IgA from *G. muris*-infected BALB/c mice occasionally binds to trophozoite protein(s) that have an approximate MW of 60 kD. Such binding has been seen when trophozoite proteins were not boiled before polyacrylamide gel electrophoresis and transfer to nitrocellulose (our usual practice has been to boil the proteins before electrophoresis) (Fig. 15.8)[71,79−81]. These findings prompt speculation that a 30 kD trophozoite antigenic target for intestinal IgA antibody is present on the organisms as a 60 kD dimer, in which the two subunits are non-covalently associated with each other. Immunoprecipitation experiments have not shown any qualitative differences between *G. muris* trophozoite proteins that are precipitated by intestinal IgA from *Giardia*-infected mice versus control mice (M. F. Heyworth, unpublished observations). Figure 15.9 shows the result of such an experiment. In this figure, it can be seen that intestinal IgA from infected BALB/c mice precipitated a 43 kD trophozoite surface protein. A surface protein of identical MW was also precipitated (though more weakly) by intestinal IgA from mice

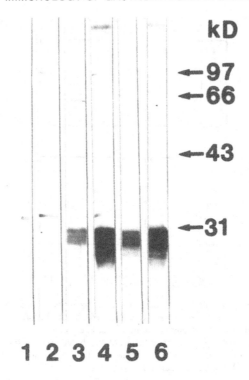

Figure 15.7 Western blots of *Giardia muris* trophozoite proteins incubated with intestinal secretions from BALB/c mice, followed by peroxidase-conjugated anti-mouse IgA[71]. Mice from which the intestinal secretions were obtained had been infected (lanes 2–6), or not infected (lane 1), with *G. muris*. Intestinal secretions were obtained at the following times after the start of *G. muris* infection: day 14 (lane 2), day 28 (lane 3), day 35 (lane 4), day 42 (lane 5), and day 49 (lane 6). Numbered arrows indicate molecular weights in kD. A broad trophozoite protein band is recognized by intestinal IgA from *Giardia*-infected mice. *G. muris*-infected nude mice were used as the source of trophozoite proteins for Figs 15.7–15.9

that had not been infected with *G. muris*. These observations suggest that the 43 kD protein is not specifically recognized by mouse intestinal IgA that is directed against *G. muris* trophozoites.

Speculation that cell-mediated immunity contributes to the clearance of *Giardia* infections is not well supported by experimental evidence. As noted above, experimental depletion of CD8 + T lymphocytes does not impair the ability of BALB/c mice to clear *G. muris* infection[62]. In addition, mice which are genetically deficient in natural killer cells eliminate the infection at the same rate as normal mice[82]. Another observation that argues strongly against lymphocyte-mediated killing of *Giardia* trophozoites is the lack of evidence that lymphocytes become attached to these organisms in the intestinal lumen of *Giardia*-infected hosts. It is well established that killing of target cells by cytotoxic (effector) lymphocytes is preceded by attachment of the effector cells to the targets[83,84]. Lymphocytes can be harvested from the intestinal lumen of *G. muris*-infected mice, along with trophozoites, but attachment of these lymphocytes to the trophozoites has not been seen (Fig. 15.10a)[85].

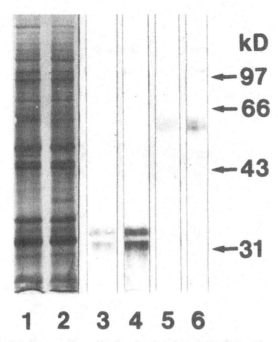

Figure 15.8 Western blots of *Giardia muris* trophozoite proteins which had been either boiled (lanes 1, 3, 4), or not boiled (lanes 2, 5, 6), before polyacrylamide gel electrophoresis and transfer to nitrocellulose[79-81]. Lanes 1 and 2 show total trophozoite proteins stained with Amido Black. Lanes 3–6 show nitrocellulose strips of trophozoite proteins which were incubated with intestinal secretions from *G. muris*-infected BALB/c mice, followed by peroxidase-conjugated anti-mouse IgA. Intestinal secretions were obtained at the following times after the start of *G. muris* infection: day 21 (lanes 3 and 5), day 28 (lanes 4 and 6). Numbered arrows indicate molecular weights in kD. One or more bands of approximate MW 60 kD are seen in lanes 5 and 6

Because macrophages can ingest *Giardia* trophozoites *in vitro* (see below), there has been speculation that such phagocytosis might represent an important effector mechanism for clearing these organisms from the mammalian intestine. Studies with *G. muris*-infected mice provide little, if any, support for this speculation. We have found that occasional phagocytic cells bearing the macrophage surface antigen Mac-1 are attached to *Giardia* trophozoites lavaged from the intestinal lumen of *G. muris*-infected mice (Fig. 15.10b,c). However, similar low numbers of Mac-1 + cells are obtainable from the intestinal lumen of *G. muris*-infected immunocompetent mice and nude mice[85]. Taken together with the fact that *G. muris* infection is persistent in nude mice, these observations militate against an effector role for intraluminal phagocytes in the elimination of *Giardia* infections. An ultrastructural study has shown that degenerating *Giardia* trophozoites are present in Peyer's patch macrophages of *G. muris*-infected mice[86]. It is conceivable that *Giardia*-specific antibody production is initiated by presentation of parasite antigens to local helper T lymphocytes and B lymphocytes, by macrophages in Peyer's patches[87-89]. Peyer's patch lymphocytes from *G. muris*-infected BALB/c mice, but not from uninfected mice, synthesize DNA in response to

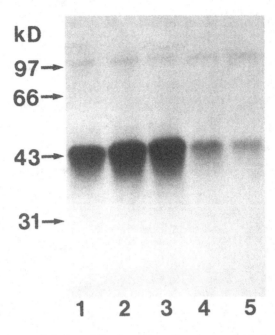

Figure 15.9 Immunoprecipitation of *Giardia muris* trophozoite proteins by intestinal IgA from BALB/c mice. Trophozoite surface proteins were labelled with ^{125}I, and precipitated by incubation with mouse intestinal secretions, followed by *Staphylococcus aureus* protein A armed with antibody directed against mouse IgA. Immunoprecipitated proteins were subjected to polyacrylamide gel electrophoresis, and gel autoradiography was then performed. Intestinal secretions were obtained from mice which had been infected (lanes 1–3), or not infected (lanes 4 and 5), with *G. muris*. The intestinal secretions from infected mice were obtained at the following times after the start of infection: day 21 (lane 1), day 28 (lane 2), and day 34 (lane 3). Numbered arrows indicate molecular weights in kD

trophozoite proteins *in vitro*[90]. This observation suggests that *G. muris* infection leads to the proliferation of Peyer's patch lymphocyte clones that have been sensitized to trophozoite antigens. Future work to identify the phenotype of such *Giardia*-responsive cells (with respect to T-cell subset markers or B-cell immunoglobulin isotype) would seem to be justified.

For reasons that are unknown, but possibly unrelated to immune responsiveness, different strains of mice clear *G. muris* infection at different rates[91]. In this connection, it was initially reported that *G. muris* infection is abnormally prolonged in C3H/He mice[55]. More recent studies, however, have not confirmed this observation. In these recent investigations, the duration of *G. muris* infection in C3H/He mice has been found to be approximately 4 weeks, i.e. similar to its duration in BALB/c mice (M. F. Heyworth, unpublished observations).

Perhaps the most important conclusion to emerge from studies with *Giardia*-infected rodents is that the immunological clearance of *Giardia* infections appears to be an antibody-dependent process.

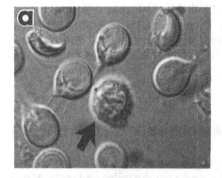
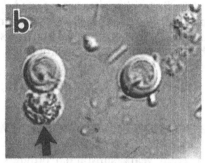
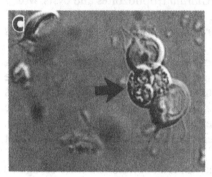

Figure 15.10 Photomicrographs of *Giardia muris* trophozoites and leukocytes (arrowed) harvested from the intestinal lumen of *G. muris*-infected mice (Nomarski optics). These cell suspensions had been incubated with monoclonal antibodies against mouse leukocyte surface antigens, and the same microscopic fields were examined by fluorescence microscopy to identify leukocyte phenotypes. **(a)** T lymphocyte (Thy-1.2+) and trophozoites from a BALB/c mouse; **(b)** and **(c)** phagocytic cells attached to trophozoites. The leukocyte in **(b)** was Mac-1+. Leukocytes and trophozoites shown in **(b)** and **(c)** were obtained, respectively, from a nude mouse and a BALB/c mouse. Figure modified from ref. 85

IN VITRO WORK USING WHOLE TROPHOZOITES

Immunological studies with whole *Giardia* trophozoites have been aimed at understanding how antibodies or phagocytes might protect against *Giardia* infections. Cytotoxicity assays have shown that trophozoite-specific antibodies kill *Giardia* trophozoites in the presence of complement. Antibodies that have this cytotoxic effect include serum antibodies from *G. muris*-infected mice, *G. muris*-immunized rabbits, and *G. lamblia*-infected human subjects[92-94]. Antibody/complement-mediated killing of trophozoites is also exerted by trophozoite-specific mouse IgG and IgM monoclonal antibodies (M. F. Heyworth, unpublished observations)[76]. However, trophozoite-specific mouse intestinal IgA is not cytotoxic to *G. muris* trophozoites, in the presence or absence of complement (M. F. Heyworth, unpublished observations). Because IgA is the only well-documented isotype of trophozoite-specific antibody at the site of *Giardia* infections, it is unlikely that antibody/complement-mediated killing contributes significantly to the clearance of trophozoites from the mammalian intestine.

There is evidence that trophozoite-specific antibodies can inhibit the attachment of *Giardia* trophozoites to intestinal epithelial cells[95,96]. In the light of this evidence, it is reasonable to postulate that coating of trophozoites with antibody facilitates their peristaltic removal from the intestine of *Giardia*-infected hosts.

Giardia trophozoites are ingested and killed by human, rabbit, and mouse macrophages *in vitro*. Such ingestion is enhanced by trophozoite-specific antibody[97-99]. As discussed above, a study of *G. muris*-infected mice suggests that intestinal luminal macrophages do not play a significant part in the clearance of *Giardia* infections[85].

BIOCHEMISTRY AND MOLECULAR BIOLOGY OF *GIARDIA* SPECIES

In recent years, substantial progress has been made in understanding the biochemistry and molecular biology of *Giardia* trophozoites and cysts. Much of the resulting literature is beyond the scope of this chapter. In the present account, issues that are pertinent to *Giardia*-specific immunological responses are discussed.

Cytoskeletal proteins are unlikely to be targets for protective antibody, because of their location in the trophozoite interior, but are among the best-characterized trophozoite proteins to date. These internal proteins include tubulin (MW 50–60 kD) and a family of structural proteins in the trophozoite adhesive disc, which are termed 'giardins'[100-104]. Interestingly, giardins have an MW of approximately 30 kD, and there is evidence that they can aggregate to form oligomers[105]. It will be recalled that trophozoite-specific antibodies from *Giardia*-infected human subjects and mice recognize one or more proteins of approximate MW 30 kD, as well as higher MW proteins in the range 70–90 kD[47-49,71,78]. Whether these trophozoite antigens include giardins is not known. Another point of interest is that proteins of MW 30–40 kD are associated with flagellar membranes of *G. lamblia* trophozoites[104,106]. Again, it is not known whether trophozoite-specific antibodies in infected hosts recognize these proteins.

Surface labelling of *G. lamblia* trophozoites with ^{125}I, followed by gel electrophoresis of solubilized trophozoite proteins, has been used to determine the MW of proteins on trophozoite surfaces. This work has shown that at least one protein of approximate MW 70–80 kD is strongly expressed on trophozoites[107,108]. Several groups of investigators have cloned and sequenced *Giardia* genes that encode trophozoite surface and cytoskeletal proteins[109-113]. It is reasonable to predict that this approach will permit the unambiguous identification and molecular description of trophozoite antigens that are recognized by protective antibodies.

It is well established that the adhesive disc of *Giardia* trophozoites enables these organisms to become attached to the host intestinal epithelium[5,6]. In addition, there is evidence that a lectin (carbohydrate-binding protein) is present on *G. lamblia* trophozoites, and that it contributes to trophozoite/epithelial attachment by interacting with carbohydrate groups on host cell glycoproteins[95,114,115]. The results of one study suggest that this lectin has an approximate MW of 30 kD[115]. Accordingly, it is conceivable that the *G. lamblia* lectin (or a putative similar molecule of *G. muris*) is part of the 30 kD antigen band recognized by Western blotting with antibodies from *Giardia*-infected hosts[21,47,71]. It is not known whether trophozoite adherence to intestinal epithelial cells can be blocked by antibody that binds exclusively to the lectin.

Proteolytic enzyme activity has been demonstrated in sonicated preparations of *G. lamblia* trophozoites[116]. Substrates for this enzyme activity include human IgA, an observation which suggests that the proteolytic enzyme(s) might help trophozoites to remain in the host intestinal lumen, by destroying trophozoite-specific IgA. However, this putative *in vivo* role for the enzyme(s) would seem to require enzyme secretion by viable trophozoites, and this has not been clearly demonstrated[116].

The question of trophozoite antigenic heterogeneity warrants brief discussion. As shown in Fig. 15.3, a *G. muris*-specific monoclonal antibody developed by the present author (mAb 2B5.3) binds to approximately 20% of *G. muris* trophozoites, but not to the other 80%[7]. This observation suggests that *G. muris* trophozoites are antigenically heterogeneous. Examination of *G. lamblia* trophozoite proteins and DNA, by protein electrophoresis, Western blotting, or restriction endonuclease analysis, has shown differences between trophozoites from different geographical locations[117,118]. Furthermore, there is evidence that the repertoire of trophozoite surface antigens can change during human and gerbil *G. lamblia* infections[48,119]. What is not yet clear is whether this antigenic variation represents *in vivo* selection of trophozoite clones that elude recognition by host antibody. Despite the existence of trophozoite antigenic heterogeneity, it should be emphasized that trophozoites from diverse sources exhibit more antigenic similarity than divergence[120,121]. Consequently, protection against *Giardia* infections by intestinal immunization with trophozoite antigens may eventually be feasible.

Acknowledgements

Grant support from the US National Institutes of Health and the Department of Veterans Affairs is gratefully acknowledged. The author is indebted to Elizabeth A. Mann for excellent clerical assistance.

References

1. Erlandsen, S. L., Bemrick, W. J. and Pawley, J. (1989). High-resolution electron microscopic evidence for the filamentous structure of the cyst wall in *Giardia muris* and *Giardia duodenalis*. *J. Parasitol.*, **75**, 787–797

2. Meyer, E. A. (1976). *Giardia lamblia*: isolation and axenic cultivation. *Exp. Parasitol.*, **39**, 101–5

3. Feely, D. E. and Erlandsen, S. L. (1985). Morphology of *Giardia agilis*: observation by scanning electron microscopy and interference reflexion microscopy. *J. Protozool.*, **32**, 691–3

4. Erlandsen, S. L. and Bemrick, W. J. (1987). SEM evidence for a new species, *Giardia psittaci*. *J. Parasitol.*, **73**, 623–9

5. Holberton, D. V. (1973). Fine structure of the ventral disk apparatus and the mechanism of attachment in the flagellate *Giardia muris*. *J. Cell. Sci.*, **13**, 11–41

6. Owen, R. L., Nemanic, P. C. and Stevens, D. P. (1979). Ultrastructural observations on giardiasis in a murine model. I. Intestinal distribution, attachment, and relationship to the immune system of *Giardia muris*. *Gastroenterology*, **76**, 757–69

7. Heyworth, M. F., Ho, K. E. and Pappo, J. (1989). Generation and characterization of monoclonal antibodies against *Giardia muris* trophozoites. *Immunology*, **68**, 341–5

8. Gillin, F. D., Reiner, D. S., Gault, M. J., Douglas, H., Das, S., Wunderlich, A. and Sauch, J. F. (1987). Encystation and expression of cyst antigens by *Giardia lamblia* in vitro. *Science*, **235**, 1040–3

9. Erlandsen, S. L., Bemrick, W. J., Schupp, D. E., Shields, J. M., Jarroll, E. L., Sauch, J. F. and Pawley, J. B. (1990). High-resolution immunogold localization of *Giardia* cyst wall antigens using field emission SEM with secondary and backscatter electron imaging. *J. Histochem. Cytochem.*, **38**, 625–32

10. Bingham, A. K. and Meyer, E. A. (1979). *Giardia* excystation can be induced *in vitro* in acidic solutions. *Nature*, **277**, 301–2

11. Hoskins, L. C., Winawer, S. J., Broitman, S. A., Gottlieb, L. S. and Zamcheck, N. (1967). Clinical giardiasis and intestinal malabsorption. *Gastroenterology*, **53**, 265–79

12. Wright, S. G., Tomkins, A. M. and Ridley, D. S. (1977). Giardiasis: clinical and therapeutic aspects. *Gut*, **18**, 343–50

13. Levinson, J. D. and Nastro, L. J. (1978). Giardiasis with total villous atrophy. *Gastroenterology*, **74**, 271–5

14. Hartong, W. A., Gourley, W. K. and Arvanitakis, C. (1979). Giardiasis: clinical spectrum and functional–structural abnormalities of the small intestinal mucosa. *Gastroenterology*, **77**, 61–9

15. Welsh, J. D., Poley, J. R., Hensley, J. and Bhatia, M. (1984). Intestinal disaccharidase and alkaline phosphatase activity in giardiasis. *J. Pediatr. Gastroenterol. Nutr.*, **3**, 37–40

16. Halliday, C. E. W., Clark, C. and Farthing, M. J. G. (1988). *Giardia*-bile salt interactions *in vitro* and *in vivo*. *Trans. R. Soc. Trop. Med. Hyg.*, **82**, 428–32

17. Buret, A., Gall, D. G. and Olson, M. E. (1990). Effects of murine giardiasis on growth, intestinal morphology, and disaccharidase activity. *J. Parasitol.*, **76**, 403–9

18. Belosevic, M., Faubert, G. M. and MacLean, J. D. (1989). Disaccharidase activity in the small intestine of gerbils (*Meriones unguiculatus*) during primary and challenge infections with *Giardia lamblia*. *Gut*, **30**, 1213–19

19. Gillon, J., Al Thamery, D. and Ferguson, A. (1982). Features of small intestinal pathology (epithelial cell kinetics, intraepithelial lymphocytes, disaccharidases) in a primary *Giardia muris* infection. *Gut*, **23**, 498–506

20. Smith, P. D., Lane, H. C., Gill, V. J., Manischewitz, J. F., Quinnan, G. V., Fauci, A. S. and Masur, H. (1988). Intestinal infections in patients with the acquired immunodeficiency syndrome (AIDS): etiology and response to therapy. *Ann. Intern. Med.*, **108**, 328–33

21. Janoff, E. N., Smith, P. D. and Blaser, M. J. (1988). Acute antibody responses to *Giardia lamblia* are depressed in patients with AIDS. *J. Infect. Dis.*, **157**, 798–804

22. Ament, M. E. and Rubin, C. E. (1972). Relation of giardiasis to abnormal intestinal structure and function in gastrointestinal immunodeficiency syndromes. *Gastroenterology*, **62**, 216–26

23. Ament, M. E., Ochs, H. D. and Davis, S. D. (1973). Structure and function of the gastrointestinal tract in primary immunodeficiency syndromes: a study of 39 patients. *Medicine (Baltimore)*, **52**, 227–48

24. Hermans, P. E., Diaz-Buxo, J. A. and Stobo, J. D. (1976). Idiopathic late-onset immunoglobulin deficiency: clinical observations in 50 patients. *Am. J. Med.*, **61**, 221–37

25. LoGalbo, P. R., Sampson, H. A. and Buckley, R. H. (1982). Symptomatic giardiasis in three patients with X-linked agammaglobulinemia. *J. Pediatr.*, **101**, 78–80

26. Nathwani, D., Morris, A. J. and Smith, C. C. (1989). Simultaneous *Streptococcus pneumoniae*, *Giardia lamblia* and *Campylobacter pylori* infection: an adult presentation of X-linked hypogammaglobulinaemia. *Scott. Med. J.*, **34**, 502

27. Korman, S. H., Granot, E. and Ramu, N. (1989). Severe giardiasis in a child during cancer therapy (Letter). *Am. J. Gastroenterol.*, **84**, 450–1

28. Bromiker, R., Korman, S. H., Or, R., Hardan, I., Naparstek, E., Cohen, P., Ben-Shahar, M. and Engelhard, D. (1989). Severe giardiasis in two patients undergoing bone marrow transplantation. *Bone Marrow Tranplant.*, **4**, 701–3

29. Roberts, D. M., Craft, J. C., Mather, F. J., Davis, S. H. and Wright, J. A. (1988). Prevalence of giardiasis in patients with cystic fibrosis. *J. Pediatr.*, **112**, 555–9

30. Ljungström, I., Stoll, B. and Islam, A. (1987). *Giardia* infection during pregnancy and lactation (Letter). *Trans. R. Soc. Med. Hyg.*, **81**, 161

31. Stevens, D. P. and Frank, D. M. (1978). Local immunity in murine giardiasis: is milk protective at the expense of maternal gut? *Trans. Assoc. Am. Phys.*, **91**, 268–72

32. Ridley, M. J. and Ridley, D. S. (1976). Serum antibodies and jejunal histology in giardiasis associated with malabsorption. *J. Clin. Pathol.*, **29**, 30–4

33. Smith, P. D., Gillin, F. D., Brown, W. R. and Nash, T. E. (1981). IgG antibody to *Giardia lamblia* detected by enzyme-linked immunosorbent assay. *Gastroenterology*, **80**, 1476–80

34. Visvesvara, G. S., Smith, P. D., Healy, G. R. and Brown, W. R. (1980). An immunofluorescence test to detect serum antibodies to *Giardia lamblia*. *Ann. Intern. Med.*, **93**, 802–5

35. Janoff, E. N., Taylor, D. N., Echeverria, P., Glode, M. P. and Blaser, M. J. (1990). Serum antibodies to *Giardia lamblia* by age in populations in Colorado and Thailand. *West. J. Med.*, **152**, 253–6

36. Birkhead, G., Janoff, E. N., Vogt, R. L. and Smith, P. D. (1989). Elevated levels of immunoglobulin A to *Giardia lamblia* during a waterborne outbreak of gastroenteritis. *J. Clin. Microbiol.*, **27**, 1707–10

37. Goka, A. K. J., Rolston, D. D. K., Mathan, V. I. and Farthing, M. J. G. (1986). Diagnosis of giardiasis by specific IgM antibody enzyme-linked immunosorbent assay. *Lancet*, **2**, 184–6

38. Gandhi, B. M., Buch, P., Sharma, M. P., Irshad, M. and Samantray, S. C. (1989). ELISA for anti-*Giardia* IgM (Letter). *Lancet*, **2**, 685

39. Isaac-Renton, J. L., Black, W. A., Mathias, R. G., Proctor, E. M. and Sherlock, C. H. (1986). Giardiasis in a group of travellers – attempted use of a serological test. *Can. J. Public Health*, **77**, 86–8

40. Miotti, P. G., Gilman, R. H., Santosham, M., Ryder, R. W. and Yolken, R. H. (1986). Age-related rate of seropositivity of antibody to *Giardia lamblia* in four diverse populations. *J. Clin. Microbiol.*, **24**, 972–5

41. Nash, T. E., Herrington, D. A., Losonsky, G. A. and Levine, M. M. (1987). Experimental human infections with *Giardia lamblia*. *J. Infect. Dis.*, **156**, 974–84

42. Briaud, M., Morichau-Beauchant, M., Matuchansky, C., Touchard, G. and Babin, P. (1981). Intestinal immune response in giardiasis (Letter). *Lancet*, **2**, 358

43. Miotti, P. G., Gilman, R. H., Pickering, L. K., Ruiz-Palacios, G., Park, H. S. and Yolken, R. H. (1985). Prevalence of serum and milk antibodies to *Giardia lamblia* in different populations of lactating women. *J. Infect. Dis.*, **152**, 1025–31

44. Nayak, N., Ganguly, N. K., Walia, B. N. S., Wahi, V., Kanwar, S. S. and Mahajan, R. C. (1987). Specific secretory IgA in the milk of *Giardia lamblia*-infected and uninfected women. *J. Infect. Dis.*, **155**, 724–7

45. Speelman, P. and Ljungström, I. (1986). Protozoal enteric infections among expatriates in Bangladesh. *Am. J. Trop. Med. Hyg.*, **35**, 1140–5

46. Istre, G. R., Dunlop, T. S., Gaspard, G. B. and Hopkins, R. S. (1984). Waterborne giardiasis at a mountain resort: evidence for acquired immunity. *Am. J. Public Health*, **74**, 602–4

47. Taylor, G. D. and Wenman, W. M. (1987). Human immune response to *Giardia lamblia* infection. *J. Infect. Dis.*, **155**, 137–40

48. Nash, T. E., Herrington, D. A., Levine, M. M., Conrad, J. T. and Merritt, J. W. (1990). Antigenic variation of *Giardia lamblia* in experimental human infections. *J. Immunol.*, **144**, 4362–9

49. Edson, C. M., Farthing, M. J. G., Thorley-Lawson, D. A. and Keusch, G. T. (1986). An 88,000-M$_r$ *Giardia lamblia* surface protein which is immunogenic in humans. *Infect. Immun.*, **54**, 621–5

50. Roberts-Thomson, I. C., Stevens, D. P., Mahmoud, A. A. F. and Warren, K. S. (1976). Giardiasis in the mouse: an animal model. *Gastroenterology*, **71**, 57–61

51. Waight Sharma, A. and Mayrhofer, G. (1988). Biliary antibody response in rats infected with rodent *Giardia duodenalis* isolates. *Parasit. Immunol.*, **10**, 181–91

52. Belosevic, M., Faubert, G. M., MacLean, J. D., Law, C. and Croll, N. A. (1983). *Giardia lamblia* infections in Mongolian gerbils: an animal model. *J. Infect. Dis.*, **147**, 222–6

53. Roberts-Thomson, I. C., Stevens, D. P., Mahmoud, A. A. F. and Warren, K. S. (1976). Acquired resistance to infection in an animal model of giardiasis. *J. Immunol.*, **117**, 2036–7

54. Stevens, D. P., Frank, D. M. and Mahmoud, A. A. F. (1978). Thymus dependency of host resistance to *Giardia muris* infection: studies in nude mice. *J. Immunol.*, **120**, 680–2

55. Roberts-Thomson, I. C. and Mitchell, G. F. (1978). Giardiasis in mice. I. Prolonged infections in certain mouse strains and hypothymic (nude) mice. *Gastroenterology*, **75**, 42–6

56. Heyworth, M. F. (1986). Antibody response to *Giardia muris* trophozoites in mouse intestine. *Infect. Immun.*, **52**, 568–71

57. Snider, D. P., Skea, D. and Underdown, B. J. (1988). Chronic giardiasis in B-cell-deficient mice expressing the xid gene. *Infect. Immun.*, **56**, 2838–42
58. Nair, K. V., Gillon, J. and Ferguson, A. (1981). Corticosteroid treatment increases parasite numbers in murine giardiasis. *Gut*, **22**, 475–80
59. Aggarwal, A., Sharma, G. L., Bhatia, A., Naik, S. R., Chakravarti, R. N. and Vinayak, V. K. (1980). Effect of corticosteroid and irradiation on experimental *Giardia lamblia* infection in mice. *Ann. Trop. Med. Parasitol.*, **74**, 369–71
60. Lewis, P. D., Belosevic, M., Faubert, G. M., Curthoys, L. and MacLean, J. D. (1987). Cortisone-induced recrudescence of *Giardia lamblia* infections in gerbils. *Am. J. Trop. Med. Hyg.*, **36**, 33–40
61. Belosevic, M., Faubert, G. M. and MacLean, J. D. (1986). The effects of cyclosporin A on the course of infection with *Giardia muris* in mice. *Am. J. Trop. Med. Hyg.*, **35**, 496–500
62. Heyworth, M. F., Carlson, J. R. and Ermak, T. H. (1987). Clearance of *Giardia muris* infection requires helper/inducer T lymphocytes. *J. Exp. Med.*, **165**, 1743–8
63. Heyworth, M. F. (1989). Intestinal IgA responses to *Giardia muris* in mice depleted of helper T lymphocytes and in immunocompetent mice. *J. Parasitol.*, **75**, 246–51
64. Snider, D. P., Gordon, J., McDermott, M. R. and Underdown, B. J. (1985). Chronic *Giardia muris* infection in anti-IgM-treated mice. I. Analysis of immunoglobulin and parasite-specific antibody in normal and immunoglobulin-deficient animals. *J. Immunol.*, **134**, 4153–62
65. Woodcock, J., Wofsy, D., Eriksson, E., Scott, J. H. and Seaman, W. E. (1986). Rejection of skin grafts and generation of cytotoxic T cells by mice depleted of L3T4+ cells. *Transplantation*, **42**, 636–42
66. Gutstein, N. L., Seaman, W. E., Scott, J. H. and Wofsy, D. (1986). Induction of immune tolerance by administration of monoclonal antibody to L3T4. *J. Immunol.*, **137**, 1127–32
67. Ledbetter, J. A. and Seaman, W. E. (1982). The Lyt-2, Lyt-3 macromolecules: structural and functional studies. *Immunol. Rev.*, **68**, 197–218
68. Anders, R. F., Roberts-Thomson, I. C. and Mitchell, G. F. (1982). Giardiasis in mice: analysis of humoral and cellular immune responses to *Giardia muris*. *Parasit. Immunol.*, **4**, 47–57
69. Snider, D. P. and Underdown, B. J. (1986). Quantitative and temporal analyses of murine antibody response in serum and gut secretions to infection with *Giardia muris*. *Infect. Immun.*, **52**, 271–8
70. Heyworth, M. F., Kung, J. E. and Caplin, A. B. (1988). Enzyme-linked immunosorbent assay for *Giardia*-specific IgA in mouse intestinal secretions. *Parasit. Immunol.*, **10**, 713–17
71. Heyworth, M. F. and Pappo, J. (1990). Recognition of a 30,000 MW antigen of *Giardia muris* trophozoites by intestinal IgA from *Giardia*-infected mice. *Immunology*, **70**, 535–9
72. Keister, D. B. (1983). Axenic culture of *Giardia lamblia* in TYI-S-33 medium supplemented with bile. *Trans. R. Soc. Trop. Med. Hyg.*, **77**, 487–8
73. Bowie, W. R., Isaac-Renton, J. L. and Prasad, N. (1988). *Giardia duodenalis*: enhanced growth in cell culture. *Trans. R. Soc. Trop. Med. Hyg.*, **82**, 433–6
74. Andrews, J. S. and Hewlett, E. L. (1981). Protection against infection with *Giardia muris* by milk containing antibody to *Giardia*. *J. Infect. Dis.*, **143**, 242–6
75. Underdown, B. J., Skea, D. L., Loney, G. M. and Snider, D. P. (1988). Murine giardiasis and mucosal immunity: a model for the study of immunity to intestinal protozoan parasites. *Monogr. Allergy*, **24**, 287–96
76. Butscher, W. G. and Faubert, G. M. (1988). The therapeutic action of monoclonal antibodies against a surface glycoprotein of *Giardia muris*. *Immunology*, **64**, 175–80
77. Mayrhofer, G. and Waight Sharma, A. (1988). The secretory immune response in rats infected with rodent *Giardia duodenalis* isolates and evidence for passive protection with immune bile. In Wallis, P. M. and Hammond, B. R. (eds), *Advances in Giardia Research*. Calgary: University of Calgary Press, pp. 49–54
78. Erlich, J. H., Anders, R. F., Roberts-Thomson, I. C., Schrader, J. W. and Mitchell, G. F. (1983). An examination of differences in serum antibody specificities and hypersensitivity reactions as contributing factors to chronic infection with the intestinal protozoan parasite, *Giardia muris*, in mice. *Aust. J. Exp. Biol. Med. Sci.*, **61**, 599–615
79. Laemmli, U. K. (1970). Cleavage of structural proteins during the assembly of the head of bacteriophage T4. *Nature*, **227**, 680–5
80. Towbin, H., Staehelin, T. and Gordon, J. (1979). Electrophoretic transfer of proteins from polyacrylamide gels to nitrocellulose sheets: procedure and some applications. *Proc. Natl.*

Acad. Sci. USA, **76**, 4350–4

81. Burnette, W. N. (1981). 'Western blotting': electrophoretic transfer of proteins from sodium dodecyl sulfate-polyacrylamide gels to unmodified nitrocellulose and radiographic detection with antibody and radioiodinated protein A. *Analyt. Biochem.*, **112**, 195–203

82. Heyworth, M. F., Kung, J. E. and Eriksson, E. C. (1986). Clearance of *Giardia muris* infection in mice deficient in natural killer cells. *Infect. Immun.*, **54**, 903–4

83. Timonen, T., Saksela, E., Ranki, A. and Häyry, P. (1979). Fractionation, morphological and functional characterization of effector cells responsible for human natural killer activity against cell-line targets. *Cell. Immunol.*, **48**, 133–48

84. Berke, G. (1980). Interaction of cytotoxic T lymphocytes and target cells. *Progr. Allergy*, **27**, 69–133

85. Heyworth, M. F., Owen, R. L. and Jones, A. L. (1985). Comparison of leukocytes obtained from the intestinal lumen of *Giardia*-infected immunocompetent mice and nude mice. *Gastroenterology*, **89**, 1360–5

86. Owen, R. L., Allen, C. L. and Stevens, D. P. (1981). Phagocytosis of *Giardia muris* by macrophages in Peyer's patch epithelium in mice. *Infect. Immun.*, **33**, 591–601

87. Keren, D. F., Holt, P. S., Collins, H. H., Gemski, P. and Formal, S. B. (1978). The role of Peyer's patches in the local immune response of rabbit ileum to live bacteria. *J. Immunol.*, **120**, 1892–6

88. Dunkley, M. L. and Husband, A. J. (1986). The induction and migration of antigen-specific helper cells for IgA responses in the intestine. *Immunology*, **57**, 379–85

89. London, S. D., Rubin, D. H. and Cebra, J. J. (1987). Gut mucosal immunization with reovirus serotype 1/L stimulates virus-specific cytotoxic T cell precursors as well as IgA memory cells in Peyer's patches. *J. Exp. Med.*, **165**, 830–47

90. Hill, D. R. (1990). Lymphocyte proliferation in Peyer's patches of *Giardia muris*-infected mice. *Infect. Immun.*, **58**, 2683–5

91. Belosevic, M., Faubert, G. M., Skamene, E. and MacLean, J. D. (1984). Susceptibility and resistance of inbred mice to *Giardia muris*. *Infect. Immun.*, **44**, 282–6

92. Belosevic, M. and Faubert, G. M. (1987). Lysis and immobilization of *Giardia muris* trophozoites *in vitro* by immune serum from susceptible and resistant mice. *Parasit. Immunol.*, **9**, 11–19

93. Heyworth, M. F. and Pappo, J. (1989). Use of two-colour flow cytometry to assess killing of *Giardia muris* trophozoites by antibody and complement. *Parasitology*, **99**, 199–203

94. Deguchi, M., Gillin, F. D. and Gigli, I. (1987). Mechanism of killing of *Giardia lamblia* trophozoites by complement. *J. Clin. Invest.*, **79**, 1296–302

95. Inge, P. M. G., Edson, C. M. and Farthing, M. J. G. (1988). Attachment of *Giardia lamblia* to rat intestinal epithelial cells. *Gut*, **29**, 795–801

96. Kaplan, B. and Altmanshofer, D. (1985). *Giardia muris* adherence to intestinal epithelium – the role of specific anti-*Giardia* antibodies. *Microecol. Ther.*, **15**, 133–40

97. Radulescu, S. and Meyer, E. A. (1981). Opsonization in vitro of *Giardia lamblia* trophozoites. *Infect. Immun.*, **32**, 852–6

98. Kaplan, B. S., Uni, S., Aikawa, M. and Mahmoud, A. A. F. (1985). Effector mechanism of host resistance in murine giardiasis: specific IgG and IgA cell-mediated toxicity. *J. Immunol.*, **134**, 1975–81

99. Hill, D. R. and Pearson, R. D. (1987). Ingestion of *Giardia lamblia* trophozoites by human mononuclear phagocytes. *Infect. Immun.*, **55**, 3155–61

100. Torian, B. E., Barnes, R. C., Stephens, R. S. and Stibbs, H. H. (1984). Tubulin and high-molecular-weight polypeptides as *Giardia lamblia* antigens. *Infect. Immun.*, **46**, 152–8

101. Holberton, D. V. and Ward, A. P. (1981). Isolation of the cytoskeleton from *Giardia*. Tubulin and a low-molecular-weight protein associated with microribbon structures. *J. Cell Sci.*, **47**, 139–66

102. Crossley, R. and Holberton, D. V. (1983). Characterization of proteins from the cytoskeleton of *Giardia lamblia*. *J. Cell Sci.*, **59**, 81–103

103. Crossley, R. and Holberton, D. (1985). Assembly of 2.5 nm filaments from giardin, a protein associated with cytoskeletal microtubules in *Giardia*. *J. Cell Sci.*, **78**, 205–31

104. Crossley, R., Marshall, J., Clark, J. T. and Holberton, D. V. (1986). Immunocytochemical differentiation of microtubules in the cytoskeleton of *Giardia lamblia* using monoclonal antibodies to α-tubulin and polyclonal antibodies to associated low molecular weight

proteins. *J. Cell Sci.*, **80**, 233–52

105. Crossley, R. and Holberton, D. V. (1983). Selective extraction with sarkosyl and repolymerization *in vitro* of cytoskeleton proteins from *Giardia*. *J. Cell Sci.*, **62**, 419–38

106. Clark, J. T. and Holberton, D. V. (1988). Triton-labile antigens in flagella isolated from *Giardia lamblia*. *Parasitol. Res.*, **74**, 415–23

107. Einfeld, D. A. and Stibbs, H. H. (1984). Identification and characterization of a major surface antigen of *Giardia lamblia*. *Infect. Immun.*, **46**, 377–83

108. Clark, J. T. and Holberton, D. V. (1986). Plasma membrane isolated from *Giardia lamblia*: identification of membrane proteins. *Eur. J. Cell Biol.*, **42**, 200–6

109. Gillin, F. D., Hagblom, P., Harwood, J., Aley, S. B., Reiner, D. S., McCaffery, M., So, M. and Guiney, D. G. (1990). Isolation and expression of the gene for a major surface protein of *Giardia lamblia*. *Proc. Natl. Acad. Sci. USA*, **87**, 4463–7

110. Upcroft, J. A., Capon, A. G., Dharmkrong-At, A., Healey, A., Boreham, P. F. L. and Upcroft, P. (1987). *Giardia intestinalis* antigens expressed in *Escherichia coli*. *Mol. Biochem. Parasitol.*, **26**, 267–76

111. Aggarwal, A. and Nash, T. E. (1989). Characterization of a 33-kilodalton structural protein of *Giardia lamblia* and localization to the ventral disk. *Infect. Immun.*, **57**, 1305–10

112. Holberton, D., Baker, D. A. and Marshall, J. (1988). Segmented α-helical coiled-coil structure of the protein giardin from the *Giardia* cytoskeleton. *J. Mol. Biol.*, **204**, 789–95

113. Peattie, D. A., Alonso, R. A., Hein, A. and Caulfield, J. P. (1989). Ultrastructural localization of giardins to the edges of disk microribbons of *Giardia lamblia* and the nucleotide and deduced protein sequence of alpha giardin. *J. Cell Biol.*, **109**, 2323–35

114. Farthing, M. J. G., Pereira, M. E. A. and Keusch, G. T. (1986). Description and characterization of a surface lectin from *Giardia lamblia*. *Infect. Immun.*, **51**, 661–7

115. Ward, H. D., Lev, B. I., Kane, A. V., Keusch, G. T. and Pereira, M. E. A. (1987). Identification and characterization of taglin, a mannose 6-phosphate binding, trypsin-activated lectin from *Giardia lamblia*. *Biochemistry*, **26**, 8669–75

116. Parenti, D. M. (1989). Characterization of a thiol proteinase in *Giardia lamblia*. *J. Infect. Dis.*, **160**, 1076–80

117. Forrest, M., Isaac-Renton, J. and Bowie, W. (1990). Immunoblot patterns of *Giardia duodenalis* isolates from different hosts and geographical locations. *Can. J. Microbiol.*, **36**, 42–6

118. Nash, T. E., McCutchan, T., Keister, D., Dame, J. B., Conrad, J. D. and Gillin, F. D. (1985). Restriction-endonuclease analysis of DNA from 15 *Giardia* isolates obtained from humans and animals. *J. Infect. Dis.*, **152**, 64–73

119. Aggarwal, A. and Nash, T. E. (1988). Antigenic variation of *Giardia lamblia* in vivo. *Infect. Immun.*, **56**, 1420–3

120. Wenman, W. M., Meuser, R. U. and Wallis, P. M. (1986). Antigenic analysis of *Giardia duodenalis* strains isolated in Alberta. *Can. J. Microbiol.*, **32**, 926–9

121. Capon, A. G., Upcroft, J. A., Boreham, P. F. L., Cottis, L. E. and Bundesen, P. G. (1989). Similarities of *Giardia* antigens derived from human and animal sources. *Int. J. Parasitol.*, **19**, 91–8

16
Intestinal nematode infections

E. S. COOPER

INTRODUCTION

Parasitic nematodes are complex metazoan organisms in which the adult, reproductive forms are long-lived. Individual worms may remain alive throughout much of the childhood of a host. To them, the gut mucosa is both a refuge and a source of sustenance, and yet it would be astonishing if they elicited no immune response or inflammation from the host. The theme of this chapter, which deals with the three most common species of human parasitic worm, hookworm, roundworm and whipworm, and the much less prevalent but potentially fatal opportunistic pathogen *Strongyloides stercoralis*, is to show that there are indeed such responses, but that they are limited and confined. Because of this, the extent of pathology, which may yet be severe, is a direct function of the area of mucosal contact between host and parasite, rather than a consequence of immunological amplification within the host among the many pathways of response to a given amount of antigen.

Although an adult nematode established in the host gut has a long life expectancy (typically months or years), the mortality of the freshly invading larvae is high. Assuming continuous exposure to infection, which means continuous exposure to contaminated soil, the normal situation in endemic areas, wave after wave of these juvenile forms will be attempting to complete their life-cycle and to become adults. It is presumably at this stage that the parasite is most vulnerable to the effects of the host immune response, and also at this stage that selection pressure on the fitness of variants within the parasite species is most intense.

Human hosts and parasitic nematodes have been together for a sufficient number of generations for considerable co-evolution to have occurred, genetically[1,2]. It is also likely that immunological adaptation within the lifetime of a host occurs. An example of this has recently been adduced by showing the slow build-up during adolescence of an IgE response to

283

schistosomiasis[3]. However, there is so far little or no direct evidence for this in the four parasites considered here. Nevertheless, the morbidity ascribed to roundworm and whipworm infection is largely a problem of childhood, although the anaemia of hookworm infection, which is not mediated by any component of the immune system, has a cumulative effect throughout life. *Strongyloides* is often acquired in childhood, but can cause disease at any age, if a detrimental change in the physiology of the host allows larval abundance to get out of control.

HISTORICAL IDEAS ON PATHOGENESIS

The idea of mutual adaptation between host and parasite, whether within the lifetime of an infection or over generations between species and strains of species, is relatively new – at least among clinicians. Until the last two or three decades the dominant view of the *cost* of a parasitic infection was one where the parasite stole nutrients from the host while possibly poisoning it through the systemic absorption of toxins, which were never identified. Watson[4] suggested that there are five basic forms of pathogenesis by parasitic worms: (1) spoliative (equivalent to food-stealing), (2) toxic, (3) traumatic, (4) mechanical, (5) irritative and inflammatory. Today, the greatest emphasis by far would be on (5), and modern concepts of cooperation between host antibodies and cells, and the final common pathways of release of chemotactic factors and inflammatory mediators, are invoked to explain the pathology.

CONSIDERATIONS FROM THE POINT OF VIEW OF POPULATION BIOLOGY

While the concept of *herd immunity* has no universally agreed definition, and seems to have little to do with modern advances in immunology, which have been largely mechanistic and at the molecular level, some consideration of the totality of the population of parasites within the total population of hosts is necessary. Such a consideration makes some sense of the variability of the burden of parasites within an individual host and of the gradation of the pathology associated with the host's response.

The ecology of the worm infections of humans is different from that of most viruses and bacteria[5]. The population of hosts is not at any one time cleanly divided into the susceptible and the immune, and the prevalence of infection does not pass through a community as a wave through time, converting the former into the latter. However, it is true that the average worm burden of adults tends to be less than that of children (Fig. 16.1)[6] and that among children themselves there is a diversity of *intensity* of infection (i.e. the number of parasites harboured) that is far greater than can be explained by random apportionment of parasites (Fig. 16.2)[6]. This distribution

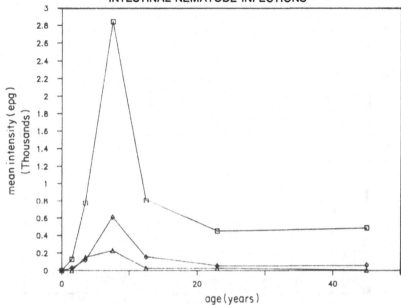

Figure 16.1 Intensity of helminth infection has a peak at a similar childhood age in different populations. The intensity of infection (here that of *Trichuris trichiura*) is the mean for each of three populations, expressed as eggs per gram of stool (epg). Although the three populations differ in mean infection intensity, the age of peak intensity is at about 8 years for all. Although the intensity declines thereafter, adults remain lightly infected throughout life. From ref. 6, with permission of the publishers

can be summarized as 'many people harbour a few parasites but a few people harbour many'. A difference among hosts in susceptibility on the basis of immunological genetics is one possible component for the explanation of this, but it is not a necessary one. Similar distributions[7] occur in, for example, the number of books per household or the number of alcoholic drinks consumed per person per day. Wherever there are self-amplifying, i.e. 'non-linear' effects (as occur with consumption of books or liquor) small differences in initial conditions, which may indeed themselves be apportioned at random, become reflected in results with a similar frequency distribution to that of parasites, aggregated among their hosts. Where a parasite reproduces within the host there is an obvious cause for non-linear dynamics and the production of a highly skewed final intensity of infection from a less diverse initial dose. However, the nematodes, apart from *Strongyloides* species, do not reproduce their adult selves within their host, and some other explanation must be sought.

There is reason to believe that for worms the distribution of infective doses is as skewed as the adult worm burdens[8]. Beyond that, explanation is lacking; although epidemiological research to find it is increasingly active. It is important to know whether the self-amplification occurs because the effects of intense parasitism themselves predispose to further infection. Possible, hypothetical, examples of such a mechanism are that iron or zinc deficiency may drive the desire to eat earth[9], so increasing the infective dose, or that

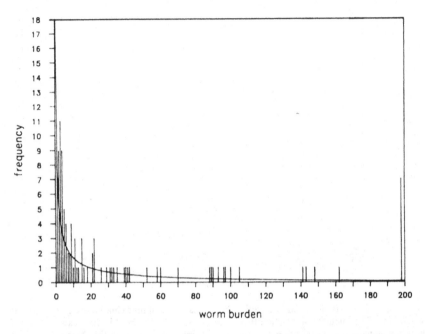

Figure 16.2 Frequency distribution of individual worm burdens in an infected population. These numbers were obtained by counting adult *Trichuris trichiura* in 4-day stool collections following anthelmintic treatment. Seven individuals had burdens in excess of 200 worms, with the greatest exceeding 1000. The continuous line is the best-fit negative binomial model[7]. From ref. 6, with permission of the publishers

malnutrition might lead to apathy exacerbating pica as simple self-gratification[10].

In case the above discussion appears arcane, we can now relate it to the chapter's theme. In every instance we shall find that what is known of inflammatory morbidity is related to the intensity of infection, that is to say the number of adult parasites harboured. Even where Type I hypersensitivity, the mechanism of anaphylaxis, is likely to be important in the mucosal response, a clear antigen–dose–effect relationship is seen. This is in contrast to other conditions considered in this book – food sensitivity, coeliac disease – where an immunopathological amplification is believed to cause damage out of proportion to the quantity of antigen, following sensitization.

Ecologically, it is considered that a stable equilibrium exists where the most intensely infected hosts pay a price in morbidity; but also contribute most to the reproduction of the parasite. This is because, despite density-dependent constraints on the fecundity of each female worm, the stool of a heavily parasitized human has a greater density of eggs and contributes more infective stages to the soil than that of a lightly parasitized host. However, the high prevalence of these infections also favours the survival of the parasites, since in the event of the loss of the heavily parasitized hosts there will remain many surviving sources of future infection. In fact, the effect of mass de-worming campaigns is generally to reduce the mean intensity of infection drastically, but the prevalence much less so; and full intensity of infection soon recovers after the intervention stops[11].

CLINICAL PATHOLOGY OF THE COMMON NEMATODE INFECTIONS

Hookworm

The two species of hookworm which parasitize the human intestinal mucosa are *Ankylostoma duodenale* and *Necator americanus*. The morphological differences between the species and the different geographical regions in which each predominates are of no clinical importance: this is why it is usual to speak of the parasite simply as hookworm. Severe iron deficiency occurs in prolonged and intense hookworm infection, and this is the principal, and sometimes the only, component widely recognized as 'hookworm disease'. However, hypoalbuminaemia is also recognized as part of the syndrome, frequently associated with oedema of the lower limbs[12].

Recently, Stephenson and her colleagues have shown, in adequately controlled studies[13], improvements in the growth of Kenyan children infected with hookworm and other intestinal parasites, following treatment with broad-spectrum anthelmintics. Moreover, they have drawn attention to literature describing studies[14,15] dating back to 1903 which associated hookworm infection with stunted growth and delayed puberty. The clinical descriptions of this neglected aspect of 'hookworm disease' include loss of appetite, although this symptom is difficult to validate and quantify. Reduced food intake is an established effect of *Nippostrongylus brasiliensis* infection in the rat[16], but such animal models need to be viewed sceptically.

Nevertheless, the effects on growth and possibly on appetite of human hookworm infection may well have their basis in intestinal inflammation, unlike the iron deficiency, which is fully explicable as direct red cell loss through the gut of the nematode. The limited evidence which exists so far on the inflammatory response can now be briefly reviewed.

There is a protein-losing enteropathy in intense hookworm infection. It is important to distinguish this from the mere loss of the plasma accompanying the red cells through the hookworms' guts. Using the oft-quoted figure[17] of 0.05 ml blood lost per worm per day, 1000 hookworms would account for some 50 ml blood loss per day, of which 35 ml or so might be plasma. Therefore, the protein content of 35 ml of plasma would be lost into the gut lumen (there to be at least partially digested and reabsorbed as nitrogenous compounds). The plasma volume is, of course, easily replaced from extracellular fluid, so the loss of the total protein content of 35 ml of plasma can be expressed as a protein clearance of 35 ml of plasma. However, using albumen labelled with ^{131}I or ^{51}Cr, clearances of over 100 ml per day have often been shown. This exudation is likely to represent inflammation, ultimately expressed as loosening of the tight junctions between the epithelial cells. A direct relationship between the extent of protein-losing enteropathy and the intensity of infection has been shown by several authors[18-20].

287

It should not be assumed that protein-losing enteropathy is the complete explanation of hypoalbuminaemia in hookworm infection. Hypoalbuminaemia due to depressed hepatic synthesis is expected as part of the systemic response to inflammation, reported in ankylostomiasis[21], and particularly in the presence of increased circulating tumour necrosis factor (TNF)[22]. The systemic cytokine profile has not been reported in hookworm infection, but we have noted high plasma concentrations of TNF in severe trichuriasis[23].

The morbid anatomy of *Ankylostoma brasiliensis* infection in dogs has, naturally, been studied[24] more thoroughly than that of hookworm in humans, although several studies of intestinal biopsies have been reported[25,26]. Several villi are drawn into the worm's buccal cavity. The epithelial cells are detached from the lamina propria, in which the capillary loops burst. There is therefore direct contact between antigenic substances from the worm, probably including proteolytic enzymes, and the macrophages and lymphocytes of the lamina propria. Nevertheless, the striking finding is a negative one: namely, that the villi not ingested by the worm usually appear normal. Immunopathology mediated by T-cell activation would have been expected to lead to villous atrophy. The histological effects of hookworm infection appear to consist only of local tissue destruction, haemorrhage within the ingested tissue and transepithelial migration of erythrocytes in adjacent tissue, as well as oedema, increased mitotic activity in the neighbouring crypts with corresponding immaturity of the cells migrating up the sides, and neutrophil infiltration of the lamina propria on the edge of the lesion. All of these effects are consistent with a local response to mechanical and chemical trauma and no thymocyte-mediated immune response needs to be invoked as an explanation. So far, there are no reports of immunohistochemical studies to confirm this inactivity. Swelling of the retroperitoneal lymph nodes has been noted[27], but its immunological basis has not been investigated.

Clinical implications

Many signs and symptoms have been ascribed to hookworms but only clear and established manifestations of the disease are set out in Table 16.1. It is very probable that Type I hypersensitivity underlies the manifestations of larval migration, but it is not established that there is any immunological mechanism behind the intestinal manifestations of mucosal attachment of

Table 16.1 Hookworm disease

Larval stage	
Skin	'Ground itch' – localized rash
Lungs	Brochitis, pneumonitis (not well established in children)
Adult in the intestine	Anorexia, pica, upper abdominal pain, diarrhoea (usually with mucus, sometimes bloody); protein-losing enteropathy
Systemic secondary effects	Iron deficiency; anaemia; hypo-albuminaemia; heart failure; acute-phase protein response; growth retardation; malabsorption/malnutrition? – not established

adult worms. However, there is clearly an inflammatory response, both local and systemic, in the broader sense of the word.

Roundworm *(Ascaris lumbricoides)*

This nematode invades the tissues only during its larval stages. The initial penetration is of second-stage larvae (i.e. they have moulted their cuticles once, inside the eggs in the soil before human infection). These penetrate the duodenal and jejunal mucosa and are found in the liver 1–4 days later. Their subsequent progress through the lungs, up the bronchial tree and back into the oesophagus is not our present concern, although it is during this time that they are at greatest risk from the host immune system. Their success at adaptation to this will be rewarded by a proportionate probability of survival to adulthood. The surviving larvae passing through the stomach for a second time are at the L4 stage. They moult for a final time in the small intestine, where they will live as adults. They appear to maintain their position in the lumen by muscular bracing: they are capable of moving back up through the alimentary canal and appearing in the mouth or upper respiratory tract. This ectopic migration is provoked by fever in the child or by the initial metabolic attack of the carbimidazole drugs[28]. Conversely, neuromuscular paralysis induced by piperazine or pyrantel leads to their rapid expulsion through the anus. The adult worms have a thick cuticle, so that the only obvious points with potential susceptibility to effective attack by luminally secreted antibody such as IgA or IgE, or effector cells such as macrophages and eosinophils, are the apertures, particularly the mouth. There is no evidence of any substantial effect here, however. The main weapon of the intestinal epithelium may be mucus, although Stephenson *et al.* have shown a reduction of intestinal mucus in piglets infected with *Ascaris suum*[29]. Goblet cell number is under T-cell control[30], so the reduction in mucus may represent a failure of cell-mediated immunity in these animals. The most effective response of the intestinal tract as a whole may be neuromuscular activity resulting in increased peristalsis tending to counteract the muscular efforts of the worms. It has been suggested that there may be a link between the immune and neuro-muscular systems in the gut, mediated by acetylcholine, substance P, vasoactive intestinal peptide, histamine, serotonin, prostaglandins or leukotrienes[31]. Increased myoelectric activity was detected in rat intestine after challenge with *Trichinella spiralis* if the host had been previously immunized[32]. The actual existence of any such mechanisms in human ascariasis have yet to be shown.

Clinical implications

See Table 16.2 for a summary of the commoner and better-established symptoms of ascariasis. During the intestinal phase of ascariasis there is really no symptomatology that can clearly be ascribed to the operation of immune or inflammatory mechanisms. All the well-founded symptoms and signs of roundworms in the gut are explicable on a mechanical basis, although

Table 16.2 Roundworm disease

Larval stage	
Lungs	Bronchitis, pneumonitis (not well established as an entity in children)
Adult in the intestine	Anorexia; abdominal pain; acute intestinal obstruction; volvulus; possible malabsorption syndrome; lactose intolerance?
Adult in ectopic site	
Bile duct	Obstructive jaundice
Pancreatic duct	Acute pancreatitis
Larynx	Asphyxia
(Many other ectopic sites and unusual presentations)	
Systemic secondary effects	Vitamin A deficiency; malnutrition? (not established)

little research has been done in the area. It has been suggested that lactose intolerance is induced by ascariasis[33], and that villous atrophy and malabsorption may occur[34], but the evidence for these as pure effects of the helminthiasis is weak and inconclusive. It is possible that the parasite has a profound influence on the intestinal microflora, mediating some of these claimed effects, but very little work has been done in this difficult area.

Trichuris trichiura

The whipworm differs from the roundworm in that it is a tissue parasite in the gut, as the adult lives with the greater part of its length buried in the colonic epithelium; but it differs from both hookworm and roundworm in having no part of its larval existence outside the intestinal mucosa. In dogs it was shown that *T. vulpis* L2 larvae could invade the crypts in the duodenum[35], but it is not known if this occurs in the human, or indeed in the dog under natural conditions, since the experimental dose that was used in the originally reported study would be exceptional in nature[6]. Probably the common site for *Trichuris* larval invasion in humans is the caecal crypts. The only further migration is up the walls of these crypts, while the larva moults and grows, until the posterior end of the adult worm bursts through the epithelium into the lumen, and the longer, finer anterior end is left snaking in an epithelial tunnel between the crypt mouths. In intense infections the whole colonic and rectal mucosa is carpeted with adult whipworms, while tangled knots of them are visible in the terminal ileum (Fig. 16.3).

Thanks to the fibreoptic colonoscope, the entire length of the colon is now accessible to inspection and biopsy, without causing significant pain or risk to the child. We have taken advantage of this to obtain the most extensive picture of the pathology surrounding a human parasitic nematode *in situ* available so far.

There is macroscopic evidence of colonic inflammation in the *Trichuris* dysentery syndrome (TDS), but it is confined to hyperaemia and oedema. Ulceration of the mucosa does not occur, and a tendency to haemorrhage (friability) is inconstant: such findings would, in contrast, be typical in ulcerative colitis.

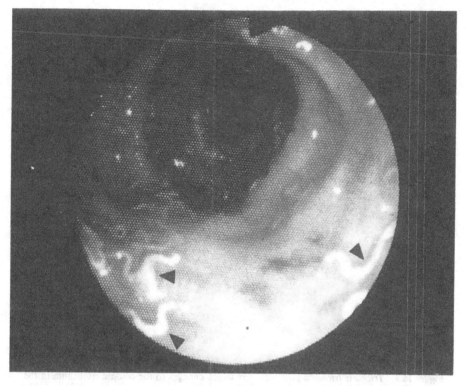

Figure 16.3 Colonoscopic visualization of *Trichuris trichiura* (arrowed) in the caecum of a child with *Trichuris* dysentery syndrome

Microscopically, in routinely stained sections, there is only one specific change and it is not of an inflammatory nature. The epithelium is flattened in the region where the adult worm lies, and appears to form a syncytium. In addition, the lamina propria is richly cellular, mostly with mononuclear cells but also with an infiltration of eosinophils in some cases. However, these changes in the lamina propria are not specific to *Trichuris* infection, for they are also seen in other children with mucoid diarrhoea from the same environment (Fig. 16.4).

What is striking is not the few positive changes but the many absences of the markers of cell-mediated immunopathology[36], in the presence of an enormous antigenic load inside the epithelial barrier of the mucosa. Intraepithelial lymphocytes are reduced in number, and so is the proportion bearing γ/δ receptors, so markedly increased in the immunopathological condition of coeliac disease. In the lamina propria the proportion of cells bearing the CD3 marker is the same in trichuriasis as in local controls, implying that there is no increase in T cell number. Lamina propria CD25+ cell numbers are also highly variable within each group of children, but with no difference between the groups. Since this implies that there is no general increase in the number of cells bearing receptors for IL2, it also implies that there is no general activation of T cells or macrophages.

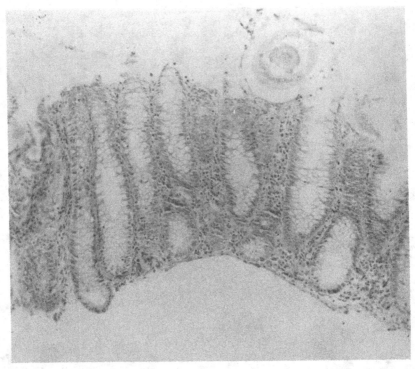

Figure 16.4 *Trichuris trichiura* produces only minor changes to the colonic epithelium in the region of the worm (H&E original magnification ×100)

The epithelium also fails to show the consequences expected of a local T cell activation: not only is the morphology undisturbed, but there is a lack of consistent expression of HLA-DR or VLA-1, both of which are characteristic of mucosal inflammation[37,38].

There are immune-mediated events taking place in the *Trichuris*-infected mucosa, however. Immunohistochemistry shows that some 10% of the lamina propria cells have membrane IgE, whereas in the children with mucoid diarrhoea from other causes the proportion is 1% or less – a 10-fold difference[39]. These cells are mucosal mast cells, as is shown by direct staining with Alcian or toluidine blue on appropriately fixed tissue, when the characteristic mast cell granules can be seen. In fact, the more superficial mast cells in trichuriasis take up relatively little stain because they are in the process of degranulating. Electron microscopy confirms this.

The assumption must be that the IgE on the cell membranes is a specific antibody to *Trichuris* soluble antigen, diffusing away from the surface or, more probably, from the oesophagus of the whipworm. Two pieces of evidence provide some support for this specificity: (1) the presence of specific IgE in the blood of *Trichuris*-infected humans[40], and (2) *in vitro* release of histamine from rectal biopsy tissue in children, which in some cases is sensitive to provocation by extremely small quantities of *Trichuris* excretory–secretory protein[39].

Table 16.3 Whipworm disease

Adult in intestine	Anorexia, pica, lower abdominal pain, dysentery (blood and mucus); rectal prolapse
Systemic secondary effects	Iron deficiency; anaemia; linear growth retardation; clubbing of fingers and toes; malnutrition?

Clinical implications

The principal consequences of intense infection by *Trichuris trichiura* are chronic diarrhoea, anaemia and stunting of growth[41] (Table 16.3). All of these are likely to be the detrimental consequences of some form of inflammatory response to the worm. They are unlikely to represent the effects of direct loss of nutrients and host substances to the worm on the outmoded model that the host's loss is the worm's gain. An adult *Trichuris trichiura* weighs, at most, 10 mg. Therefore, a burden of 1000 whipworms, which would be associated with all the clinical features of the *Trichuris* dysentery syndrome[42,43], represents less than 10 g of nematode tissue. This should not pose significant metabolic competition to the 10 or 20 kg homeothermic child who is its host.

The mechanism of blood loss in severe trichuriasis is likely to be both by gross loss from the inflamed rectum and by passage of red cells across the entire colonic epithelium[35], rendered highly permeable by the anaphylactic inflammation. The mechanism of growth retardation is unknown, but may be related to the increased concentration of circulating cytokines associated with an inflammatory plasma protein response (Cooper and MacDonald, unpublished data). Cytokines including IL-6 and TNF[22] are possibly derived from the excess of macrophages in the colonic mucosa of children with the *Trichuris* dysentery syndrome[22].

Strongyloides stercoralis

This small worm differs from the pathogens considered above in many significant ways, as an animal, as a parasite and as an agent of disease. An immature form, the L3 larva, appears to be the repository of an extraordinary versatility in life strategy. It is filariform (i.e. very slim) and penetrates the human colonic mucosa, passes via the lymphatics or directly into venous blood, through the alveolae into the bronchial tree, up to the larynx and across to the pharynx, down the oesophagus, through the stomach and into the duodenum, where it can mature into an adult female form. This worm grows to a length of 2.2 mm with a width of 45 µm, and lives embedded between enterocytes. The adult reproduces parthenogenetically, yielding what is by parasite standards a modest progeny, between 20 and 50 eggs a day. These have thin walls and hatch rhabdtidiform larvae while still within the small intestine. Some of these pass through the anus in this form, but others moult to reach the L3 stage, ready to penetrate the colonic epithelium again. This auto-infective, non-sexual life cycle can continue indefinitely, in fact throughout a human lifetime.

The L3 larva is as capable of entering this cycle through the skin of the host as through the colonic epithelium. This can occur in the perianal area or the buttocks, but it can also occur in any cutaneous region from contact with soil, where the filariform larva is also capable of existence. In the soil the ontogeny of L3 larvae may be by moulting from the L1 larvae passed through a host's anus (homogonic development) or it may be from L1 forms that hatched from ova produced by sexual reproduction of adult *Strongyloides* in the soil (heterogonic development). The existence of the heterogonic development has led many to speak of a 'free-living life cycle'. However, this is not strictly correct, since this is to suppose that the heterogonically developed L3 larvae can proceed on through the L4 stage to male or female adult forms with indefinite numbers of repetitions, without renewal from rhabditiform larvae shed by a host: this has not been shown. If there is a true free-living cycle then the gloomy implication for environmental control of this parasite is obvious.

Humans are not the only host of *Strongyloides stercoralis*; apes, dogs and cats are also involved[44]. This is remarkable, and unlike any of the other parasitic nematode species, which show host-specificity. In the other helminthiases the pathology, and in particular the immunopathology, differs when inter-species cross-infection does occur, as, for example, with toxocariasis (equivalent to ascariasis in dogs, but causing visceral larva migrans and ocular larva migrans in humans). It is estimated that 1% of the dogs of the eastern United States is infected with *S. stercoralis*. This is very much the same order of prevalence as in the humans of Jamaica. This brings out another difference between strongyloidiasis and ascariasis, trichuriasis, and hookworm: the prevalence of the parasitosis is generally much lower. In one part of Brazil a prevalence of 60% has been claimed[45], and high prevalences may be reached in institutions, such as mental asylums, but community prevalences of less than 5% are more the rule, even in areas where intestinal parasitoses in general greatly exceed 50%. In the Second World War prisoners of war in Southeast Asia who were described 35 years later[46], only 30% were infected, although the prolonged circumstances under which they were originally exposed would have been expected to give the parasite every opportunity for an initial invasion.

This brings us to the heart of the set of immunological paradoxes posed by strongyloidiasis. In those ex-prisoners of war who were still infected by *Strongyloides* 35 years later many auto-infective cycles must have taken place, and yet there was neither such an immune defence as to lead to parasite extinction nor such reproductive amplification of parasite numbers as to lead to disseminated larval invasion. How is such a precise regulation of parasite abundance achieved? We have no idea. Furthermore, strongyloidiasis is the only human helminthiasis in which we have clear evidence that there *is* immunological regulation of parasite abundance. This comes from clinical observations of the disastrous effects of immunosuppression[47]. If there has been, as suggested at the beginning of this chapter, such coevolution of host and parasite as to lead to a distribution of parasites within hosts that tends towards the equilibrium least costly to both species, then it is extremely difficult to see how *Strongyloides* can lack host-specificity to the extent that

294

it does. The picture makes most sense if we regard *Strongyloides* in humans differently from the other worms, as a truly *opportunistic* pathogen.

In 1964 Bras *et al.* described as representative 10 cases of disseminated strongyloidiasis in Jamaica[48]. Four of these patients were in their teens. Six had died and only one had fully recovered. All were severely undernourished. This is quite different from the picture today in Jamaica, where over the past few years we have been seeking out cases to study, with some difficulty, and have encountered none so severe, least of all in young people. Nevertheless, prevalence was estimated at 1% by Bras *et al.* in 1964, and at 3.6% in a community survey in 1987[49], so the difference does not seem to be one of prevalence. Nutritional status and life expectancy, however, have improved enormously over the period[50]. It seems reasonable to speculate that immunodepression associated with poor nutrition was a factor in the failure of the patients of the 1960s to control the larval dissemination.

An association of strongyloidiasis with infection by the retrovirus, HTLV1, has been described. This virus is endemic in the Caribbean and in the Ryuku islands of Japan, among other places, and is the subject of much current research. The mechanism whereby the retrovirus infection, which is itself one principally of T cells, favours chronic strongyloidiasis is as yet unknown. *Strongyloides* infection has a general association with eosinophilia, but in severe or disseminated infection the eosinophil count tends to be depressed[51]. In HTLV1 infection serum IgE concentration and blood eosinophil counts tend to be low, also[52]. The higher the eosinophil count the greater the success in parasitological cure with thiabendazole[53] (Terry, S. I., personal communication), which suggests a partially effective defence function of the IgE–eosinophil system against this parasite in the gut. Cell-mediated immune function is thought to be involved in protection against larval dissemination, since a group of conditions associated with this catastrophe have deficiency of cell-mediated immunity as their common denominator (Table 16.4). Antibody dependence of cell-mediated cytotoxicity is also a possibility, since disseminated strongyloidiasis has also been described in hypogammaglobulinaemia[54]. There have been reports of disseminated strongyloidiasis in AIDS[55], but generally the lack of association has been the more striking[56]. This leads one

Table 16.4 Risk factors for hyperinfection and disseminated strongyloidiasis

Immunosuppression	Corticosteroids; organ transplantation; other immunosuppressive chemotherapy; radiation therapy
Immunodepression	Hypogammaglobulinaemia; autoimmune diseases
Infections	Leprosy; tuberculosis; (AIDS)
Gastrointestinal abnormalities	History of gastrectomy with blind loop (Billroth); antacid therapy (cimetidine); malabsorption; delayed intestinal transit time
Malignancies	Leukaemias; lymphomas; solid tumours with ectopic ACTH production
Miscellaneous	Severe malnutrition; early childhood; pregnancy (?)

From ref. 47, with permission.

to question whether a simple shortage of CD4 + cells alone can account for susceptibility to disseminated strongyloidiasis.

Clinical implications: strongyloidiasis as a purely gastroenterological disease

A number of symptoms are ascribed to the state of chronic infection of the small bowel with *Strongyloides*. However, many of them fall into the general class of symptoms common to huge numbers of people, infected and uninfected. Examples are the sensation of fullness, abdominal pain, diarrhoea alternating with constipation, etc. Others, particularly related to malabsorption and steatorrhea, have not been linked to strongyloidiasis with the necessary rigour. What is needed is a comparison of frequencies of symptoms, signs and pathological findings in unbiased samples of infected and uninfected members of a general population in the tropics. The reports of malabsorption and villous atrophy in strongyloidiasis are similar to those in hookworm infection, which, as discussed above, are not clear-cut. They are also at variance with histopathological pictures of adult *Strongyloides in situ* (Fig. 16.5), in which the absence of an inflammatory response to the nematode is quite striking.

There is one feature of chronic strongyloidiasis which is reported consistently by radiologists[57], and that is rigidity of the duodenal loop. This is thought to indicate healing of duodenitis by fibrosis. It is possible that secondary bacterial invasion plays a part in this.

SUMMARY AND CONCLUSIONS

Even after generations of coexistence, human populations remain susceptible to gut nematodes throughout life. There may be some diminution in susceptibility during life, and genetic differences in susceptibility on an immunological basis among individuals, but these effects have not yet been shown and are likely to be relatively small. Despite this there is great variance in intensity of infection, a far greater variance than can be explained on a model of random apportionment. The characteristic highly skewed frequency distribution suggests a non-linear relationship between present intensity of infection and rate of acquisition of more parasites, the explanation of which is still unknown. Very limited morbidity in numerous, lightly infected, people, and a trade-off between host morbidity and infectivity in the relatively few intensely infected people, could explain a stable equilibrium of parasitism in a human population in a contaminated environment. A direct relationship between infecting dose and inflammatory response is necessary to sustain this equilibrium, and this requires that immunological sensitization and amplification of inflammation in the mucosa be in some way severely limited.

In spite of this, parasitic worms do elicit inflammatory effects from the mucosa surrounding the area with which they are in direct contact. Mediators which lead to oedema, increased mucus production and possibly also neuromuscular changes appear to be released. The mechanisms inducing the

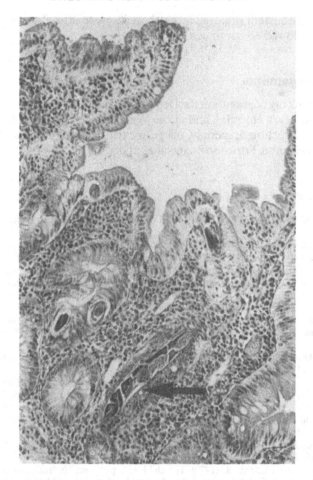

Figure 16.5 *Strongyloides stercoralis* in the jejunum. Note the worm head (arrowed) buried in the lamina propria, but despite some local inflammation there are still tall villi (H&E, original magnification ×100)

release are likely to comprise: (1) non-immunologically, direct physical and chemical trauma; (2) immunologically, reactions involving IgE, mast cells and eosinophils, i.e. local anaphylaxis. Humoral changes probably also occur, consisting of cytokine circulation and secondary changes in plasma proteins (the 'acute phase response'). Specific antibody to worm antigens is also found in the blood, but its protective role in intestinal helminthiasis appears to be limited or unconvincing.

Finally, it may appear from the many uncertain or negative statements on the role of gut immunology in worm infections in this chapter that this largely unresearched field has little future. The answer to that contention lies in an appreciation of the enormous worldwide prevalences of these infections. Hookworm is estimated currently to infect 700–900 million people[58], *Ascaris* 1000 million[59], whipworm 550–800 million[6] and *Strongyloides* 50–100 million[44]. The current situation in which we know so little about pathogenesis cannot be allowed to continue.

Acknowledgements

I wish to thank my colleagues at the Department of Paediatric Gastroenterology, St Bartholomew's Hospital, and at the Wellcome Trust Centre for Research in Parasitic Infection, Imperial College, for their collaboration and teaching; also the Wellcome Trust for financial support.

References

1. Anderson, R. M. and May, R. M. (1982). Coevolution of hosts and parasites. *Parasitology*, **85**, 411–26
2. Behnke, J. M. and Barnard, C. J. (1990). Coevolution of parasites and hosts: host-parasite arms races and their consequences. In Behnke, J. M. (ed.), *Parasites: Immunity and Pathology*. London: Taylor & Francis, pp. 1–22
3. Hagan, P., Blumenthal, U. J., Dunn, D., Simpson, A. J. G. and Wilkins, H. A. (1991). Human IgE, IgG4 and resistance to infection with *Schistosoma haematobium*. *Nature*, **349**, 243–5
4. Watson, J. M. (1960). *Medical Helminthology*. London: Baillière, Tindall & Cox
5. Anderson, R. M. (1982). The population dynamics and control of hookworm and roundworm infections. In Anderson, R. M. (ed.), *Population Dynamics of Infectious Diseases*. London: Chapman & Hall, pp. 69–108
6. Bundy, D. A. P. and Cooper, E. S. (1989). *Trichuris* and trichuriasis in humans. *Adv. Parasitol.*, **28**, 107–73
7. Bliss, C. A. and Fisher, R. A. (1953). Fitting the negative binomial distribution to biological data and a note on the efficient fitting of the negative binomial. *Biometrics*, **9**, 176–200
8. Wong, M. S., Bundy, D. A. P. and Golden, M. H. N. (1991). The rate of ingestion of *Ascaris lumbricoides* and *Trichuris trichiura* eggs in soil and its relationship to infection in two children's homes in Jamaica. *Trans. R. Soc. Trop. Med. Hyg.*, **85**, 89–91
9. Halstead, J. A. (1968). Geophagia in man: its nature and nutritional effects. *Am. J. Clin. Nutr.*, **21**, 1384–93
10. Millican, F. and Lourie, R. (1970). The child with pica and his family. In Anthony, C. J. and Koupernick, C. (eds), *The Child in the Family*. New York: Wiley, pp. 176–93
11. Anderson, R. M. and May, R. M. (1982). Population dynamics of human helminth infections: control by chemotherapy. *Nature*, **297**, 557–563
12. Variyam, E. P. and Banwell, J. G. (1982). Nutrition implications of hookworm infection. *Rev. Infect. Dis.*, **4**, 830–5
13. Stephenson, L. S., Latham, M. C., Kurz, K. M., Kinoti, S. N. and Brigham, H. (1989). Treatment with a single dose of albendazole improves growth of Kenyan schoolchildren with hookworm, *Trichuris trichiura*, and *Ascaris lumbricoides* infections. *Am. J. Trop. Med. Hyg.*, **41**, 78–87
14. Smillie, W. G. and Augustine, D. L. (1926). Hookworm infestation. The effect of varying intensities on the physical condition of schoolchildren. *Am. J. Dis. Child.*, **31**, 151–68
15. Keller, A. E., Googe, H. B., Cotrell, H. B., Miller, D. G. and Harvey, R. H. (1935). Clinical study under controlled conditions of 1,083 children with hookworm. *J. Am. Med. Assoc.*, **105**, 1670–5
16. Crompton, D. W. T., Walters, D. E. and Arnold, S. E. (1981). Changes in the food intake and body weight of protein-malnourished rats infected with *Nippostrongylus brasiliensis* (Nematoda). *Parasitology*, **82**, 23–38
17. Roche, M. and Layrisse, M. (1966). The nature and causes of 'hookworm anaemia'. *Am. J. Trop. Med. Hyg.*, **15**(6), Part 2
18. Hodes, P. J. and Keefer, G. P. (1945). Hookworm disease: a small intestinal study. *Am. J. Roentgenol. Radium Ther. Nucl. Med.*, **54**, 728–42

19. Blackman, V., Marsen, P., Banwell, J. G. and Craggs, M. H. (1965). Albumin metabolism in hookworm anaemia. *Trans. R. Soc. Trop. Med. Hyg.*, **59**, 472–82

20. Areekul, S., Devakul, K., Chantachum, Y., Boonanyanta, C., Egoromaiphol, S. and Viravan, C. (1971). Gastrointestinal protein loss in patients with hookworm infection. *J. Med. Assoc. Thailand*, **34**, 28–32

21. Blom, M., Prag, J. B. and Norredam, K. (1979). α_1-Acid glycoprotein, α_1-antitrypsin, and ceruloplasmin in human intestinal helminthiasis. *Am. J. Trop. Med. Hyg.*, **28**, 76–83

22. Grimble, R. F. (1989). Cytokines: their relevance to nutrition. *Eur. J. Clin. Nutr.*, **43**, 217–30

23. Cooper, E., Spencer, J., Murch, S., Venugopal, S., Hanchard, B., Bundy, D. and MacDonald, T. T. (1990). *Bulletin de la Societe Francaise de Parasitologie*, Suppl. 2, p. 347

24. Kalkofen, U. P. (1974). Intestinal trauma resulting from feeding activities of *Ancylostoma caninum*. *Am. J. Trop. Med. Hyg.*, **23**, 1046–53

25. Tandon, B. N., Das, B. C., Saraya, A. K. and Geo, M. G. (1966). Functional and structural studies of the small bowel in ankylostomiasis. *Br. Med. J.*, **1**, 714–16

26. Burman, N. N., Sehgal, A. K., Chakravarti, R. N., Sodhi, J. G. and Chuttani, R. N. (1970). Morphological and absorption studies in hookworm infestation (ankylostomiasis). *Indian J. Med. Res.*, **58**, 317–25

27. Miller, T. A. (1979). Hookworm infection in man. *Adv. Parasitol.*, **17**, 315–83

28. Chanco, P. P. and Vidad, J. Y. (1978). A review of trichuriasis, its incidence, pathogenesis and treatment. *Drugs* (Suppl.), **15**, 87–93

29. Stephenson, L. S., Pond, W. G. and Nesheim, L. C. (1980). Nutrient absorption, growth and intestinal pathology in young pigs experimentally infected with 15-day-old larvae. *Exp. Parasitol.*, **49**, 15–25

30. Miller, H. R. P. and Nawa, Y. (1979). *Nippostrongylus brasiliensis*: intestinal goblet cell response in adoptively immunized rats. *Exp. Parasitol.*, **47**, 81–90

31. Castro, G. A. (1990). Intestinal pathology. In Behnke, J. M. (ed.), *Parasites: Immunity and Pathology*. London: Taylor & Francis, pp. 283–316

32. Palmer, J. M. and Castro, G. A. (1986). Anamnestic stimulus-specific myoelectric responses associated with intestinal immunity in the rat. *Am. J. Physiol.*, **250**, G266–73

33. Taren, D. L., Nesheim, M. C., Crompton, D. W. T. and Holland, C. (1987). Contribution of ascariasis to poor nutritional status in children from Chiriqui province, Republic of Panama. *Parasitology*, **95**, 615–22

34. Tripathy, K., Duque, E., Bolanos, O., Lotero, H. and Mayoral, L. G. (1972). Malabsorption syndrome in ascariasis. *Amer. J. Clin. Nutr.*, **25**, 1276–87

35. Miller, M. J. (1947). Studies on the life cycle of *Trichuris vulpis*, the whipworm of dogs. *Can. J. Research D*, **25**, 1–11

36. MacDonald, T. T., Choy, M.-Y., Spencer, J., Richman, P. I., Diss, T., Hanchard, B., Venugopal, S., Bundy, D. A. P. and Cooper, E. S. (1991). Histopathology and immunohistochemistry of the caecum in children with the *Trichuris* dysentery syndrome. *J. Clin. Pathol.*, **44**, 194–9

37. Selby, W. S., Janossy, G., Mason, D. Y. and Jewell, D. P. (1983). Expression of HLA-DR antigens by colonic epithelium in inflammatory bowel disease. *Clin. Exp. Immunol.*, **53**, 614–18

38. MacDonald, T. T., Horton, M. A., Choy, M.-Y. and Richman, P. I. (1990). Increased expression of the laminin/collagen receptor (VLA-1) on epithelium of inflamed human intestine. *J. Clin. Pathol.*, **43**, 313–15

39. MacDonald, T. T., Whyte, C. A. M., Spencer, J., Cromwell, O., Whitney, P., Venugopal, S., Bundy, D. A. P. and Cooper, E. S. (1991). Immediate hypersensitivity in the colon of children chronically parasitised with the whipworm, *Trichuris trichiura*. *Lancet* (In press)

40. Lillywhite, J. E., Bundy, D. A. P., Didier, J. M., Cooper, E. S. and Bianco, A. E. (1991). Humoral immune responses in human infection with the whipworm *Trichuris trichiura*. *Parasit. Immunol.*, **13**, 491–6

41. Copper, E. S., Bundy, D. A. P., MacDonald, T. T. and Golden, M. H. N. (1990). Growth suppression in the *Trichuris* dysentery syndrome. *Eur. J. Clin. Nutr.*, **44**, 285–91

42. Cooper, E. S. and Bundy, D. A. P. (1987). Trichuriasis. *Clin. Trop. Med. Commun. Dis.*, **2**, 629–43

43. Gilman, R. H., Chong, Y. H., Davis, C., Greenberg, B., Virik, H. K. and Dixon, H. B. (1983). The adverse consequences of heavy *Trichuris* infection. *Trans. R. Soc. Trop. Med. Hyg.*, **77**, 432–8

44. Grove, D. I. (1989). Strongyloidiasis. In Warren, K. S. and Mahmoud, A. A. F. (eds), *Tropical and Geographical Medicine*, 2nd edn. New York: McGraw-Hill, pp. 393–9

45. Faria, J. (1972). Prevalencia de *Strongyloides stercoralis* em escolares de 7–14 años na cidade do Salvador. *Gazetim Mèdico da Bahia*, **72**, 59–63
46. Grove, D. I. (1980). Strongyloidiasis in Allied ex-prisoners of war in South-East Asia. *Br. Med. J.*, **280**, 598–601
47. Genta, R. M. (1987). Strongyloidiasis. *Clin. Trop. Med. Commun. Dis.*, **2**, 645–65
48. Bras, G., Richards, R. C., Irvine, R. A., Milner, P. F. A. and Ragbeer, M. M. S. (1964). Infection with *Strongyloides stercoralis* in Jamaica. *Lancet*, **2**, 1257–60
49. Speed, J. C., Culpepper, V., Thompson, D. E., Henson, R., Wint, B. and Bundy, D. A. P. (1987). A community-based study of gastrointestinal helminth and protozoan infection in Western Jamaica. *W.I. Med. J.*, **36**, 73–5
50. Sinha, D. P. (1988). *Children of the Caribbean 1945–1984*. Kingston: Caribbean Food & Nutrition Institute/UNICEF
51. Carvalho, E. M., Andrade, T. M., Andrade, J. A. and Rocha, H. R. (1983). Immunological features in different forms of strongyloidiasis. *Trans. R. Soc. Trop. Med. Hyg.*, **77**, 346–9
52. Matsumoto, T., Miike, T., Mizoguchi, K., Yamaguchi, K., Takatsuki, K., Hosada, M., Kawabe, T. and Yodo, J. (1990). Individuals infected with HTLV1. *Clin. Exp. Immunol.*, **81**, 207–11
53. Terry, S. I., Blattner, W., Neva, F. A., Murphy, C. P., Golden, M. H. N., Hanchard, B., Robinson, R. and Morgan, O. S. (1989). Coincidental HTLV1 infection influences outcome of treatment of strongyloidiasis. *W.I. Med. J.*, **38** (Suppl. 1), 36
54. Shelhammer, J. H., Neva, F. A. and Finn, D. R. (1982). Persistent strongyloidiasis in an immunodeficienc patient. *Am. J. Trop. Med. Hyg.*, **31**, 746–51
55. Maayan, S., Wormser, G. P., Widerhorn, J., Sy, E. R., Kim, H. and Ernst, J. A. (1987). *Strongyloides stercoralis* hyperinfection in a patient with the acquired immune deficiency syndrome. *Am. J. Med.*, **83**, 945–8
56. Dutcher, J. P., Marcus, S. L., Tanowitz, H. B., Wittner, M., Fuks, J. Z. and Wiernik, P. H. (1990). Disseminated strongyloidiasis in a patient with acquired immune deficiency syndrome and Burkitt's lymphoma. *Cancer*, **66**, 2417–20
57. Louisy, C. L. and Barton, C. J. (1971). The radiological diagnosis of *Strongyloides stercoralis* enteritis. *Radiology*, **98**, 535–41
58. Walsh, J. A. and Warren, K. S. (1979). Selective primary health care: an interim strategy for disease control in developing countries. *N. Engl. J. Med.*, **301**, 967–74
59. Pawlowski, Z. S. (1989). Ascariasis. In Warren, K. S. and Mahmoud, A. A. F. (eds), *Tropical and Geographical Medicine*, 2nd edn. New York: McGraw-Hill, pp. 393–9

Index

301